THE WASHINGTON MANUAL™

Gastroenterology `Subspecialty Consult`

Second Edition

Editor

C. Prakash Gyawali, MD, MRCP
Associate Professor of Medicine
Division of Gastroenterology
Washington University School of Medicine
St. Louis, Missouri

Series Editors

Katherine E. Henderson, MD
Instructor in Medicine
Department of Internal Medicine
Division of Medical Education
Washington University School of Medicine
Barnes-Jewish Hospital
St. Louis, Missouri

Thomas M. De Fer, MD
Associate Professor of Internal Medicine
Washington University School of Medicine
St. Louis, Missouri

D0757240

 Wolters Kluwer | Lippincott Williams & Wilkins
Health
Philadelphia · Baltimore · New York · London
Buenos Aires · Hong Kong · Sydney · Tokyo

Acquisitions Editor: Ave McCracken
Managing Editor: Michelle LaPlante
Project Manager: Bridgett Dougherty
Marketing Manager: Kimberly Schonberger
Manufacturing Manager: Kathleen Brown
Design Coordinator: Risa Clow
Cover Designer: Joseph DePinho
Production Service: Aptara, Inc.

Second Edition

Library of Congress Cataloging-in-Publication Data

The Washington manual gastroenterology subspecialty consult. — 2nd ed. / editor, C. Prakash Gyawali.
  p. ; cm.
  Includes bibliographical references and index.
  ISBN 978-0-7817-9150-2 (pbk. : alk. paper)
  1. Gastroenterology—Handbooks, manuals, etc. 2. Digestive organs—Diseases—Handbooks, manuals, etc.
I. Gyawali, C. Prakash. II. Title: Gastroenterology subspecialty consult.
  [DNLM: 1. Digestive System Diseases—diagnosis—Handbooks. 2. Digestive System Diseases—therapy—
Handbooks. WI 39 W319 2008]
  RC802.W37 2008
  616.3'3—dc22

                                                                                    2008001357

The Washington Manual™ is an intent-to-use mark belonging to Washington University in St. Louis to which international legal protection applies. The mark is used in this publication by LWW under license from Washington University.

Care has been taken to confirm the accuracy of the information present and to describe generally accepted practices. However, the authors, editors, and publisher are not responsible for errors or omissions or for any consequences from application of the information in this book and make no warranty, expressed or implied, with respect to the currency, completeness, or accuracy of the contents of the publication. Application of this information in a particular situation remains the professional responsibility of the practitioner; the clinical treatments described and recommended may not be considered absolute and universal recommendations.

The authors, editors, and publisher have exerted every effort to ensure that drug selection and dosage set forth in this text are in accordance with current recommendations and practice at the time of publication. However, in view of ongoing research, changes in government regulations, and the constant flow of information relating to drug therapy and drug reactions, the reader is urged to check the package insert for each drug for any change in indications and dosage and for added warnings and precautions. This is particularly important when the recommended agent is a new or infrequently employed drug.

Some drugs and medical devices presented in this publication have Food and Drug Administration (FDA) clearance for limited use in restricted research settings. It is the responsibility of health care providers to ascertain the FDA status of each drug or device planned for use in their clinical practice.

To purchase additional copies of this book, call our customer service department at **(800) 638-3030** or fax orders to **(301) 223-2320**. International customers should call **(301) 223-2300**.

Visit Lippincott Williams & Wilkins on the Internet: http://www.lww.com. Lippincott Williams & Wilkins customer service representatives are available from 8:30 am to 6:00 pm, EST.

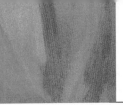

Table of Contents

PART II. APPROACH TO SPECIFIC DISEASES

Contributing Authors

Sumeet Asrani, MD
Resident in Internal Medicine
Department of Medicine
Washington University School of Medicine
St. Louis, Missouri

Riad Azar, MD
Assistant Professor of Medicine
Division of Gastroenterology
Washington University School of Medicine
St. Louis, Missouri

Brian B. Borg, MD
Fellow in Gastroenterology
Division of Gastroenterology
Washington University School of Medicine
St. Louis, Missouri

Walter W. Chan, MD
Resident in Internal Medicine
Department of Medicine
Washington University School of Medicine
St. Louis, Missouri

Matthew A. Ciorba, MD
Instructor in Medicine
Division of Gastroenterology
Washington University School of Medicine
St. Louis, Missouri

Jeffrey S. Crippin, MD
Professor of Medicine
Division of Gastroenterology
Washington University School of Medicine
St. Louis, Missouri

Dayna S. Early, MD
Associate Professor of Medicine
Division of Gastroenterology
Washington University School of Medicine
St. Louis, Missouri

C. Prakash Gyawali, MD
Associate Professor of Medicine
Division of Gastroenterology
Washington University School of Medicine
St. Louis, Missouri

Christina Y. Ha, MD
Fellow in Gastroenterology
Division of Gastroenterology
Washington University School of Medicine
St. Louis, Missouri

Michael J. Hersh, MD
Fellow in Gastroenterology
Division of Gastroenterology
Washington University School of Medicine
St. Louis, Missouri

Julie A. Holinga, MD
Resident in Internal Medicine
Department of Medicine
Washington University School of Medicine
St. Louis, Missouri

Dustin G. James, MD
Fellow in Gastroenterology
Division of Gastroenterology
Washington University School of Medicine
St. Louis, Missouri

Sreenivasa Jonnalagadda, MD
Associate Professor of Medicine
Division of Gastroenterology
Washington University School of Medicine
St. Louis, Missouri

Manreet Kaur, MD
Fellow in Gastroenterology
Division of Gastroenterology
Washington University School of Medicine
St. Louis, Missouri

Thomas A. Kerr, MD
Fellow in Gastroenterology
Division of Gastroenterology
Washington University School of Medicine
St. Louis, Missouri

Kevin M. Korenblat, MD
Assistant Professor of Medicine
Division of Gastroenterology
Washington University School of Medicine
St. Louis, Missouri

Sonal Kumar, MD
Resident in Internal Medicine
Department of Medicine
Washington University School of Medicine
St. Louis, Missouri

Vladimir Kushnir, MD
Resident in Internal Medicine
Department of Medicine
Washington University School of Medicine
St. Louis, Missouri

Mauricio Lisker-Melman, MD
Professor of Medicine
Division of Gastroenterology
Washington University School of Medicine
St. Louis, Missouri

Anne K. Nagler, MD
Attending in Internal Medicine
Department of Medicine
Washington University School of Medicine
St. Louis, Missouri

Yume P. Nguyen, MD
Fellow in Gastroenterology
Division of Gastroenterology
Washington University School of Medicine
St. Louis, Missouri

T. J. Paradowski, MD
Resident in Internal Medicine
Department of Medicine
Washington University School of Medicine
St. Louis, Missouri

Daniel A. Ringold, MD
Fellow in Gastroenterology
Division of Gastroenterology
Washington University School of Medicine
St. Louis, Missouri

Deborah C. Rubin
Professor of Medicine
Division of Gastroenterology
Washington University School of Medicine
St. Louis, Missouri

Gregory S. Sayuk, MD
Assistant Professor of Medicine
Division of Gastroenterology
Washington University School of Medicine
St. Louis, Missouri

Anil B. Seetharam, MD
Resident in Internal Medicine
Department of Medicine
Washington University School of Medicine
St. Louis, Missouri

Pari M. Shah, MD
Resident in Internal Medicine
Department of Medicine
Washington University School of Medicine
St. Louis, Missouri

Somal S. Shah, MD
Resident in Internal Medicine
Department of Medicine
Washington University School of Medicine
St. Louis, Missouri

Anisa Shaker, MD
Fellow in Gastroenterology
Division of Gastroenterology
Washington University School of Medicine
St. Louis, Missouri

Vilaas Shetty, MD
Resident in Internal Medicine
Department of Medicine
Washington University School of Medicine
St. Louis, Missouri

Sanjay Sikka, MD
Fellow in Gastroenterology
Division of Gastroenterology
Washington University School of Medicine
St. Louis, Missouri

Shelby A. Sullivan
Instructor in Medicine
Division of Gastroenterology
Washington University School of Medicine
St. Louis, Missouri

Babac Vahabzadeh, MD
Resident in Internal Medicine
Department of Medicine
Washington University School of Medicine
St. Louis, Missouri

Chairman's Note

Medical knowledge is increasing at an exponential rate, and physicians are being bombarded with new facts at a pace that many find overwhelming. The Washington Manual™ Subspecialty Consult Series was developed in this context for interns, residents, medical students, and other practitioners in need of readily accessible practical clinical information. They, therefore, meet an important unmet need in an era of information overload.

I would like to acknowledge the authors who have contributed to these books. In particular, the series editors, Katherine E. Henderson, MD and Thomas M. De Fer, MD, for their oversight of the project. I'd also like to recognize Melvin Blanchard, MD, Chief of the Division of Medical Education in the Department of Medicine at Washington University for his guidance and advice. The efforts and outstanding skill of the lead authors are evident in the quality of the final product. I am confident that this series will meet its desired goal of providing practical knowledge that can be directly applied to improving patient care.

Kenneth S. Polonsky, MD
Adolphus Busch Professor
Chairman, Department of Medicine
Washington University School of Medicine
St. Louis, Missouri

Preface

Gastroenterology is a unique field wherein advanced technologies and diagnostic modalities have to be effectively meshed with clinical evaluation of the patient for an accurate diagnosis. This makes the discipline broad and challenging, and requires that the physician be well informed and clinically astute. Most gastrointestinal ailments start with simple symptoms and signs, and accurate interpretation of these can lead to appropriate diagnostic tests and a conclusive diagnosis.

Management of gastrointestinal disorders has changed substantially in the past decades, and newer therapeutic options, both pharmacologic and interventional, have led to better patient outcomes. The identification of *Helicobacter pylori* as an important cause of peptic ulcer disease has led to effective eradication therapies and reduction in the recurrence of peptic ulcers, but nonsteroidal anti-inflammatory drugs are gaining importance in the causation of peptic ulcers in the elderly. Genetic testing is now available for several gastrointestinal disorders, including hemochromatosis, cystic fibrosis, and certain hereditary colon cancer syndromes. Identification of the adenoma-carcinoma sequence has led to effective screening and surveillance strategies for colon cancer and Barrett's esophagus. It is important for the novice entering the medical field as well as the experienced practitioner to keep abreast of advances in the field.

The objective of *The Washington Manual Gastroenterology Subspecialty Consult* is for the reader to obtain a synopsis of gastrointestinal symptoms and signs, common gastrointestinal ailments encountered in clinical practice, and up-to-date approaches to investigation and management, taking advances in the field into consideration. The chapters have been written and updated by internal medicine residents and gastroenterology fellows with gastroenterology faculty supervision and, therefore, represent the "trainee eye view" of gastrointestinal disorders. Bulleted key points highlight the salient features of each chapter. The descriptions of each symptom, sign, and disorder are not meant to be exhaustive; instead, they provide an abbreviated update with references to a more descriptive source in the literature.

I would like to dedicate this manual to the memory of my mentor, teacher, colleague, and friend, Ray E. Clouse, MD, Professor of Medicine and Psychiatry, and gastroenterologist *extraordinaire*, who passed away in August 2007 after a valiant battle with cancer. I owe most of my gastroenterology knowledge, writing skills, and academic career as a whole to Dr. Clouse's mentorship and guidance, and I miss him terribly.

CPG

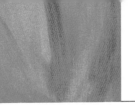

Dysphagia and Odynophagia

Michael J. Hersh

1

INTRODUCTION

Background

Dysphagia is defined as the sensation of impediment in movement of food from mouth to stomach. Patients report a sensation of obstruction of food passage through the oropharynx or esophagus or of food "sticking" in the chest. It must be distinguished from **odynophagia**, which means pain during swallowing. Dysphagia and odynophagia may coexist in the same patient. **Globus** is the sensation of a lump or fullness in the throat without difficulty swallowing. Finally, some patients may complain of an inability to swallow, or **aphagia**. Aphagia typically occurs when a food bolus becomes impacted in the esophagus, thus blocking the passage of any ingested solids or liquids.

Classification

A thorough history is extremely important in differentiating between oropharyngeal and esophageal dysphagia. Based on the patient's history, a diagnostic evaluation may be chosen to further assess the cause for dysphagia.

- **Oropharyngeal dysphagia** results from defects in the oral and pharyngeal phases of swallowing. These disorders cause difficulties with preparing the food for swallowing or with transferring a bolus of food from the oral cavity into the esophagus. Patients with oropharyngeal dysphagia may report the sensation of food sticking in the back of the throat, difficulty initiating a swallow, or coughing, choking, drooling, or nasal regurgitation during the swallow. The discomfort typically is reported within 1 second of initiating a swallow.
- **Esophageal dysphagia** results from defects in the esophageal phase of swallowing. Patients may describe the sensation of food sticking in the throat or chest, retrosternal chest pain, or regurgitation soon after swallowing. It is important to further delineate the cause for esophageal dysphagia, specifically whether the dysphagia is a result of a structural or neuromuscular disorder. Initially, structural disorders usually cause dysphagia to solid foods, but may later include liquids as well. Patients with neuromuscular disorders commonly report dysphagia to both solids and liquids from the onset of symptoms.

CAUSES

Pathophysiology

Normal swallowing, one of the most intricate neuromuscular actions performed by the human body, can be divided into three distinct phases: oral, pharyngeal, and esophageal.

The oral and pharyngeal phases involve the striated or voluntary muscles of the mouth and pharynx. The initiation of a swallow is under direct neurologic control. The swallowing control center, which resides in the medulla, can be activated by either the cerebral cortex (volitional swallowing) or by afferent impulses from the oropharynx (reflexive swallowing).

Oral Phase

The oral phase begins as the food bolus is mechanically prepared by the muscles of the jaw, face, and tongue. It is then propelled posteriorly and superiorly by the tongue and palate. As the bolus passes the anterior tonsillar pillars, the pharyngeal phase begins.

Pharyngeal Phase

The pharyngeal phase continues with the soft palate closing the nasopharynx. The tongue base and pharyngeal constrictors continue to propel the bolus posteriorly. The lips and jaw remain closed, fixing the upper attachments of the suprahyoid muscles to allow elevation of the larynx and closure of the laryngeal valves (the epiglottis and vocal cords). This enhances airway protection and opens the upper esophageal sphincter (UES). At rest, the UES acts as a barrier against entry of air into the esophagus and regurgitation of material from the esophagus into the pharynx. This entire process takes <1 second.

Esophageal Phase

The esophageal phase begins with the entry of a food bolus into the esophagus. When the bolus reaches the esophagus, the UES closes and the bolus is propelled toward the stomach by coordinated muscular contractions. Primary peristalsis in striated muscles is initiated by the act of swallowing via the central program generator in the medulla. Through multiple, complicated control mechanisms, these coordinated contractions are propagated through the striated muscle and into the smooth muscle of the more distal esophagus. Secondary peristalsis occurs as a response to esophageal distension from the presence of retained or refluxed material. The lower esophageal sphincter (LES) is a combination of esophageal smooth muscle and crural diaphragm. The LES relaxes with swallowing and peristaltic contractions through the actions of the vagus nerve to allow passage of the food bolus into the stomach.

PRESENTATION

Evaluation

Oropharyngeal Dysphagia

Oropharyngeal dysphagia is most commonly a manifestation of a systemic disorder. The evaluation should begin with a thorough history and physical examination aimed at identifying any underlying illness. A careful neurologic examination, including direct observation of the patient swallowing water, may also be helpful. Table 1-1 lists some of the more frequent causes of oropharyngeal dysphagia.

The best initial study for suspected oropharyngeal dysphagia is a **modified barium swallow (MBS)**. An MBS is a radiographic study in which the oral and pharyngeal phases are observed in real time while the patient swallows barium of varying consistencies, such as thin liquids, thick liquids, and barium cookies or crackers. This study helps to identify abnormalities of the oropharyngeal phases and may direct therapy. Patients may tolerate

TABLE 1-1	CAUSES OF OROPHARYNGEAL DYSPHAGIA

Neuromuscular Disorders

Cerebrovascular accident
Parkinson's disease
Amyotrophic lateral sclerosis
Poliomyelitis
Polymyositis
Myasthenia gravis
Brain tumors
Hypothyroidism
Abnormal upper esophageal sphincter relaxation

Structural Lesions

Neoplasm
Inflammation (pharyngitis, radiation)
Plummer-Vinson syndrome
Cervical hyperostosis
Thyromegaly
Lymphadenopathy
Prior oropharyngeal surgery
Zenker's diverticulum

certain consistencies better than others, and the diet can be modified accordingly. If structural lesions are identified, then direct laryngoscopy should be performed for further evaluation.

Esophageal Dysphagia

When esophageal dysphagia is suspected, an **upper endoscopy** is useful as the initial test, because it allows for direct visualization of the esophagus and permits tissue biopsy and dilation of structural narrowings if found. An alternate test is the **esophagogram (barium swallow)**, most useful when subtle strictures or narrowings are suspected, or when road mapping of a tight or complicated stricture is desired before endoscopic evaluation. Esophagograms also commonly reveal structural esophageal abnormalities, such as tumors, webs, rings, or strictures. The addition of a solid bolus, such as a barium marshmallow or pill, aids in the detection of subtle abnormalities. Motility disorders, such as achalasia, diffuse esophageal spasm, and scleroderma esophagus, have typical esophagogram findings, but **esophageal manometry** is typically required for a definitive diagnosis. Manometry is considered when no structural or obstructive process is identified on upper endoscopy or barium esophagogram in patients presenting with dysphagia. Manometry involves the passage of a thin catheter through the nose, down the esophagus and past the LES. Pressure measurements are then obtained over the full length of the esophagus, including the UES and LES, both at rest and during a swallow. Manometry is the gold standard for the diagnosis of achalasia. Other primary and secondary motor disorders can also be diagnosed using manometry. Table 1-2 lists some common causes of esophageal dysphagia.

TABLE 1-2	CAUSES OF ESOPHAGEAL DYSPHAGIA

Structural Causes

Benign stricture
Esophageal cancer
Schatzki ring
Esophageal webs
Foreign bodies
Extrinsic (vascular, cervical osteoarthritis, adenopathy)

Motility Disorders

Achalasia
Scleroderma
Hypertensive lower esophageal sphincter
Diffuse esophageal spasm
Chagas' disease
Nutcracker esophagus

MANAGEMENT

Treatment

Oropharyngeal Dysphagia

When possible, treatment of oropharyngeal dysphagia should be directed at the underlying disorder. Many patients, however, have irreversible or progressive neurologic diseases, which can lead to worsening oropharyngeal dysphagia. Consultation with a speech therapist is often helpful to provide modifications in eating behaviors and food consistency. Despite these interventions, some patients will continue to experience oropharyngeal dysphagia placing them at a high risk of aspiration or inadequate caloric intake. If significant improvement in oropharyngeal dysphagia is not expected, alternative sources of nutritional support should be pursued. Options may include a nasogastric feeding tube, gastrostomy tube, or jejunostomy tube. These can be placed by a gastroenterologist, radiologist, or surgeon, depending on the particular health care center.

Esophageal Dysphagia

As noted, management of esophageal dysphagia should be tailored to the underlying disorder. Endoscopic therapies, including dilation of strictures and disruption of esophageal rings, can be helpful in the management of structural causes of esophageal dysphagia. Empiric endoscopic dilation with a large caliber dilator is often performed in patients wherein a definitive etiology for esophageal-type dysphagia is not apparent on routine investigation. This approach may result in symptomatic improvement of varying durations. Obstructing tumors can be treated with dilation or by placement of an endoscopic stent. Some motility disorders are amenable to endoscopic therapy, including botulinum toxin injection into the LES in disorders of LES relaxation. Surgical myotomy and pneumatic dilation are durable options in achalasia. Gastrostomy tube placement may be indicated in patients with large, obstructing esophageal tumors that are not amenable to dilation or stent placement. (See Chapter 12, Esophageal Disorders, for a discussion on the specific management of common esophageal disorders.)

KEY POINTS TO REMEMBER

- Dysphagia, or difficulty swallowing, must be differentiated from odynophagia, which is painful swallowing.
- Oropharyngeal dysphagia results from defects in the oral and pharyngeal phases of swallowing. Patients may experience food sticking in their throat, difficulty initiating a swallow, or coughing, choking, drooling, or nasal regurgitation during the swallow.
- Esophageal dysphagia results from defects in the esophageal phase of swallowing. Patients may describe the sensation of food sticking in the throat or chest, retrosternal chest pain, or regurgitation soon after swallowing.
- Structural disorders usually cause dysphagia to solid foods initially, but later include liquids as well. Patients with neuromuscular disorders commonly report dysphagia to both solids and liquids from the initiation of symptoms.
- The best initial study for suspected oropharyngeal dysphagia is a modified barium swallow.
- Upper endoscopy is useful as the initial test in evaluating esophageal dysphagia, or it may be used to evaluate abnormal imaging, such as an esophagram.

REFERENCES AND SUGGESTED READINGS

Clouse RE, Richter JE, Heading RC, et al. Functional esophageal disorders. *Gut* 1999;45(Suppl 2):II31–II36.

Cook IJ, Kahrilas PJ. AGA technical review on management of oropharyngeal dysphagia. *Gastroenterology* 1999;116(2):455–478.

Pandolfino JE, Kahrilas, PJ. AGA technical review on the clinical use of esophageal manometry. *Gastroenterology* 2005;128:209–224.

Schechter GL. Systemic causes of dysphagia in adults. *Otolaryngol Clin North Am* 1998;31(3):525–535.

Shapiro J. Evaluation and treatment of swallowing disorders. *Compr Ther* 2000;26 (3):203–209.

Spechler SJ. AGA technical review on treatment of patients with dysphagia caused by benign disorders of the distal esophagus. *Gastroenterology* 1999;117(1):233–254.

Spieker MR. Evaluating dysphagia. *Am Fam Physician* 2000;61(12):3639–3648.

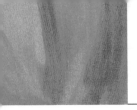

Nausea and Vomiting

2

Babac Vahabzadeh and C. Prakash Gyawali

INTRODUCTION

Nausea refers to the feeling of an imminent urge to vomit and is usually sensed in the throat or epigastrium. **Vomiting** (or emesis), in turn, denotes the forceful ejection of upper gastrointestinal (GI) contents through the mouth. It is important to distinguish these symptoms from regurgitation and rumination. **Regurgitation** is the passive retrograde flow of esophageal contents into the mouth, commonly seen in gastroesophageal reflux. **Rumination** is the effortless regurgitation of recently ingested food into the mouth, followed by rechewing and swallowing. These two conditions have very different causes and therapy.

Nausea, which can precede the act of emesis, can occur concurrently with emesis or on its own. Generally, altered autonomic activity and decreased function of the upper GI tract accompany severe nausea. The act of emesis is a highly coordinated event requiring the integration of both central and peripheral nervous systems.

EPIDEMIOLOGY

Nausea and vomiting frequently prompt consultation with a gastroenterologist. These conditions contribute significantly to increased hospital costs and physician visits. It is important to note that medication-induced, systemic, metabolic, and even neurologic causes may be more common than upper gut mucosal causes for nausea and vomiting (Table 2-1); therefore, upper endoscopic examination may not be revealing if performed as the first investigation in many situations. Intra-abdominal inflammatory disorders (e.g., cholecystitis, pancreatitis, and appendicitis, to name a few) and bowel obstruction are important causes of nausea and vomiting, however, and imaging studies can help diagnose these conditions under appropriate clinical situations. Pregnancy is an important cause of nausea and vomiting, especially in the early months when it may not be immediately apparent that the patient is pregnant.

Etiology and Pathophysiology

Initiation of Emesis

The vomiting center, located in the dorsal portion of the lateral reticular formation, serves as the point of integration and initiation of emesis. Afferent stimuli are received by the vomiting center from a variety of sources. The vestibular system, particularly the labyrinthine apparatus located in the inner ear, sends afferent signals through the vestibular nucleus and the cerebellum to the vomiting center. Peripheral neural pathways from the GI tract play a large role in the initiation of emesis. Afferent vagal fibers project to the nucleus tractus solitarius (NTS) and from there to the vomiting center. Serotonergic pathways are also believed

TABLE 2-1 — DIFFERENTIAL DIAGNOSIS OF NAUSEA AND VOMITING

Medications

Chemotherapy: cisplatinum, dacarbazine,
  nitrogen mustard
Analgesics
Oral contraceptives
Cardiovascular: digoxin, antiarrhythmics,
  beta-blockers, antihypertensives, calcium
  channel blockers
Antibiotics: erythromycin, tetracycline,
  sulfonamides
Sulfasalazine
Azathioprine
Antiparkinsonian agents
Theophylline

Infections

Gastroenteritis
Viral: rotavirus, Norwalk virus, adenovirus,
  reovirus
Bacterial: *Staphylococcus aureus*,
  Salmonella, Bacillus cereus, and
  Clostridium perfringens (toxins)
Systemic nongastrointestinal infections

Other Disorders

Pregnancy
Uremia
Diabetic ketoacidosis
Addison's disease
Postoperative nausea and vomiting
Cardiac ischemia or infarction

Gastrointestinal and Peritoneal Disorders

Peptic ulcer disease
Appendicitis
Hepatitis
Mesenteric ischemia
Pancreatitis
Cholecystitis
Gastric outlet obstruction
Small bowel obstruction
Gastroparesis
Nonulcer dyspepsia

Central Nervous System Disorders

Increased intracranial pressure:
  tumor, hemorrhage, pseudotumor
  cerebri
Migraine
Psychogenic vomiting
Cyclic vomiting syndrome

Anorexia Nervosa

Bulimia nervosa
Labyrinthine disorders

to play a large role in peripheral stimulation via 5-hydroxytryptamine-3 (5-HT_3) receptors located on the afferent vagal nerves. The chemoreceptor trigger zone, located in the area postrema on the floor of the fourth ventricle, is a major mediator of the initiation of emesis. A number of drugs and toxins activate the zone via dopamine D_2, muscarinic M_1, histaminergic H_1, serotonergic 5-HT_3, and vasopressinergic receptors. A number of metabolic abnormalities also affect the trigger zone. Once activated, efferent signals are sent on to the vomiting center, where the physical act of emesis is initiated.

Mechanisms of Emesis

Efferent pathways from the vomiting center serve to initiate the mechanism of vomiting. Important pathways include the phrenic nerves to the diaphragm, the spinal nerves to the abdominal musculature, and visceral efferent vagal fibers to the larynx, pharynx, esophagus, and stomach.

The act of emesis involves a coordinated sequence of events that include the abdominal wall musculature and the muscular walls of the GI tract. While the gastroesophageal sphincter and the gastric body relax, a combination of forceful contractions of the abdominal wall muscles, diaphragm, and gastric pylorus causes the expulsion of gastric contents into the esophagus. Reverse peristalsis propels these contents into the mouth, while reflex closure of the glottis prevents aspiration and elevation of the soft palate prevents reflux into the nasopharynx.

Medications

Antiparkinsonian agents (e.g., L-dopa, bromocriptine), nicotine, digoxin, and opiate analgesics produce nausea and vomiting through direct action on receptors in the chemoreceptor trigger zone. Nonsteroidal anti-inflammatory drugs (NSAID) and antibiotics, such as erythromycin, stimulate peripheral afferent pathways to activate the vomiting center directly. Chemotherapeutic agents frequently cause nausea and vomiting through several mechanisms. Acute vomiting, usually caused by agents such as cisplatinum, nitrogen mustard, and dacarbazine, is generally mediated through serotonergic pathways, both centrally and peripherally. Both delayed and anticipatory vomiting are serotonin independent.

Infections

Viral gastroenteritis is a common cause of acute nausea and vomiting, particularly in the pediatric population. Causative agents include rotavirus, Norwalk virus, reovirus, and adenovirus. Bacterial infections with *Staphylococcus aureus*, *Salmonella*, *Bacillus cereus*, and *Clostridium perfringens* are commonly associated with "food poisoning." Enterotoxins act both centrally and peripherally. Miscellaneous infectious processes, such as otitis media, meningitis, and acute hepatitis, also commonly produce nausea and vomiting.

Gastrointestinal and Peritoneal Disorders

Dyspepsia is often caused by gastroesophageal reflux disease or peptic ulcer disease, but is also frequently functional in nature. Functional disorders constitute a large percentage of cases of chronic nausea and vomiting. Alterations in motility may be present but correlate poorly with symptoms. Gastroparesis, a situation where there is failure or near failure of gastric emptying, is associated with a multitude of systemic disorders, notably diabetes mellitus, systemic lupus erythematous (SLE), scleroderma, and amyloidosis. Intestinal or gastric outlet obstruction often causes nausea that is relieved with vomiting.

Inflammation of any viscus can cause nausea and vomiting through activation of afferent pathways. Pancreatitis, appendicitis, cholecystitis, and biliary pain (colic) are common causes. Peritoneal inflammation is usually associated with severe abdominal pain.

Central Nervous System Disorders

Increased intracranial pressure from any cause (malignancy, infection, cerebrovascular accident, hemorrhage) can induce emesis with or without nausea. Labyrinthine disorders, including labyrinthitis, tumors, Ménière's disease, and motion sickness, are common causes of nausea and vomiting.

Endocrine and Metabolic Disorders

Uremia, diabetic ketoacidosis, and hypercalcemia are postulated to cause nausea and vomiting through direct action on the area postrema. Parathyroid, thyroid, and adrenal disease act by disruption of GI motility. The nausea of pregnancy deserves special mention. It occurs in approximately 70% of women during the first trimester. The symptoms typically peak around the ninth week and subside by the end of the first trimester. The cause of nausea in pregnancy is likely related to fluctuations in hormones, as the symptoms parallel the rise and fall of beta-human chorionic gonadotropin (hCG) levels. Hyperemesis gravidarum complicates 1% to 5% of pregnancies, causing intractable vomiting. This condition is serious and can result in an inability to gain weight or in significant weight loss.

PRESENTATION

History

Acute vomiting suggests infection, medication- or toxin-induced cause, or an accumulation of toxins as in uremia or diabetic ketoacidosis. Chronic vomiting, defined as emesis for $\geq$1 month, suggests a chronic medical or psychiatric condition.

Timing can also suggest an etiology such as the following:

- Vomiting that occurs within minutes of a meal can be caused by an obstructive process in the proximal GI tract.
- Inflammatory conditions generally produce vomiting approximately 1 hour after meals.
- Vomiting from gastroparesis can occur several hours after a meal, and is typically associated with weight loss.
- Early morning vomiting often occurs with first-trimester pregnancy and uremia.

Vomiting of undigested foods may suggest an esophageal process, such as achalasia, whereas vomiting of partially digested foods suggests gastric retention caused by obstruction or gastroparesis. Blood or the appearance of "coffee grounds" in the emesis indicates an upper GI bleed. Bile rules out the possibility of obstruction proximal to the duodenal papilla. Foul odor can indicate a more distal obstruction, fistula, or bacterial overgrowth.

Abdominal pain is commonly associated with nausea and vomiting and may indicate an inflammatory condition, such as appendicitis or pancreatitis. Diarrhea or fever suggests an infectious process. Weight loss occurs with chronic vomiting. Mental status changes and headache may indicate meningitis or other central nervous system (CNS) pathology. Vertigo and tinnitus suggest a labyrinthine process.

Physical Examination

Assessment of volume status should be the initial focus of the physical examination. Orthostatic hypotension and tachycardia indicate hypovolemia and should be corrected immediately with volume resuscitation. Examination of the oropharynx may reveal loss of dental enamel, often found in bulimia. Abdominal tenderness suggests an inflammatory condition, and rebound tenderness suggests peritonitis. Absence of bowel sounds is consistent with intestinal ileus, whereas obstruction classically presents with high-pitched, hyperactive bowel sounds. Hepatomegaly or a tender liver edge may indicate hepatitis. Neurologic examination can reveal signs of meningitis and other CNS disorders.

MANAGEMENT

Diagnostic and Laboratory Evaluation

Laboratory tests should include the following:

- Basic metabolic panel evaluating for hyponatremia and elevated blood urea nitrogen (BUN) and creatinine, which are seen with dehydration. Hypokalemia and contraction alkalosis are also seen with prolonged vomiting and dehydration and result from a hyperaldosterone state.
- Liver chemistries, which may reveal acute hepatitis or cholestasis.
- Elevated lipase and amylase indicating pancreatitis.
- Complete blood count (CBC), which is useful to rule out blood loss with decreased hemoglobin and hematocrit. An elevated white blood cell count suggests an infectious process.
- Urine or serum beta-hCG levels in women of reproductive age with acute vomiting to exclude pregnancy.

Initial diagnostic testing should include radiographic evaluation with flat and upright plain films of the abdomen. The presence of air–fluid levels and small bowel dilatation demonstrates obstruction. Free air under the diaphragm indicates bowel perforation. Small bowel follow-through with barium contrast can further evaluate for subtle obstruction and mucosal lesions. Computed tomography (CT) of the abdomen may be useful in evaluating the liver, pancreas, and biliary system, as well as small and large intestines. Esophagogastroduodenoscopy (EGD) and colonoscopy allow direct visualization of GI mucosa. Further potential diagnostic studies include gastric emptying scans, GI manometry, and electrogastrography.

Treatment

Orthostatic hypotension and sinus tachycardia are signs of hypovolemia (with loss of approximately 10% of circulating blood volume) and should be corrected immediately with administration of intravenous (IV) fluids. Patients with severe comorbid conditions should be hospitalized, because dehydration may be more severe in these patients. Emesis caused by peptic ulcer disease can be treated by acid suppression and eradication of *Helicobacter pylori*. Many inflammatory conditions, such as appendicitis and cholecystitis, as well as mechanical small bowel or gastric outlet obstruction, require surgical intervention. Antiemetic and promotility agents are useful for symptomatic relief. Patients with chronic functional vomiting syndromes may benefit from low-dose antidepressants, especially tricyclic antidepressants. It is important to note that many patients with acute, self-limited nausea and vomiting may only require observation, antiemetics, and hydration.

Antiemetic Medications

Antihistamines

Antihistamines are useful for symptomatic relief. Meclizine (25 mg PO QID) is used for labyrinthitis, whereas promethazine (12.5–25 mg PO/IM/IV q6h) is very useful in treating the nausea caused by uremia.

Anticholinergics

Scopolamine (1.5-mg patch every 3 days) is used for the nausea of motion sickness. Scopolamine may be prescribed in the form of a transdermal patch.

Dopamine Receptor Antagonists

Prochlorperazine (5–10 mg PO/IM/IV q6h) and chlorpromazine (10–50 mg PO/IM q8h) are commonly used for both chronic and acute vomiting. Side effects, which are caused by the action on dopamine receptors throughout the CNS, include drowsiness, insomnia, anxiety, mood changes, confusion, dystonic reactions, tardive dyskinesia, and parkinsonian symptoms.

5-HT$_3$ Receptor Antagonists

Included in the class of 5-HT$_3$-receptor antagonists are ondansetron (4–8 mg PO/IV q8h) and granisetron (1 mg PO q12h), which are very useful in nausea caused by chemotherapeutic agents, particularly cisplatin.

Miscellaneous Agents

Corticosteroids and cannabinoids exert potent antiemetic effects in patients having chemotherapy. Aprepitant, which selectively antagonizes human substance P or neurokinin 1 receptors, is used for prevention of chemotherapy related nausea and vomiting.

Prokinetic Medications

- Metoclopramide (5–20 mg PO QID), which acts on both 5-HT$_4$ and peripheral dopamine receptors, is used for chemotherapy-induced nausea. Although used for poor gastric emptying from any cause, including gastroparesis, its promotility action is subject to tachyphylaxis with continued use. Its antiemetic properties, through its central action, may allow suppression of nausea and vomiting despite continued use. Jitteriness, tremors, and parkinsonian side effects limit its long-term use.

- Erythromycin, a macrolide antibiotic, is a motilin receptor agonist that improves gastric emptying but without significant suppression of nausea. It can be administered IV for acute gastric distension to stimulate gastric emptying. Its promotility action is subject to tachyphylaxis, and therefore, it is not useful for long-term management.
- Cisapride is no longer available in the United States because of its proarrhythmic effects.
- Domperidone, also a peripheral dopamine receptor antagonist, is a potent prokinetic agent but is not currently available in the United States.
- Tegaserod, a 5-HT$_4$ receptor agonist, primarily used in the treatment of irritable bowel syndrome, has modest promotility action in the stomach, and can be used to improve gastric emptying. This medication, however, is currently not available for routine use since postmarketing surveillance revealed a statistically significant risk of cardiovascular events over placebo.

REFRACTORY NAUSEA AND VOMITING

Nausea and vomiting is considered refractory if investigation fails to reveal a treatable etiology, and if routine measures do not result in symptomatic improvement. Two patterns of symptoms are recognized. The first is chronic persistent nausea and vomiting, occurring on a daily or frequent basis. This symptom pattern is similar to other functional syndromes, and benefit can be expected with use of neuromodulators, including tricyclic antidepressants, selective serotonin reuptake inhibitors (SSRI), and to a lesser extent, bupropion, buspirone, and sumatriptan. The second pattern is cyclic nausea and vomiting. This disorder is unique in that short periods of violent and unrelenting nausea and vomiting are separated by symptom-free intervals during which patients are relatively asymptomatic. Associated complaints during symptom "attacks" include upper abdominal pain, diarrhea, flushing, and sweating. Some patients report a prodrome lasting several minutes to hours. Current understanding of this condition links it to migraine and, therefore, treatments as for migraine, both abortive and prophylactic, have been found to be of benefit in reducing the intensity and frequency of attacks. Abortive therapy could include triptans during the prodromal period, and combinations of antiemetic medications, anxiolytics, and narcotic analgesics, in addition to IV hydration, during symptomatic periods. Prophylactic approaches include tricyclic antidepressants as first-line medications, but also antiepileptic medications, such as zonisamide, levetiracetam, or even topiramate.

- Low-dose tricyclic antidepressants, such as oral amitriptyline or nortriptyline (10–50 mg at bedtime) are useful in functional vomiting syndromes. These agents can also be used in patients with predominantly dyspeptic symptoms even in the presence of gastric emptying delays, especially if the clinical picture suggests a dyspepsia predominant picture rather than gastroparesis with impairment of nutrition. Tricyclic antidepressants are also useful in chronic persistent nausea and vomiting, and are useful early option prophylactic medications for cyclic vomiting syndrome.
- Selective serotonin reuptake inhibitors, which are generally used for depression and anxiety disorders, may also block presynaptic serotonin receptors on sensory vagal fibers, helping with control of functional nausea and vomiting. Although anecdotal reports are available, systematic studies are lacking; however, these agents are sometimes better tolerated in small doses compared with tricyclic antidepressants. Their role in cyclic nausea and vomiting has not been established.
- Bupropion, an inhibitor of neuronal uptake of norepinephrine and dopamine, is used to treat depression and may additionally help relieve nausea and vomiting. It

can be considered if side effects from tricyclic antidepressants (especially anticholinergic effects, sexual side effects, and weight gain) are poorly tolerated.

- Buspirone, an anxiolytic drug that binds to serotonin and dopamine receptors, may secondarily help correct symptoms in refractory cases. This can be considered especially in functional dyspepsia associated with nausea and vomiting.
- Sumatriptan activates 5-HT$_1$ receptors and is used as an abortive therapy for migraines. It can be used as part of abortive therapy early during a cyclic vomiting attack, especially during the prodrome.
- Zonisamide, an antiepileptic agent, has multiple mechanisms of action, including blockade of voltage-dependent sodium and T-type calcium channels as well as binding to the γ-aminobutyric acid (GABA) receptor and facilitating dopaminergic and serotoninergic neurotransmission. These broad actions help in the continuing cessation of symptoms in patients with cyclic nausea and vomiting as second-line prophylactic therapy if use of tricyclic antidepressants fails to control symptoms or is not tolerated.
- Levetiracetam, another antiepileptic drug with a less well-understood mechanism of action, appears to inhibit bursts of neuronal firing without affecting normal neuronal excitability. It may also be of benefit as second-line prophylactic therapy in cyclic vomiting syndrome.
- Gastric stimulator, a device that delivers electrical stimulation through electrodes implanted into the gastric wall, can be an option for patients with refractory persistent nausea and vomiting. It does not appear to improve gastric emptying and, therefore, may not benefit advanced gastroparesis wherein impaired gastric emptying leads to weight loss and nutritional issues.
- Enteral feeding through jejunostomy tubes (and rarely, short-term parenteral nutrition) are considered a last resort in refractory nausea and vomiting, especially where significant weight loss results from the symptomatic state or from impaired gastric emptying.

KEY POINTS TO REMEMBER

- The chemoreceptor trigger zone, located in the area postrema on the floor of the fourth ventricle, is a major mediator of the initiation of emesis.
- Viral gastroenteritis is a common cause of acute nausea and vomiting, particularly in the pediatric population.
- Functional disorders constitute a large percentage of cases of chronic nausea and vomiting.
- Acute vomiting suggests infection, medication- or toxin-induced cause, or an accumulation of toxins as in uremia or diabetic ketoacidosis. Chronic vomiting, occurring for ≥1 month, suggests a chronic medical or psychiatric condition.
- Orthostatic hypotension and tachycardia indicate hypovolemia and should be corrected immediately with volume resuscitation.
- Dopamine receptor antagonists (prochlorperazine, chlorpromazine) are commonly used for both chronic and acute vomiting.
- Cyclic vomiting syndrome is a unique disorder characterized by stereotypic nausea and vomiting with symptomfree intervals in between attacks. Treatments as for migraine appear of benefit to patients with this condition.

REFERENCES AND SUGGESTED READINGS

Clouse RE, Sayuk GS, Lustman PJ, et al. Zonisamide or levetiracetam for adults with cyclic vomiting syndrome: a case series. *Clin Gastroenterol Hepatol* 2007;5(1):44–48.

Lance LW, Anthony M. Some clinical aspects of migraine. *Arch Neurol* 1966;15:356–361.

Prakash C, Lustman PJ, Freedland KE, et al. Tricyclic antidepressants for functional nausea and vomiting: clinical outcome in 37 patients. *Dig Dis Sci* 1998;43:1951–1956.

Quigley EMM, Hasler WL, Parkman HP. AGA technical review on nausea and vomiting. *Gastroenterology* 2001;120:263–286.

Quigley EMM. Gastric and small intestinal motility in health and disease. *Gastroenterol Clin North Am* 1996;25:113–145.

Talley NJ, Phillips SF. Non-ulcer dyspepsia: potential causes and pathophysiology. *Ann Intern Med* 1988;108:865–879.

Talley NJ, Silverstein MD, Agreus L, et al. AGA technical review: evaluation of dyspepsia. *Gastroenterology* 1998;114:582–595.

Watcha MF, White PF. Postoperative nausea and vomiting: its etiology, treatment and prevention. *Anesthesiology* 1993;78:403–406.

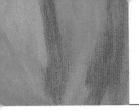

Diarrhea

Dustin G. James

INTRODUCTION

Background

The evaluation of diarrhea, especially chronic forms, requires a thorough understanding of gastrointestinal pathophysiology. Despite this, the cause of diarrhea will sometimes remain elusive. Most cases of acute diarrhea resolve, however, without intervention and do not require an exhaustive evaluation. In addition, many cases of chronic diarrhea are not associated with significant health-related adverse outcomes and can be controlled symptomatically. This chapter provides insight into the causes of diarrhea, suggesting appropriate therapy when warranted.

Definition

The best working definition of **diarrhea** is an increased liquidity or decreased consistency of stools. Experts consider increased frequency of bowel movements, specifically more than three stools per day, as part of this definition. Definitions that incorporate stool weight alone are no longer used. The intestine and colon are highly efficient in reabsorption of water. Nearly 10 L of intestinal fluid enters the jejunum on a daily basis, of which 1 L is passed into the colon. The colon further limits the fluid loss in the stool to only 100 mL/day. Diarrhea results from the inability of the digestive tract to perform this reabsorptive function.

Classification

The first step in the evaluation of diarrhea is to distinguish acute diarrhea (lasting <14 days) from chronic diarrhea (lasting >4 weeks). Most forms of acute diarrhea are infectious and do not come to medical attention. Chronic diarrhea is a more nebulous disorder, with multiple contributing processes. A detailed history and physical examination, coupled with subsequent medical testing, can narrow the diagnostic potential to a limited number of diagnoses based on pathophysiology. It is important to note that many processes that result in chronic diarrhea involve more than one mechanism.

Osmotic Diarrhea

Osmotic diarrhea results from large amounts of poorly absorbed solute in the intestinal lumen. Osmotic diarrhea has **two clinical hallmarks:** (a) the diarrhea ceases with fasting, and (b) the stool osmotic gap is abnormally elevated. The stool osmotic gap can be determined by measuring the stool [Na1] and [K1] and using the following formula:

$$\text{Stool osmotic gap} = 290 - 2 \, (Na^+ + K^+)$$

The stool osmotic gap, which is akin to the serum anion gap, detects the presence of non-measured stool osmols. Under normal circumstances, the body maintains equal fecal and serum osmolality, which is approximately 290 mOsm/kg. The presence of a poorly absorbed substance within the intestinal lumen requires that additional water be retained in the stool to maintain this value and, consequently, an osmotic gap can be measured. Osmotic gap values <50 mOsm/kg are considered normal, whereas values >125 mOsm/kg are consistent with a pure osmotic diarrhea. Indeterminate values are less helpful. The most common causes of osmotic diarrhea are disaccharidase deficiencies (e.g., lactose intolerance), excessive intakes of sugar substitutes (e.g., hexitol), or foods high in fructose, and laxative abuse. Disaccharidase deficiency results in the delivery of poorly absorbed carbohydrate molecules to the colon. These molecules not only contribute to an osmotic load, but provide a substrate for colonic fermentation by enteric bacteria, leading to increased gas production and acidic pH. Lactase deficiency is the most common disaccharidase deficiency, affecting nearly three-fourths of nonwhites and one-fourth of whites worldwide.

Secretory Diarrhea

Secretory diarrhea occurs when intestinal secretion overcomes the absorptive capability of the small intestine and colon. Because intestinal secretion is a constant process, diarrhea is incessant regardless of fasting state or time of day. Large amounts of watery diarrhea (1–10 L/24 hours) with a normal stool osmotic gap are typical. Examples of secretory diarrhea include infections, such as cholera; bile salt diarrhea (wherein bacterial breakdown of bile acids stimulates secretion from colonic mucosa); endocrine tumors, such as VIPomas and gastrinomas; and medications, such as selective serotonin reuptake inhibitors (SSRI). Although chloride-secreting colonic villous adenomas hold great interest for gastroenterologists, they are a very rare cause of secretory diarrhea.

Inflammatory Diarrhea

Disruption of the integrity and function of the gastrointestinal mucosa results in inflammatory diarrhea. Inflammation and ulceration impair the absorptive and digestive functions of normal mucosa. In addition, inflammation itself often elaborates mucus, proteins, fluid, and blood into the bowel lumen, adding to stool volume. Infectious colitis and inflammatory bowel disease (IBD) are common causes of this type of diarrhea. Clinical indicators of inflammatory diarrhea include nocturnal diarrhea and systemic signs, such as fatigue or fever.

Steatorrhea

Steatorrhea or fatty diarrhea is diarrhea of malabsorption. Any process that affects digestion and absorption of fats, ranging from celiac disease to pancreatic insufficiency, can lead to steatorrhea. In addition, inadequate contact time of bowel contents with the digestive juices and absorptive intestinal mucosa can also contribute. Examples include short gut syndrome, inappropriate bolus feeds through a small bowel feeding tube, or increased intrinsic motility from hyperthyroidism or erythromycin administration. Further, altered intestinal motility from a broad range of disease processes predisposes individuals to bacterial overgrowth, which causes diarrhea by bacterial deconjugation of bile acids within the small bowel, preventing adequate micelle formation and leading to fat malabsorption. Common risk factors include diabetes, scleroderma, small bowel diverticulosis, and immune deficiency states such as IgA deficiency. Clinical clues to fatty diarrhea include foul-smelling stool, often with oil droplets in the toilet water, or stool that adheres to the toilet bowel despite repeated flushing.

Irritable Bowel Syndrome

Irritable bowel syndrome deserves some mention because it is an important cause of chronic diarrhea in many patients. Current clinical definitions require a pain aspect to this syndrome that distinguishes it from many other causes of chronic diarrhea. Clues for functional disease include lack of noctural symptoms, disease duration >1 year, and lack of significant weight loss.

ACUTE DIARRHEA

Acute diarrhea is defined as diarrhea persisting <2 weeks. Worldwide, more than 2 billion people experience at least one episode of acute diarrhea each year. As a result of poor sanitation and limited access to health care, acute infectious diarrhea remains one of the most common causes of death in developing countries, accounting for >5 million childhood deaths per year. In the United States, nearly 100 million people are affected by acute diarrhea annually. Nearly half of these individuals must limit their activities, 250,000 require hospitalization, and approximately 3000 people die. Most deaths occur in the debilitated and the elderly. Most cases of acute diarrhea are mild and are caused by self-limited processes, lasting <5 days. Nearly 90% of cases require no diagnostic evaluation and respond to simple rehydration therapy.

Causes

Differential Diagnosis
The most common causes of acute diarrhea are infectious agents, toxins, and medications (Table 3-1). Less common causes include radiation colitis, ischemic colitis, fecal impaction, ingestion of poorly absorbable sugars, and pelvic inflammation.

Presentation

History
A careful history and physical examination narrow the differential diagnosis and help the evaluating physician decide if further diagnostic workup is necessary. Key points to address are character and duration of the diarrhea and a detailed medication history, including

TABLE 3-1	CAUSES OF ACUTE INFECTIOUS DIARRHEA
Viruses	Enterotoxigenic *E. coli*
Adenovirus	*Yersinia*
Norwalk virus	**Parasites**
Rotavirus	*Entamoeba histolytica*
Bacteria	*Giardia lamblia*
Campylobacter	*Cyclospora* (90% patients with
Salmonella	significant fatigue)
Shigella	*Isospora*
Clostridium difficile	*Cryptosporidium*
Escherichia coli O157:H7	**HIV+ Patient**
(Shiga toxin)	Microsporidia
Vibrio (cellulitis in cirrhotic	Cytomegalovirus
patients)	*Mycobacterium avium intracellulare*

HIV+, human immunodeficiency virus positive.

laxatives, antibiotics, and over-the-counter medications. Recent travel to endemic areas may suggest traveler's diarrhea. Recent immigration from a developing country or an immune-compromised state raises the possibility of a parasitic infection. Numerous sick contacts or a marked rise in regional cases of a diarrheal illness raise the possibility of a food-related outbreak. Time from ingestion of food to onset of symptoms is useful in distinguishing causes. A short incubation time (<6 hours) suggests a preformed toxin-induced food poisoning (e.g., *Staphylococcal aureus*), whereas a longer time (up to 3 days) suggests an enteroinvasive infection (e.g., Shigella, *Escherichia coli*).

Noninflammatory diarrhea often results in watery, nonbloody diarrhea associated with periumbilical cramps, bloating, nausea, or vomiting. This type of diarrhea is usually caused by disruption of normal absorption or a secretory process in the small intestine, such as that seen with certain bacterial toxins. In most cases, the diarrhea is mild. It may, however, become voluminous, ranging from 10 to 200 mL/kg/24 hours, which can result in dehydration and electrolyte abnormalities.

Inflammatory diarrhea often presents with fever and with blood in the stool. The infectious agents preferentially involve the colon, leading to a small-volume diarrhea defined as <1 L/day. Abdominal pain and tenesmus can be present. Because these infectious agents are often invasive, fecal leukocytes can be present. The initial clinical presentation of IBD may be unmasked by acute infectious diarrhea.

Physical Examination
A complete physical examination should be performed, paying particular attention to volume status and signs of severe abdominal tenderness or peritonitis. Hospitalization is necessary in cases of dehydration, toxicity, or marked abdominal pain.

Management
Diagnostic Evaluation
Most cases of acute diarrhea are mild and self-limited. Patients with signs of inflammatory diarrhea with high fever (>38.5°C), bloody diarrhea, or abdominal pain should be promptly evaluated, however. Patients with orthostatic hypotension, presyncope, excess thirst, dry mouth, oliguria, or profuse watery diarrhea should receive aggressive volume resuscitation. The frail and elderly, as well as patients with an immunodeficiency state, require urgent evaluation.

Stool bacterial cultures have a sensitivity of only 40% to 60%, although the yield can be improved by sending at least three samples. Many enteropathogens are reportable, and reporting requirements are available through the Centers for Disease Control (CDC) website. Patients with a history of recent antibiotic use should have their stool analyzed for *Clostridium difficile* toxin. Any patient whose diarrhea persists >10 days should have three stool samples sent for ova and parasites. Certain laboratories only test a limited panel of ova and parasites with specific pathogen assays. If extensive evaluation for ova and parasites is desired, microscopic examination of the stool is warranted. Sigmoidoscopy may be useful in cases of severe proctitis or suspected *C. difficile* colitis. In protracted cases, endoscopic examination with biopsy is helpful in distinguishing infectious diarrhea from ischemic colitis or IBD. A stool wet mount examination should be considered in sexually active male homosexuals or in the setting of travel to endemic areas to look for amebiasis. Any sexually active patient in whom acute proctitis is suspected should have a rectal swab cultured to rule out chlamydia, *Neisseria gonorrhea*, and herpes simplex virus.

Treatment
Patients with uncomplicated, mild, acute diarrhea are treated with oral fluids containing carbohydrates and electrolytes. Outpatients can be instructed to take such over-the-counter products as Gatorade or AllSport to improve volume status. Although the carbohydrate load is greater and the sodium is lower than that of World Health Organization

(WHO) oral rehydration solutions, these are often easier to obtain and are well tolerated. Patients may find further comfort with bowel rest or a change to a clear liquid or bland diet that avoids high-fiber foods, fats, milk products, caffeine, and alcohol. Some patients develop a transient, acquired mucosal digestive insufficiency following an acute gastroenteritis. This phenomenon often manifests as persistent diarrhea, abdominal cramps, and bloating until normal mucosal enzymatic activity is restored. A subset of patients with an acute gastroenteritis develop a chronic postinfectious IBS.

In cases of severe diarrhea, intravenous (IV) fluids may be necessary when the patient is dehydrated. In these cases, Lactated ringers or 0.9% normal saline should be given in adequate amounts to restore volume depletion and to keep up with ongoing losses.

In cases of mild to moderate diarrhea, antidiarrheal agents are safe and may improve patient comfort. Patients with bloody diarrhea, high fever, or systemic toxicity should not be given antidiarrheal agents. Anticholinergic agents are absolutely contraindicated in acute diarrhea because of the rare, but dreaded complication of toxic megacolon. If the decision to use an antidiarrheal agent is made, loperamide is recommended. Initially, 4 mg of loperamide is given PO followed by 2 mg after each loose stool up to a maximum daily dose of 16 mg. In patients with suspected traveler's diarrhea, 30 mL of bismuth subsalicylate given QID may reduce symptoms through its anti-inflammatory and antibacterial properties. The enteral antibiotic rifaximin (Xifaxan) (400 mg PO TID × 3 days), or probiotics may lessen the duration and severity of the illness. The lack of regulations and consensus on probiotic formulations limits enthusiasm for this therapy at present time.

Empiric treatment with antibiotics is only recommended in cases of suspected invasive bacterial infection, suggested by high fever, tenesmus, bloody diarrhea, or fecal leukocytes. The drug of choice is a fluoroquinolone for 5 to 7 days. Alternative antibiotics include trimethoprim-sulfamethoxazole (TMP-SMX) or erythromycin. In patients with *Salmonella* infection, treatment is reserved for those with evidence of systemic toxicity or with disease states that predispose to sepsis. Treatment consists of a fluoroquinolone such as Ciprofloxacin (500 mg) PO BID for 7 days, or zithromycin (500 mg) PO daily for 3 days. If *Giardia* is suspected, metronidazole may be given. Antibiotic treatment is also recommended in infectious diarrhea caused by amebiasis, cholera, *C. difficile*, *Shigella*, traveler's diarrhea, and sexually transmitted diseases (STDs), such as chlamydia, gonorrhea, herpes simplex virus, and syphilis. Antibiotics are not recommended for patients with *E. coli* O157:H7, because they have not been shown to hasten recovery or decrease the contagious period. In fact, their use may precipitate the hemolytic–uremic syndrome, especially in pediatric patients.

CHRONIC DIARRHEA

Chronic diarrhea persists ≥4 weeks and usually requires diagnostic evaluation. Chronic diarrhea has an estimated prevalence of 3% to 5%. There are a wide variety of causes, but a careful and detailed history and physical examination, along with selective testing, often yield an accurate diagnosis. In contrast to acute diarrhea, chronic diarrhea often has a noninfectious etiology. The exception is patients who are human immunodeficiency virus positive (HIV+) with low CD4 counts. In these patients, infectious causes are common. The lack of simple diagnostic tools and directed treatment, however, often relegate these patients to symptomatic therapy.

Causes

Differential Diagnosis
Table 3-2 lists the classes and most common causes of chronic diarrhea.

TABLE 3-2 CAUSES OF CHRONIC DIARRHEA

Secretory Diarrhea

Carcinoid syndrome
Vasoactive intestinal polypeptide tumor
Zollinger-Ellison syndrome
Medullary thyroid carcinoma
Mastocytosis
Villous adenoma of the colon
Microscopic colitis

Inflammatory Diarrhea

Inflammatory bowel disease
Infectious colitis
Radiation enterocolitis
Eosinophilic enterocolitis
Chronic ischemic colitis

Osmotic Diarrhea

Disaccharidase deficiency
High sugar substitute ingestion
Laxative abuse

Steatorrhea

Pancreatic insufficiency
Bacterial overgrowth
Celiac sprue
Whipple's disease
Short bowel syndrome
Abetalipoproteinemia
Protein losing enteropathy

Altered Intestinal Motility

Irritable bowel syndrome
Hyperthyroidism
Diabetes mellitus
Fecal impaction (overflow diarrhea)
Enteric Fistula
Amyloidosis

Presentation

History and Physical Examination

As in acute diarrhea, a comprehensive history is important to help direct the diagnostic workup. It is important to elicit the onset, duration, pattern, aggravating factors (paying special attention to diet and medications), and relieving factors as well as characteristics of the patient's stool. Care is taken to distinguish whether the stools are watery, bloody, or fatty. Patients should be questioned about fever, pain, presence or absence of fecal incontinence, and weight loss. A history of diabetes, thyroid problems, or other autoimmune disorders may be pertinent. Often, patients with Crohn's disease may have a long history of nonspecific gastrointestinal or extraintestinal complaints. A complete surgical history may also provide clues to the etiology (e.g., gastric surgery, bowel resections, or cholecystectomy). Nocturnal diarrhea that wakes a patient at night and a family history of celiac disease should be elicited. Weight loss can occur in all types of chronic diarrhea, often secondary to a patient's volitional effort to decrease intake in order to decrease diarrhea. Significant weight loss (>10 lb) is more worrisome and often points to nutrient malabsorption. In most cases, the physical examination is less revealing than the patient's history, but it should focus on volume status and evidence of malnutrition, often manifested as skin rashes or neuropathies.

Management

Diagnostic Evaluation

A complete blood count (CBC) may reveal anemia suggesting blood loss or malnutrition. Leukocytosis favors an inflammatory cause, whereas eosinophilia may suggest a parasitic infection or eosinophilic gastroenteritis. Serum chemistry screening may identify coexistent liver disease and electrolyte abnormalities. Very low levels of serum albumin in the absence of urine protein raise the possibility of a protein-losing enteropathy. Tests of thyroid function should be performed to evaluate for hyperthyroidism. In nearly two-thirds of cases, the cause of a patient's chronic diarrhea remains unclear after the initial history, physical examination, and basic laboratory work have been completed. Therefore, before pursuing an extensive evaluation, it is often appropriate to initiate a therapeutic trial if a specific diagnosis is suggested. If the patient's diarrhea resolves with empiric treatment, the diagnosis is essentially confirmed and no further workup is necessary. If symptoms persist, however, further studies should be performed.

Stool Studies

Quantitative stool analysis often provides information about the severity and type of diarrhea, helping to guide further investigations. The following studies may be useful:

- **Stool osmotic gap:** Secretory diarrheas typically have osmotic gaps <50 mOsm/kg, whereas osmotic diarrheas have osmotic gaps >125 mOsm/kg.
- **Stool pH:** A pH <5.6 suggests carbohydrate malabsorption.
- **Fecal occult blood testing:** The presence of occult blood suggests mucosal damage, including IBD, infectious colitis, malignancy, or some cases of celiac disease.
- **Fecal leukocytes:** The presence of leukocytes is consistent with an inflammatory diarrhea.
- **Stool fat measurement:** The presence of excess stool fat suggests malabsorption or maldigestion as the cause of diarrhea. This can be performed by Sudan stain on a single stool specimen or a 24-hour collection while the patient consumes >100 g of fat per day. Normal fat absorption is 95% efficient, so <5 g of fat in the stool sample is normal.
- **Stool culture:** Although it is less common as a cause of chronic diarrhea, infectious diarrhea has occasionally been implicated.
- **Stool for ova and parasites:** Three samples should be sent for examination of ova and parasites.
- **Laxative screening:** This screen should be reserved for patients in whom the diagnosis of laxative misuse is suspected. New assays that detect laxatives in the urine are especially useful in surreptitious cases.

The type of diarrhea can typically be classified based on the results of the initial evaluation and stool studies. Further diagnostic evaluation is dictated by the type of diarrhea. For instance, in cases of ongoing, unexplained diarrhea, endoscopy is warranted for small bowel biopsy to exclude villous atrophy in celiac disease, and colon biopsy to exclude microscopic colitis.

Chronic Secretory Diarrhea

Patients with secretory diarrhea typically experience watery diarrhea, and stool studies reveal a normal osmotic gap. Several studies should be performed to evaluate this process further. Mucosal diseases should be excluded by endoscopic studies, including flexible sigmoidoscopy or colonoscopy and small bowel biopsy by upper endoscopy. A small bowel magnetic resonance enterography can be considered to detect structural and inflammatory disease of the small bowel that eludes endoscopic detection. Specific testing for peptide-secreting tumors should be performed if the clinical situation suggests this diagnosis. Serum levels of vasoactive intestinal peptide, gastrin, calcitonin, pancreatic polypeptide, somatostatin, tryptase, and urinary excretion of 5-hydroxyindoleacetic acid can be measured, and followed up with appropriate imaging tests, if indicated.

Chronic Inflammatory Diarrhea

Patients with an inflammatory disorder may have fecal leukocytes or blood in the stool sample. In addition, other clues include anemia, leukocytosis, and hypoalbuminemia.

In these cases, microbiologic studies, including *C. difficile* toxin, colonic biopsy, or both may be helpful, depending on the clinical scenario. Colonoscopy or flexible sigmoidoscopy may be indicated for structural evaluation or biopsy to rule out IBD or other chronic inflammatory conditions, such as chronic ischemic colitis. Chronic food allergies may be a cause of chronic diarrhea, although no consensus recommendations are available.

Chronic Osmotic Diarrhea

A stool osmotic gap >125 mOsm/kg suggests osmotic diarrhea. In most patients with osmotic diarrhea, the cause is either carbohydrate malabsorption or ingestion of magnesium-containing salts. A lactose-free diet should be tried, because this is the most common cause of carbohydrate malabsorption. If necessary, breath tests can be obtained to evaluate for specific types of carbohydrate malabsorption. Review all medications to evaluate for inadvertent magnesium ingestion. Finally, if surreptitious laxative use is suspected, urine analysis for laxatives can be performed.

Chronic Steatorrhea

If stool studies suggest excess fat, then evaluate for causes of malabsorption. An initial examination includes imaging of the small bowel to exclude findings such as small bowel diverticula or strictures that predispose to bacterial overgrowth. Endoscopic examination of the upper gastrointestinal tract is also warranted to exclude findings that lead to inadequate small bowel activity, such as sprue or inflammation, and to exclude rare disorders, such as Ménétrièr's disease associated with protein-losing enteropathy or *Tropheryma whipplei* infection. Finally, tests of pancreatic insufficiency, such as determination of fecal elastase concentration, should be performed when the diagnosis remains elusive. In cases of villous atrophy, follow-up serology is recommended to confirm celiac disease with anti-tissue transglutaminase antibody and a determination of serum IgA levels, because up to 10% of patients with celiac disease will be IgA deficient and have a false–negative result.

Treatment

Treatment of chronic diarrhea depends on the cause. All patients with chronic diarrhea require careful attention to volume status and electrolytes. Many patients require replacement of fat-soluble vitamins, especially those with chronic steatorrhea. Chronic diarrhea can be cured if the cause is parasitic, dietary, or related to an offending medication. In cases of bacterial overgrowth, clinical response to antibiotics is often rapid and excellent, although cyclic antibiotics are often necessary unless the predisposing cause for bacterial overgrowth has been addressed. In case of bile acid malabsorption, an adsorptive agent, such as cholestyramine, is helpful. The recommended dose of cholestyramine is 4 g PO TID.

When a specific etiology for chronic diarrhea is not found, empiric therapy may be helpful. For mild to moderate watery diarrhea, mild opiates, such as oral loperamide (4 mg, up to 16 mg/day) or diphenoxylate plus atropine (Lomotil) (two tablets PO QID), are often beneficial. Other, more potent options include combinations of opiates with antispasmodics, such as tincture of opium with belladonna or hyocyamine. Anti-motility agents should be used with caution in patients with severe IBD because of the potential complication of toxic megacolon. Finally, in cases of severe secretory diarrhea, octreotide (a somatostatin analog) may be given subcutaneously to decrease the volume of diarrhea. Octreotide may also have a role in acute postoperative diarrhea. In this scenario, a fluid-filled bowel is often mistaken for a postoperative ileus. Clues to this diagnosis are abdominal distention on examination in the presence of significant diarrhea. Cross-sectional imaging reveals a distended, fluid-filled bowel. Symptoms resolve rapidly with decompression by a nasogastric tube and initiation of subcutaneous octreotide, such as 50 μg BID.

KEY POINTS TO REMEMBER

- Diarrhea is generally caused by an imbalance of water and electrolyte transport within the gut, often as a result of impaired absorption, increased secretion, or both.
- Most cases of acute diarrhea are mild and are caused by self-limited processes, lasting <5 days.
- Alarm symptoms in acute diarrhea include evidence of dehydration, systemic toxicity, and overt bleeding. These may warrant hospital admission, investigation, and specific therapy. Otherwise, nearly 90% of cases require no diagnostic evaluation and respond to simple oral rehydration therapy.
- Osmotic diarrhea has two clinical hallmarks that help lead to its diagnosis: the diarrhea ceases with fasting and the stool osmotic gap is abnormally elevated.
- Patients with bloody diarrhea, high fever, or systemic toxicity should not be given antidiarrheals. Anticholinergic agents are absolutely contraindicated in acute diarrhea because of the rare complication of toxic megacolon.
- Patients with Shiga-like *E. coli* infection (0157:H7) should not receive antibiotics given the risk of precipitating hemolytic-uremic syndrome.
- Chronic diarrhea persists ≥4 weeks and usually requires diagnostic evaluation. In contrast to acute diarrhea, chronic diarrhea often has a noninfectious cause in a normal immune state.
- Quantitative stool analysis often provides information about the severity and type of diarrhea, helping to guide further investigations.
- Secretory diarrheas typically have osmotic gaps <50 mOsm/kg, whereas osmotic diarrheas have osmotic gaps >125 mOsm/kg.
- In mild to moderate watery diarrhea, mild opiates, such as loperamide or diphenoxylate, are often beneficial. Other, more potent options include tincture of opium and belladonna.

REFERENCES AND SUGGESTED READINGS

Afzalpurkar RG, Schiller LR, Little KH, et al. The self-limited nature of chronic idiopathic diarrhea. *N Engl J Med* 1992;327:1849–1852.

Bertomeu A, Ros E, Barragan V, et al. Chronic diarrhea with normal stool and colonic examinations: organic or functional? *J Clin Gastroenterol* 1991;13:531–536.

Bruckstein AH. Diagnosis and therapy of acute and chronic diarrhea. *Postgrad Med* 1989;86:151–159.

Donowitz M, Kokke FT, Saidi R. Evaluation of patients with chronic diarrhea. *N Engl J Med* 1995;332:725–729.

Eherer AJ, Fordtran JS. Fecal osmotic gap and pH in experimental diarrhea of various causes. *Gastroenterology* 1992;103:545–551.

Fine KD, Schiller LR. AGA technical review on the evaluation and management of chronic diarrhea. *Gastroenterology* 1999;116:1464–1486.

Thielman NM, Guerrant RL. Acute infectious diarrhea. *N Engl J Med* 2004;350:38–47.

Zins BJ, Tremaine WJ, Carpenter HA. Collagenous colitis: mucosal biopsies and association with fecal leukocytes. *Mayo Clin Proc* 1995;70:430–433.

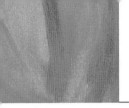

Constipation

4

Christina Y. Ha

INTRODUCTION

Constipation is often defined as a decrease in stool frequency to fewer than three bowel movements per week. Many patients who complain of constipation have other associated symptoms including passage of hard stools, straining, unproductive urges, and the sensation of incomplete evacuation. To address the varied components of constipation, a consensus definition for constipation was created (Table 4-1).

Constipation is the most common gastrointestinal (GI) complaint in the general population. Studies indicate up to 27% of the population may have constipation at any given time. Constipation is responsible for more than 2.5 million physician visits per year and more than $1 billion dollars is spent annually on laxatives in the United States. Epidemiologic studies reveal that women tend to have more self-reported constipation than men, and the prevalence of constipation increases with age. Risk factors for constipation include physical inactivity, malnutrition, restricted diets, polypharmacy, recent abdominal or pelvic surgery, travel, and known comorbid conditions.

Recognition of constipation is important, because chronic constipation can lead to fecal impaction, pudendal nerve damage, fecal incontinence, rectal prolapse, stercoral ulcers with perforation or bleeding, volvulus, hemorrhoids, and anal fissures. Severe constipation associated with abdominal pain can lead to unnecessary surgeries, such as appendectomy, hysterectomy, or ovarian cystectomy.

CAUSES

Constipation involves disordered fecal movement through the colon and anorectal region. Inadequate intake of fiber and fluid is the common precipitant, but cannot be considered an etiologic factor, because repletion of fiber and adequate fluid intake will only modestly improve bowel movement frequency. Impairment of fecal transit can also be caused by mechanical obstruction, metabolic conditions, myopathies, neuropathies, medications, or disorders of colorectal motility, such as slow-transit constipation and pelvic floor dysfunction (Table 4-2). Slow transit constipation is an idiopathic form of constipation resulting from slow transit of contents from the proximal to distal colon and rectum. Pelvic floor dysfunction occurs when the puborectalis and anal sphincter muscles fail to relax with attempted defecation, leading to an inability to defecate at the level of the anorectum; colonic transit to the rectum is otherwise normal in this disorder.

TABLE 4-1	DIAGNOSTIC CRITERIA FOR FUNCTIONAL CONSTIPATION

At least 12 weeks (with symptom onset within the past 6 months) of two or more of the following:

- Straining with >25% of defecations
- Lumpy or hard stools with >25% of defecations
- Sensation of incomplete evacuation with >25% of defecations
- Sensation of anorectal obstruction or blockage with >25% of defecations
- Manual maneuvers to facilitate >25% of defecations
- More than three defecations per week

Loose stools are absent

Insufficient criteria for diagnosis of irritable bowel syndrome (IBS)

No organic disorder present as cause of change in bowel habits

Modified from Longstreth GF, Thompson WG, Chey WD, et al. Functional bowel disorders. *Gastroenterology.* 2006;130:1480–1491, with permission.

PRESENTATION

History

Obtaining a careful history is important to establish what the patient specifically means by "constipation" and can help differentiate between organic and functional causes of constipation. A well-performed history elicits whether the patient has infrequent stools, hard stools, sense of incomplete evacuation, and straining, as well as the duration of symptoms. Lifelong symptoms suggest abnormal gut transit, such as colonic inertia, chronic idiopathic intestinal pseudo-obstruction, or rarely, a congenital disorder such as

24 hr
metanephrines

TABLE 4-2	DIFFERENTIAL DIAGNOSIS OF CONSTIPATION
Endocrine	Diabetes mellitus, hypothyroidism, pregnancy, pheochromocytoma
Metabolic	Uremia, hypercalcemia, hypokalemia, hypomagnesemia, porphyria, heavy metal poisoning
Neurogenic	Hirschsprung's disease, Chagas' disease, Parkinson's disease, spinal cord injuries or tumors, autonomic neuropathy, intestinal pseudo-obstruction, stroke, multiple sclerosis
Myopathies	Scleroderma, amyloidosis, myotonic dystrophy
Structural	Colon cancer, stricture, external compression, rectocele, fissure, hemorrhoids
Medications	See Table 4-3
Other	Irritable bowel syndrome, anal spasm, rectal prolapse, depression, low-fiber diet, sedentary lifestyle, slow-transit constipation, pelvic floor dysfunction

TABLE 4-3	MEDICATIONS CAUSING CONSTIPATION
Analgesics	Narcotics, NSAIDs
Anticholinergics	Antidepressants, antihistamines, antipsychotics, antispasmodics, antiparkinsonian drugs
Antidiarrheals	Loperamide, bismuth subsalicylate
Antihypertensives	Calcium-channel blockers, clonidine, hydralazine, diuretics
Cation-containing	Iron, antacids (aluminum based), sucralfate, calcium-containing medicines, barium, arsenic, lead, mercury, bismuth, lithium
Resins	Cholestyramine, polystyrene

NSAID, nonsteroidal anti-inflammatory drug.

Hirschsprung's disease. Later onset implies acquired disorders that can include functional constipation.

Associated symptoms may help narrow the differential diagnosis. If the patient reports cold intolerance and weight gain, hypothyroidism must be considered. The triad of kidney stones, confusion, and constipation suggests hypercalcemia. Current diuretic use or vomiting may predispose to constipation through hypokalemia and ileus. Esophageal dysmotility along with constipation is often seen in systemic sclerosis. Colon cancer can present with obstructive symptoms, but this is typically a late manifestation; important questions include a history of weight loss, bloody stools, family history of colon cancer, and prior screening colonoscopy. Abdominal pain, bloating, and psychiatric history point toward irritable bowel syndrome (IBS). Excessive straining, digital anorectal manipulation, or utilizing perineal or vaginal pressure to allow passage of stool suggests possible pelvic floor dysfunction. Finally, a thorough medication history must be taken, because medications are often the culprit. Discontinuation may lead to resolution of constipation without unnecessary tests. A list of some medications that cause constipation is found in Table 4-3.

Physical Examination

The physical examination serves to look for gastrointestinal and nongastrointestinal causes of constipation. For example, the presence of a thyroid goiter or peripheral neuropathies may suggest an endocrine or neurologic etiology.

Auscultation for the presence and frequency of bowel sounds; palpation for presence of distention, masses, or retained stool; and examination for previous surgeries are important. The digital examination can detect internal hemorrhoids, fissures, or masses. Anorectal neuromuscular function can be assessed by checking the sphincter tone at rest and with a squeeze. Perineal sensation should be assessed along with anal wink to evaluate reflex contraction of sphincter. Gaping of the anal canal on immediate withdrawal of the finger may suggest external anal sphincter denervation. Asking the patient to strain may reveal rectal prolapse or, in a female patient, the presence of a rectocele. Significant pain on rectal examination may imply a fissure. Finally, the stool should be tested for occult blood.

MANAGEMENT

Diagnostic Testing

Initial laboratory tests include basic chemistry panel with glucose, calcium, thyroid-stimulating hormone, and complete blood count. These tests are relatively inexpensive and can exclude many of the treatable disorders or prompt an evaluation for colon cancer. More specific tests for endocrinopathies, metabolic disorders, or collagen vascular disorders should be performed only with a high suspicion for specific disorders.

Imaging studies are often required but not always necessary. An obstructive series may indicate stool retention, megacolon, or bowel obstruction. Barium radiographs can be performed if plain x-rays are suggestive of megacolon, megarectum or structural disease with luminal narrowing.

Flexible sigmoidoscopy or colonoscopy is performed when there is no obvious cause for new-onset constipation, especially in patients more than 50 years of age. Warning symptoms or signs, such as weight loss, anemia, bloody stools, family history of colon cancer, or hemoccult-positive stools, should prompt a full colonoscopy to evaluate for colon cancer. Hemorrhoids may be detected as well as fissures, which can cause pain leading to secondary retention of stool. Sometimes, brownish-black discoloration of the bowel mucosa is seen, termed **melanosis coli.** It is caused by chronic anthraquinone laxative use (e.g., senna, cascara), suggesting long-standing constipation.

Colonic motility tests are useful in patients with long-standing constipation if empiric treatment has been unsuccessful and the aforementioned tests have been unrevealing. In manometric studies, pressure transducers can be placed in the sigmoid colon and rectum followed by insertion and inflation of a balloon. Various pressures are recorded at different segments of the distal bowel, and the patient's symptoms are then recorded (pain, urge to expel the balloon). In IBS, patients have low compliance of the bowel wall and, thus, low tolerability to the inflation of the balloon as opposed to megarectum, in which the opposite occurs. Although defecography is rarely done, it may identify puborectalis dysfunction, abnormal perineal descent, or rectoceles. Colonic transit studies may identify idiopathic slow-transit constipation. Radiopaque markers are ingested and transit time monitored by serial radiographs.

Treatment

Acute, short-lived constipation can usually be successfully managed with a short course of a laxative after appropriate initial evaluation has been completed. Specific management may be available if investigation reveals a treatable condition.

In chronic idiopathic constipation, if a specific diagnosis is not made after investigation, several options exist for management. Dietary approaches are first-line interventions for patients with mild or moderate symptoms. A diet high in fiber through foods such as bran, fruits, and vegetables (beans, lentils) may be helpful to increase stool bulk and promote bowel movements. Fiber supplementation can begin at 10 g/day and increase by approximately 5 g/day each week to a total intake of approximately 25 g/day. It is important to instruct patients to maintain adequate hydration during trials of increased fiber, otherwise constipation might worsen. Bloating, abdominal distention, and flatulence can result from increased fiber intake. These symptoms are usually self-limited and resolve with continued use. Patients who cannot meet these requirements can use fiber supplements such as methylcellulose, calcium polycarbophil, or psyllium.

Pharmacologic options may be required if dietary modifications fail to relieve constipation, or in moderate to severe constipation. More than 700 products are available. They are generally effective with minimal side effects provided that they are not abused. Mechanical obstruction and fecal impaction should be ruled out before beginning a laxative regimen.

- **Saline laxatives** create an osmotic gradient in the GI tract, bringing fluid into the bowel lumen. Examples are magnesium citrate, phosphate, or sulfate. Adverse effects include dehydration, abdominal cramping, and magnesium toxicity (avoid in renal dysfunction).
- **Stimulant laxatives** are the most frequently prescribed laxatives. They work by increasing colonic motility (anthraquinones work by increasing fluid and electrolyte content in the distal ileum and colon). Examples are senna and bisacodyl. Adverse effects include abdominal cramping, cathartic colon, and melanosis coli (senna, cascara).
- **Emollient laxatives** consist of mineral oils and docusate salts. Mineral oil penetrates the stool and softens it, whereas the docusate salts lower surface tension of stool and allow more water in the stool. Examples are docusate sodium and mineral oil. Adverse effects include malabsorption of fat-soluble vitamins and lipid pneumonia if aspirated.
- **Hyperosmolar laxatives** consist of nonabsorbable sugars, such as lactulose, sorbitol, and mixed electrolyte solutions (polyethylene glycol); they work by osmotically increasing fluid in bowel lumen. Adverse effects include electrolyte imbalance, dehydration, and incontinence because of potency.
- **Enemas** using tap water, saline, mineral or cottonseed oil, and sodium phosphate cause reflex evacuation of luminal contents. Adverse effects include mechanical trauma and damage to rectal mucosa with chronic use.
- **5-hydroxytryptamine-4 (5-HT$_4$) receptor agonists**, specifically tegaserod, have demonstrated efficacy in treating patients with constipation-predominant IBS where abdominal pain and bloating are often present between bowel movements. Tegaserod stimulates gut motility through the cholinergic pathways, leading to improved bowel habits as well as decreased visceral hypersensitivity. Concerns regarding potentially increased cardiac adverse events, however, led to its withdrawal from the market in March 2007, but it is anticipated that the agent will be available with restrictions in the future.
- **Lubiprostone**, a chloride-channel activator that increases intestinal water secretion, is one of the newer agents on the market for treatment of constipation. Recent studies suggest improved bowel habits with lubiprostone versus placebo with predominant adverse effects being nausea and diarrhea. No head-to-head comparisons have been made of lubiprostone with other agents for treatment of severe constipation, however.
- **Methylnaltrexone**, a peripherally acting mu-receptor antagonist, has been used to treat patients with opioid-related constipation. By not crossing the blood–brain barrier, methylnaltrexone can promote bowel movements without decreasing the pain-relieving effects of narcotics. Studies have indicated a significantly favorable response to methylnaltrexone versus placebo.

Nonpharmacologic Treatments

- **Biofeedback** is often used to treat patients with pelvic floor dysfunction because laxatives tend to be ineffective treatments for this disorder. Patients can be retrained to relax their pelvic floor muscles and restore normal anorectal synergy during defecation. This process has been demonstrated to be effective in relieving obstructive symptoms and increasing stool frequency.
- **Surgical treatment** of chronic constipation is reserved only for the patient who has failed prolonged and repeated trials of laxatives, prokinetic agents, and dietary modifications. In this select population, usually patients with colonic inertia, a total colectomy with ileorectal anastomosis can be performed.

KEY POINTS TO REMEMBER

- Complications of constipation include hemorrhoids, anal fissures, rectal prolapse, ischemic colitis, volvulus, fecal impaction, stercoral ulcers, and fecal incontinence.
- The presence of warning symptoms or signs, such as weight loss, anemia, blood in stools (gross or occult), age (>50 years), or family history of colon cancer, should prompt colonoscopy to exclude colon cancer.
- A careful medication history should be obtained before embarking on an involved workup of constipation.
- Fecal impaction and mechanical obstruction should be excluded before proceeding with the use of laxatives.
- When recommending increased fiber intake, maintenance of adequate hydration is key, or the constipation could worsen.
- Patients with pelvic floor dysfunction may benefit from a trial of biofeedback to retrain pelvic floor muscles to relax because laxatives tend to be ineffective to treat this disorder.

REFERENCES AND SUGGESTED READINGS

Ambizas EM, Ginzburg R. Lubiprostone: a chloride channel activator for treatment of chronic constipation. *Ann Parmacother* 2007;41(6):957–964.

Brandt L, Prather C, Quigley E, et al. Systematic review on the management of chronic constipation in North America. *Am J Gastroenterol* 2005;100(S1):S5–S22.

Locke GR, Pemberton JH, Phillips SH. AGA technical review on constipation. *Gastroenterology* 2000;119(6):1766–1778.

Longstreth GF, Thompson WG, Chey WD, et al. Functional bowel disorders. *Gastroenterology* 2006;30:1480–1491.

Shaiova L, Rim F, Friedman D, et al. A review of methylnaltrexone, a peripheral opioid receptor antagonist, and its role in opioid-induced constipation. *Palliative Support Care* 2007;5(2):161–166.

Wald A. Approach to the patient with constipation. In: Yamada T, ed. *Textbook of Gastroenterology*. Philadelphia: Lippincott Williams & Wilkins; 1999.

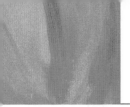

Abdominal Pain

5

Daniel A. Ringold

INTRODUCTION

Abdominal pain represents one of the most common complaints for which patients seek medical attention. The ability to diagnose and treat abdominal pain accurately and efficiently is important to internists, gastroenterologists, and surgeons. A general understanding of abdominal anatomy and physiology is important in creating a differential diagnosis. Further, because multiple disorders can result in the perception of pain in the abdomen, an orderly approach is critical to avoid unnecessary testing and potentially harmful delays in diagnosis.

CAUSES

Pathophysiology

Several means exist by which noxious stimuli result in the sensation of pain within the abdomen. The specific characteristics for each type of pain help in identifying the underlying disease process. The two principal mechanisms of pain on which this chapter focuses are parietal pain and visceral (somatic) pain. Other important mechanisms include ischemia, musculoskeletal pain, referred pain, metabolic derangements, neurogenic pain, and functional pain. It is important to note that a single diseased organ can produce pain through multiple mechanisms.

Parietal Pain

The parietal peritoneum lining the abdominal cavity is innervated by somatic nerve fibers. The pain caused by irritation of the parietal peritoneum, therefore, is usually sharp, well-localized, and lateralizes to the site of irritation. The most frequent stimulus is inflammation, often from an inflamed adjacent organ. Other stimuli that can irritate the parietal peritoneum are blood, gastric acid, or stool. The pain is constant and is worse with motion of the peritoneum. Pain severity depends on the specific irritating agent and the rate of development. There is often associated reflex muscle spasm of the abdominal muscles, referred to as *involuntary guarding*.

Visceral Pain

Noxious stimuli affecting the abdominal viscera result in the perception of visceral pain. This can result from traction on the peritoneum, distention of a hollow viscus, or muscular contraction, often against an obstructed lumen. The pain fibers innervating the visceral structures are bilateral, so pain is typically perceived in the midline. As opposed to parietal pain, visceral pain is dull and poorly localized. The pain is often intermittent or colicky, but it can be constant. There are often associated autonomic symptoms such as nausea, vomiting, diaphoresis, or pallor.

TABLE 5-1	CAUSES OF ABDOMINAL PAIN			
Inflammatory Conditions	**Mechanical**	**Ischemic**	**Metabolic**	**Other**
Cholecystitis	Small or large bowel obstruction	Mesenteric ischemia	Diabetic ketoacidosis	Thoracic disorders
Pancreatitis	Volvulus	Splenic infarction	Uremia	Herpes zoster
Appendicitis	Biliary obstruction	Testicular torsion	Porphyria	SLE
Diverticulitis	Ureteral stones	Ovarian cyst torsion	Lead poisoning	Musculoskeletal disorders
Hepatitis	Ruptured aortic aneurysm	Incarcerated hernia		Functional abdominal pain
PID	Ruptured ectopic pregnancy			
Peptic ulcer	Intussusception			
Gastroenteritis				
Spontaneous bacterial peritonitis				
Acute colitis				
Pyelonephritis				
Acute cholangitis				

PID, pelvic inflammatory disease; SLE, systemic lupus erythematosus.

Differential Diagnosis

The list of diagnoses that can cause abdominal pain is extensive and includes inflammatory, mechanical, ischemic, metabolic, and neurologic conditions. This emphasizes the need for a careful and systematic history and physical examination to narrow the possible diagnoses. Table 5-1 lists some of the common causes of abdominal pain.

Presentation

A thorough, detailed history and physical examination are the keys to efficient evaluation of the patient with abdominal pain. An accurate diagnosis can be made in most patients with only a meticulous history and physical examination.

History

An organized approach to the history is essential. Attempts should be made to identify the pain's onset, duration, character, location, severity, exacerbating or alleviating factors, and associated symptoms. Other key features of the history should include underlying medical conditions, prior surgeries, current medications, substance abuse, recent travel, and family history. Some general principles regarding these aspects of the history are described here.

Onset of Pain

Severe pain that begins abruptly may indicate an intra-abdominal catastrophe, including ruptured abdominal vasculature or perforated viscus. Pain that develops rapidly over minutes suggests inflammation or luminal obstruction. Gradual onset over a few hours may also suggest inflammation.

Duration

Pain caused by irritation of the parietal peritoneum is constant, whereas obstruction of a hollow viscus results in crampy or colicky pain that waxes and wanes.

Character

Parietal pain is usually severe and well-localized, whereas the pain associated with visceral noxious stimuli is dull or gnawing and poorly localized.

Location

Pain location is often the most important characteristic. Because the parietal peritoneum is supplied by somatic nerves, pain is perceived in the area where the peritoneum is irritated. Visceral pain is usually midline and poorly localized, but the location may provide useful information regarding the involved organ. Radiation of the pain may also help identify the affected organ. Table 5-2 lists the commonly affected organs and the corresponding perceived areas of pain.

Severity

Severe pain suggests ruptured abdominal viscus or vasculature structure. Pain that is severe in the setting of a benign examination may suggest mesenteric ischemia.

Exacerbating and Alleviating Factors

Pain caused by inflammation of the peritoneum is worse with coughing or movement. Pain from peptic ulcer disease is often relieved immediately after eating or taking antacids, but it can worsen 1 to 2 hours after eating. In contrast, both ischemic and biliary pains are often brought on soon after eating. The pain associated with pancreatitis is classically relieved by bending forward or curling up in the fetal position.

TABLE 5-2	ORGAN INVOLVEMENT AND PERCEIVED LOCATION OF PAIN
Esophagus	Chest, epigastrium
Stomach	Epigastrium
Small intestine	Periumbilical region
Colon	Lower abdomen
Gallbladder	Right upper quadrant, radiation to scapula, shoulder, back
Liver	Right upper quadrant
Kidney or ureter	Costovertebral angle, flank, radiation to groin
Bladder	Suprapubic region
Aorta	Mid-back region

Associated Symptoms

Nausea, vomiting, diaphoresis, hematemesis, hematochezia, melena, diarrhea, obstipation, hematuria, and fever may further focus the diagnostic evaluation.

Physical Examination

As with the history, an organized approach to the examination, particularly that of the abdomen, increases the likelihood of an accurate diagnosis. In addition, focusing on key extra-abdominal physical examination findings is crucial because they may provide valuable clues as to the diagnosis. An exhaustive review of all the signs is beyond the scope of this chapter. However, several points deserve emphasis.

Vital Signs

Particular attention must be given to frequent hemodynamic monitoring. The presence of tachycardia or orthostatic hypotension suggests significant volume depletion and should prompt an immediate search for the underlying cause (hemorrhage, vomiting, diarrhea, or third-spacing). Tachycardia may be the only sign of impending hemodynamic collapse in a patient with a vascular catastrophe. Fever suggests an inflammatory process, often infectious. Tachypnea is often the earliest sign of sepsis.

General Appearance

Much information can be determined by observing the patient's general appearance. Patients with peritonitis often lie very still, whereas those with renal colic often writhe in bed. Patients with acute inflammatory or vascular disorders frequently appear toxic. Generalized pallor suggests severe anemia, possibly from acute blood loss.

Abdominal Examination

Because patients with acute abdominal pain are very apprehensive, it is important to take a gentle, reassuring approach to the abdominal examination. The abdomen should be examined with the patient's knees and hips flexed to relax the abdominal muscles. First, the abdomen should be visually inspected for surgical scars, distention, bulging flanks, or other obvious abnormalities. Next, auscultate for the presence or absence of bowel sounds or bruits. Gentle pressure with the stethoscope allows assessment of tenderness without alarming the patient. Palpation should begin at the site furthest away from the area of pain and additionally noting any visceral enlargement or masses. The presence or absence of guarding, rigidity, or rebound tenderness should be noted, because these may signify peritoneal irritation. Peritoneal inflammation is best determined by light percussion on the abdomen, gently shaking the bed, or asking the patient to cough. Finally, all patients with acute abdominal pain should have rectal examinations performed; female patients should have pelvic examinations performed in addition.

MANAGEMENT

Diagnostic Evaluation

Because most patients with acute abdominal pain can be diagnosed with a careful history and physical examination, further diagnostic evaluation should be targeted to the clinical scenario. Excessive, undirected testing increases the costs and may cause unnecessary delays in diagnosis and treatment. Specific tests deserve special mention.

Blood Tests

A complete blood count should be ordered in all patients to evaluate for leukocytosis or anemia. Electrolytes and liver chemistries should also be obtained. Amylase and lipase estimations are useful for suspected pancreatic disease, but these values can be elevated in other conditions, such as bowel obstruction or perforation. Lactate levels may be helpful for suspected bowel infarction, but a normal lactate level does not exclude intestinal ischemia. Finally, all female patients of childbearing age should have pregnancy excluded with a urine or serum beta-human chorionic gonadotropin (β-hCG).

Standard Radiography

Not all patients with acute abdominal pain require plain or upright films of the abdomen. Abdominal x-rays are useful, however, for diagnosing perforated viscus (identified as free air under the diaphragm), ileus, or bowel obstruction. Abdominal films may also demonstrate the calcific changes associated with chronic pancreatitis as well as calcium-containing renal stones. Additionally, some features of intestinal inflammation, such as colonic "thumbprinting," may be perceived on abdominal x-ray films. The sensitivity of abdominal radiography in the diagnosis of abdominal pathology in the setting of acute abdominal pain is about 10%, however. Regardless, abdominal films are safe, relatively inexpensive, and can usually be performed quickly.

Ultrasonography

Transabdominal ultrasound is useful for patients with suspected biliary tract disease, including acute cholecystitis, biliary pain, and choledocholithiasis. It also allows for the rapid diagnosis of abdominal aortic aneurysms. Its sensitivity and specificity, however, are limited by operator and interpreter experience. Ultrasound is safe and can be performed at the bedside in most cases.

Computed Tomography

Abdominal computerized tomography (CT), especially with rapid spiral scanning techniques, provides a powerful imaging tool. It allows "three-dimensional" imaging of the entire abdomen and pelvis and is less operator-dependent than is ultrasound. It is the most sensitive test for identifying a perforated viscus and is useful for suspected cases of bowel obstruction, intra-abdominal abscess, appendicitis, ruptured aortic aneurysm, necrotizing pancreatitis, and diverticulitis. Care, however, must be used in selecting patients for abdominal CT. The test is costly and may unnecessarily delay diagnosis and treatment, especially in patients who require urgent surgery. In addition, the use of iodinated contrast dye is associated with nephrotoxicity and carries a small risk of anaphylactic reaction.

Magnetic Resonance Imaging

In recent years, magnetic resonance imaging (MRI) has emerged as a powerful tool in the diagnosis of GI disorders. It is a multiplanar imaging modality using the different intrinsic soft-tissue contrast properties to distinguish areas with different degrees of enhancement. It can detect subtle lesions that do not conform to organ contours with high sensitivity. MRI is an excellent modality in the evaluation and differentiation of liver and pancreatic lesions. For instance, magnetic resonance cholangiopancreatography (MRCP) has become the noninvasive imaging modality of choice for evaluating abnormalities of the biliary and pancreatic ducts. MRI is also highly sensitive in evaluating the mesenteric vessels in suspected ischemia. Recently, MR enterography has been used to image the small bowel and colon to detect inflammation, strictures, and fistulae. One of the major advantages of MRI is that it is safer than CT in children, teenagers, and pregnant women because of lack of ionizing radiation. Secondly, the intravenous contrast medium typically used (gadolinium) carries a minimal risk of nephrotoxicity, and generally can be used in patients with renal insufficiency. One of the main drawbacks of MRI is that it cannot be used in patients with permanent pacemakers, defibrillators, and aneurysm clips. Because most MRI devices consist of a closed tube with opening on the ends, it is not well suited for patients with severe claustrophobia. In addition to being more costly, MRI studies are generally more time-consuming and require greater patient cooperation than CT scans, making them less desirable in urgent settings.

KEY POINTS TO REMEMBER

- A careful, detailed history and physical examination are the keys to efficient evaluation of the patient with abdominal pain. An accurate diagnosis can be made in most patients with only a meticulous history and physical examination.
- The pain caused by irritation of the parietal peritoneum is usually well localized and lateralizes to the site of irritation.
- Visceral pain is dull and poorly localized. There are often associated autonomic symptoms, including nausea, vomiting, diaphoresis, or pallor.
- Peritoneal inflammation is best determined by light percussion on the abdomen, gently shaking the bed, or asking the patient to cough. Rebound tenderness is less specific for peritoneal inflammation.

REFERENCES AND SUGGESTED READINGS

Ahn SH, Mayo-Smith WW, Murphy BL, et al. Acute non-traumatic abdominal pain in adult patients: abdominal radiography compared with CT evaluation. *Radiology* 2002;225:159–164.

Fauci A, ed. *Harrison's Principles of Internal Medicine*. 16th ed. New York: McGraw-Hill; 2005:1725–1729.

Flasar MH, Cross R, Goldberg E. Acute abdominal pain. *Prim Care Clin Office Pract* 2006;33:659–684.

Ginsberg GG, Kochman ML. *Endoscopy and Gastrointestinal Radiology*. 1st ed, Philadelphia: Mosby; 2004:111–133.

Sleisenger MH, Fordtran JS. *Gastrointestinal Disease: Pathophysiology, Diagnosis, Management*. 8th ed. Philadelphia: WB Saunders; 2002:71–82.

Wolfe MM. *Therapy of Digestive Disorders*. 2nd ed. Philadelphia: WB Saunders; 2006:961–968.

Yamada T, ed. *Textbook of Gastroenterology*. 4th ed, Philadelphia: Lippincott Williams & Wilkins; 2003:781–801.

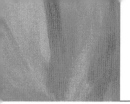

Acute Gastrointestinal Bleeding

6

Sonal Kumar

INTRODUCTION

Acute gastrointestinal bleeding (GIB) is generally defined as bleeding that occurs anywhere in the digestive tract. GI bleeding can be further classified into upper GI bleeding (UGIB) or lower GI bleeding (LGIB). **UGIB** is defined as bleeding that occurs from a source proximal to the ligament of Treitz, whereas **LGIB** originates distal to the ligament of Treitz. Regardless of the location in the digestive tract, GI bleeding is a significant cause of morbidity and mortality in the United States. Recent studies have estimated the yearly hospitalization rate for UGIB at approximately 100 to 200 per 100,000 population, with nearly half of these hospitalizations occurring in individuals older than 60 years of age. Unlike UGIB, LGIB tends to be slow and intermittent. Several studies have revealed that the incidence of lower GI bleeds is much less compared with upper GI bleeds (anywhere from one-fifth to one-third as frequent). The annual incidence of LGIB is 20 to 27 per 100,000 population. LGIB is also more common with increasing age with a >200 times increase from the third to the ninth decades. Approximately 80% of all acute episodes of GIB, in both the upper and lower GI tracts, require only supportive care and resolve spontaneously without any intervention. Mortality rates from UGIB have remained steady, however, ranging from 6% to 12%, accounting for 10,000 to 20,000 deaths in the United States annually; mortality rates from LGIB is <5%.

CAUSES

Peptic Ulcer Disease

Peptic ulcer disease (PUD) is the most common cause of upper GI hemorrhage, although more recent data suggest that the incidence of PUD-related bleeding may be decreasing. Mortality rates remain around 20%, however, whereas rebleeding rates are around 14%. Risk factors include *Helicobacter pylori* infection, nonsteroidal anti-inflammatory drug (NSAID) use, and hypersecretion of gastric acid, as in Zollinger-Ellison syndrome. In patients taking NSAIDs, cofactors such as age (>75 years), concurrent coronary artery disease, previous GIB, and past PUD may be independent risk factors for ulcer bleeding. Bleeding can occur without previous dyspepsia. Ulcers are most commonly located in the duodenal bulb and stomach, but can also occur in the esophagus, pyloric channel, duodenal loop, jejunum, and Meckel's diverticulum. Duodenal ulcers are strongly associated with *H. pylori* infection. The organism disrupts the mucosal barrier and has an inflammatory effect on gastric and duodenal mucosa. NSAID use also predisposes patients to ulcer hemorrhage because of its effect on cyclooxygenase-1, which leads to impaired mucosal defense toward acid secretion. Ulcers located on the lesser curve of the stomach and posteroinferior wall of the duodenal bulb and are >2 cm in size have been demonstrated to rebleed with greater frequency.

Erosions

An erosion can be defined as a 3- to 5-mm break in the mucosa that does not penetrate the muscularis mucosa. Gastric erosions are most commonly related to medications, such as NSAIDs or aspirin, which can cause a hemorrhagic gastropathy within 24 hours of administration in certain situations. Gastric erosions can also be seen in situations of severe physiologic stress (burns, sepsis, trauma, surgery, shock, or respiratory, renal or liver failure). The pathophysiology behind stress ulcers is thought to be related to gastric hypoperfusion as a result of splanchnic vasoconstriction during physiologic stress. Hypoperfusion causes mucosal injury by disrupting the supply of oxygen and other nutrients along with disrupting the removal of waste products.

Variceal Bleeding

Variceal bleeding most commonly occurs from esophageal varices but can also result from gastric and duodenal varices. Varices may be seen in patients who have portal hypertension of any cause. Most patients, however, have underlying liver cirrhosis. In the United States, alcoholic cirrhosis is the most common cause of portal hypertension. Other causes of portal hypertension include mechanical obstruction from portal or hepatic vein thrombosis, congenital hepatic fibrosis, or schistosomiasis. Regardless of the cause, portosystemic collateral circulations usually form at junctions of squamous and columnar mucosa to decompress the portal circulation. These collateral circulations enlarge to form varices. Of note, the portosystemic gradient must be >12 mm Hg for varices to form. Approximately one-third of patients with cirrhosis have at least one variceal hemorrhage and about 20% of all patients with cirrhosis and varices have GIB. Red or blue color and larger size of the varix (>5 mm) predict a greater risk of rupture and subsequent hemorrhage. Mortality from a single variceal bleed is 30% to 50%. Of those patients who survive the initial episode, 60% to 70% die within 1 year. This high mortality rate is caused both by the high risk of rebleeding and the comorbid conditions and complications that patients with varices often have (hepatic coma, septicemia, liver decompensation, renal failure, and aspiration). Gastric varices can occur in the setting of portal hypertension or after injection sclerotherapy of esophageal varices. Isolated gastric varices may be seen with splenic vein thrombosis. Bleeding risk is similar to that of esophageal varices.

Portal Gastropathy

Portal gastropathy caused by cirrhosis may be a mechanism of nonvariceal bleeding in patients with portal hypertension. There is congestion of the gastric mucosa from dilated arterioles and venules mainly in the gastric fundus and cardia. Erythema, petechiae, multiple bleeding areas, vascular ectasias, and congestion are hallmarks of portal gastropathy. Endoscopic evaluation often shows a mottled or mosaic pattern.

Mallory-Weiss Tear

Mallory-Weiss tears, which occur from mucosal disruption at the gastroesophageal junction, are evidenced by longitudinal ulcerations. Bleeding ensues when an underlying venous or arterial plexus is exposed by the tear. They generally are preceded by prolonged episodes of retching or vomiting (typically after an alcohol binge). The hemorrhage may be brisk but is self-limited (80%–90%), and the tear usually heals within a few days. Continued vomiting, however, can lead to esophageal rupture (Boerhaave's syndrome). Comorbid portal hypertension confers a risk of more massive bleeding from Mallory-Weiss tears.

Esophagitis

Esophagitis is a common condition that often results from gastroesophageal reflux when gastric contents are regurgitated into the esophagus. Esophagitis can also result from infection (candida, herpes simplex, cytomegalovirus [CMV]), radiation therapy, or medications (quinidine, tetracycline, alendronate), but rarely causes severe bleeding. The most common symptoms of esophagitis are heartburn, nausea, epigastric discomfort, and chest pain.

Arteriovenous Malformations

Arteriovenous malformations (AVM) are defects of the circulatory system, including vascular ectasias, angiomas, and angiodysplasias. Those that occur in the small intestine are generally believed to be congenital in nature. The result is a complex tangle of arteries and veins connected by one or more fistulae. The vascular complex is known as the nidus, which is lacking a capillary bed and, therefore, arteries directly drain into veins. The draining veins are known to dilate secondary to the high-velocity blood flow and can eventually rupture, resulting in a bleed. AVMs include Dieulafoy lesions (an ectatic vessel that erodes through the mucosa), hemorrhagic telangiectasias (seen in Osler-Weber-Rendu syndrome), and those associated with chronic renal failure. Noncongenital lesions are also common causes of subacute GIB with slow, intermittent blood loss. These angiodysplastic lesions are usually multiple, <5 mm in diameter, and involve primarily the cecum and right colon, but can also be found in the stomach. Most are degenerative lesions associated with aging. Two thirds of patients with colonic angiodysplasia are older than 70 years of age. One theory of pathogenesis is that repeated, partial, intermittent obstruction of the submucosal veins where they pierce the muscle layers of the colon leads to dilation and tortuosity of the veins. Eventually, the entire arteriolar-capillary-venular unit dilates, creating a small arteriovenous communication. Because active bleeding is infrequently identified and because these lesions appear to be common in the elderly without a significant blood loss history, definitive diagnosis is difficult. If no other source of GIB is identified in a patient with recurrence of persistent GIB sufficient to require transfusions or cause significant anemia, the presence of angiodysplasia is an indication for treatment. The diagnosis of vascular ectasias can be made by colonoscopy or angiography. Both diagnostic modalities frequently identify the lesions without demonstrating active bleeding. The diagnostic sensitivity of colonoscopy is 80%, with 90% specificity. The earliest angiographic sign is a densely opacified, dilated, tortuous, slowly emptying intramural vein. A vascular tuft represents a more advanced lesion, and an early-filling vein, which reflects an arteriovenous communication, is a late sign.

Aortoenteric Fistulas

Fistulas generally occur after aortic graft surgery and, although the point of intestinal breach can be anywhere from the esophagus to the colon, it usually involves the third or fourth part of the duodenum. Often, the fistulas can be difficult to diagnose because visualization of the graft eroding through the intestinal wall is uncommon. The classic "herald bleed" is a small bleed that can occur days to weeks before massive fatal hemorrhage. Secondary fistulas have been described in the distal small bowel and colon.

Hemobilia

Hemobilia is hemorrhage into the biliary tract. This is usually caused by trauma, but can also be seen in malignant tumors, cholelithiasis, acalculous inflammatory disease, or vascular disorders.

Hemosuccus Pancreaticus

Hemosuccus pancreaticus is a rare cause of hemorrhage in the GI tract. It is caused by a bleeding source in the pancreas, pancreatic duct, or structures adjacent to the pancreas, such as the splenic artery. It usually occurs in patients with chronic pancreatitis, pseudocyst, pancreatic cancer, aneurysms of the splenic artery, or trauma. Hemosuccus pancreaticus results in hemorrhage into the pancreatic duct.

Diverticular Bleeding

Diverticular bleeding is the most common cause of major lower GI hemorrhage caused by the high prevalence of diverticulosis in the Western world. Bleeding occurs in only 3% of patients with diverticulosis. Diverticula form at sites of weakness in the muscle wall of the colon where arteries penetrate the muscularis layer to reach the mucosa and submucosa. Bleeding presumably results from rupture of a colonic artery into the diverticular sac. Diverticular bleeding presents with acute, painless, maroon to bright red hematochezia, although melenic stools may occur. Among the 75% to 80% of patients in whom bleeding ceases, 25% to 35% have repeated episodes of diverticular hemorrhage. If the initial bleeding ceases spontaneously, no further therapy is indicated because bleeding does not recur in most patients.

Neoplasms

Benign and malignant neoplasms of the colon are common lesions that occur predominantly in the elderly. Major hemorrhage from a colonic polyp or carcinoma is uncommon. The diagnosis is made by colonoscopy or barium enema, and treatment is colonoscopic or surgical excision, as appropriate.

Anorectal Disease

Hemorrhoids and anal fissures are probably the most common causes of minor intermittent lower GIB. The characteristic clinical history of hemorrhoidal bleeding is bright red blood on the toilet tissue or around the stool but not mixed in the stool. Bleeding often occurs with straining or passage of hard stool. A similar history is common in patients with bleeding from anal fissures, with the exception that anal fissures are often painful. Only rarely is the amount of bleeding sufficiently severe to cause iron deficiency anemia or sufficiently acute and severe to require transfusions. Massive hemorrhage from simple hemorrhoids is rare, but can occur from rectal varices in patients with portal hypertension. Perianal disease is treated with sitz baths, bulk-forming agents, avoidance of straining, and ointments or suppositories. It is unknown if actual therapeutic benefit is obtained with locally applied medications containing lubricants and hydrocortisone, but many patients report symptomatic relief. When bleeding or other symptoms continue to be troublesome, hemorrhoidal banding, coagulation techniques, or surgery may be indicated.

Meckel's Diverticulum

Meckel's diverticulum is the most frequent congenital anomaly of the intestinal tract, with an incidence of 0.3% to 3.0% in autopsy reports. It develops from incomplete obliteration of the vitelline duct, leaving an ileal diverticulum. Patients present with painless bleeding that may be melenic or bright red. The diagnosis can be made by radiolabeled technetium scanning. Barium filling of the diverticulum may occur, especially with enteroclysis. Mesenteric angiography may demonstrate the site of bleeding. Surgical excision is the treatment of choice.

Inflammatory Bowel Disease

Inflammatory bowel disease usually causes a small to moderate degree of bleeding, although rarely it can be massive. The blood is usually mixed in with the stool and is associated with other symptoms of the disease, such as diarrhea, tenesmus, and pain. The diagnosis and treatment of this bleeding depend on management of the underlying disorder.

Ischemic Colitis

Ischemic colitis is a common entity in the elderly population. It is usually caused by "low-flow states" and small vessel disease rather than by large vessel occlusion. Any segment of the colon might be involved, although most commonly the splenic flexure, descending colon, and sigmoid colon are involved. The typical presentation is mild, crampy abdominal pain localized to the lower left side, followed within 24 hours by rectal bleeding or bloody diarrhea. The blood loss is characteristically minimal, although massive bleeding has been described rarely. Plain abdominal films may show the classic "thumb-printing" lesion of the colon. The diagnosis is best made by colonoscopy and biopsy. Most cases resolve spontaneously with observation and medical support. Surgery is reserved for the rare circumstance of clinical deterioration with fever and rising leukocyte count or persistent hemorrhage.

Infectious Colitis

Infectious colitis caused by *Campylobacter jejuni*, *Shigella* species, invasive *Escherichia coli* or *E. coli* O157:H7, or *Clostridium difficile* often presents with bloody diarrhea. The degree of blood loss is rarely significant. The diagnosis is made by sigmoidoscopy with biopsy and stool culture. Treatment is determined by the specific pathogen.

Radiation-induced Enteritis

Radiation injury is a chronic or recurrent problem that may follow irradiation immediately or present several years later. Radiation impairs the normal course of repopulation of surface epithelium within the GI tract. The loss of absorptive surface can often lead to malabsorption and diarrhea, but microulcerations can also form. These microulcerations can coalesce and form bigger lesions and eventually result in a GI bleed. The blood loss is rarely massive, but can cause iron deficiency or the need for intermittent blood transfusion. The diagnosis is made by the history of irradiation and with endoscopic biopsy confirmation.

Colonic Ulcers

Colonic ulcers are increasingly recognized as causes of acute LGIB. Although not classically associated with colonic ulcers, NSAID use can cause discrete ulcers throughout the colon.

Intussusception

Intussusception may present with maroon stools and is almost always accompanied by crampy abdominal pain. Uncommon in adults, it usually has a leading point, such as a polyp or malignancy. Patients often present with bloody stools mixed with mucous, often described as "currant jelly." The diagnosis may be suggested by plain abdominal films and a sausage-shaped mass found during physical examination. Barium enema may be useful for diagnosis; in children, it may be used for therapeutic reduction. Treatment of intussusception in adults is usually surgical.

PRESENTATION

History

A careful history should be taken in the setting of acute gastrointestinal bleeding to decipher the source of the bleed. History should include specifics of hematemesis, melena, or hematochezia. Clues to bleeding severity include duration of bleeding, and stool color, frequency, and volume. Abrupt hematochezia (within 24 hours of presentation) associated with hemodynamic instability or bleeding that has occurred over several days that causes the patient to complain of dizziness or other orthostatic symptoms suggests major blood loss and the need for quick resuscitation. Associated symptoms, including abdominal pain, recent change in bowel habits, fever, or weight loss, may point to specific diagnoses. Chronic abdominal pain or dyspeptic symptoms points toward PUD. Liver disease and chronic alcohol use are important risk factors for variceal hemorrhage. A history of vomiting or retching suggests a Mallory-Weiss tear. A recent history of anorexia or weight loss may indicate an underlying malignancy. Other relevant medical history includes previous bleeding (diverticulosis, hemorrhoids, ulcers, varices, or angiodysplasia), recent polypectomy, past abdominal surgeries, inflammatory bowel disease, history of radiation therapy to the abdomen or pelvis, trauma, coagulation disorders, immune status, and malignancies. Current medications should also be reviewed, with particular attention to NSAID use, acetylsalicylic acid (ASA) and anticoagulants. Also, the presence or absence of chest pain, palpitations, dyspnea on exertion, lightheadedness, or orthostatic symptoms should be determined. Chest pain may suggest a superimposed myocardial infarction or dissecting aneurysm, whereas a history of abdominal vascular surgery adds aortoenteric fistula to the differential diagnosis.

Physical Examination

Vital signs are the most important aspect of the physical examination. Tachycardia and hypotension suggest a hemodynamically significant bleed that requires prompt diagnosis and therapy. Evaluation for orthostatic hypotension should also be performed. Stigmata of chronic liver disease and portal hypertension (i.e., telangiectasias, ascites, splenomegaly) should be closely evaluated. Abdominal tenderness, rebound, and guarding should also be determined. Digital rectal examination can provide useful information to the color and consistency of stools and presence or absence of hemorrhoids or masses. Use of color-coded cards is helpful in determining the actual color of stools. It is important to note that stool may remain guaiac positive for up to 2 weeks after a GI bleed.

MANAGEMENT

Resuscitation

- Evaluate for possible causes of hemorrhage during or after hemodynamic stabilization. Signs of hypovolemia (i.e., hypotension, tachycardia, pallor, agitation) necessitate immediate repletion of intravascular volume.
- Intravascular volume should be restored initially with either isotonic saline or lactated Ringer's solution. Two large-bore ($\geq$18-gauge) intravenous (IV) lines should be in place at all times. Centrally inserted, triple lumen catheters do not confer any advantage over peripheral IV lines in terms of rate of fluid administration. Vasopressors should be avoided because hypotension is secondary to hypovolemia. Rate of IV fluid administration is dictated by the degree of hypovolemia. Rarely, patients bleed at a rate such that special equipment (so-called rapid-infuser) may be required to keep up with blood loss.
- Blood transfusion with packed red cells is the method of choice for volume resuscitation in patients with severe GI hemorrhage. All patients who are admitted for GIB should be typed and crossed, and crossmatched blood should be transfused when possible. In the case of catastrophic bleeding, however, O-negative units should be used without delay. The target hematocrit is 25%, although in patients with coronary disease, a hematocrit of 30% is desirable. Care must be taken not to over transfuse patients with variceal hemorrhage because of the risk of inducing hemorrhage from overdistending the varices. Coagulopathy should be corrected with fresh frozen plasma (FFP) in the unstable patient, but subcutaneous vitamin K (5–10 mg) can be used if the patient is hemodynamically stable. Heparin drips and other anticoagulants should be discontinued and protamine used for reversal, if necessary. If the patient is at risk for aspiration, consider endotracheal intubation to protect the airway. It is often required for management of variceal bleeding.

Laboratory Analysis

Initial studies should include a complete blood count (CBC), serum electrolytes, coagulation profile, and type and crossmatch. Hemoglobin and hematocrit must be followed through the entire hospital stay. Initial hematocrit does not reflect the amount of blood loss because blood volume is contracted. Once blood volume is restored, usually in the form of IV fluid administration, hematocrit begins to fall. Platelet transfusions are given if the platelet count is <50,000 cells/μL. Basic metabolic panels may demonstrate a blood urea nitrogen (BUN) level elevated out of proportion to creatinine. This is owing to both hypovolemia and increased absorption of blood. Patients older than 50 years of age, patients who have a history of heart disease or patients who report chest pain or palpitations with the bleeding episode should have an electrocardiogram.

Diagnosis

Nasogastric Lavage

An NG lavage should be performed if an upper GI source of bleeding is suspected. Positive gastric aspirate indicates that bleeding has occurred proximal to the jejunum. Negative aspirate does not preclude UGIB and, if suspicion of UGIB remains despite a negative NG lavage, then upper endoscopy should be performed. An aspirate is considered positive if fresh blood or "coffee ground" material is present. There is no utility in testing for occult blood (gastroccult) in gastric aspirate. NG lavage serves two purposes. First, it can be used to assess rapidity and severity of bleeding by determining how much water is required to clear the aspirate. Second, it clears the endoscopic field of blood, clots, and particulate matter, thus ensuring clear visualization and facilitating accurate diagnosis and treatment. The NG tube does not need to be left in place, especially if bleeding is not brisk and the lavage rapidly clears with water or saline.

Upper Endoscopy

Esophagogastroduodenoscopy is the preferred method for evaluating patients with UGIB. Endoscopy allows direct visualization of the mucosa and identification of the bleeding site. Early endoscopy (i.e., within 24 hours of admission) has not been demonstrated to decrease mortality. Total cost, length of hospitalization, and need for emergent surgery have all been greatly reduced, however, largely because of the therapeutic options available to the endoscopist. It is important that the hemodynamically unstable patient be adequately volume resuscitated and any coagulopathy be corrected before performing upper endoscopy. Morbidity and mortality from upper endoscopy have been reported at 1% and 0.1%, respectively. Contraindications include an agitated patient, perforated viscus, and severe cardiopulmonary disease. Definitive diagnosis is made when active bleeding, stigmata of bleeding, or significant lesions are seen. Of patients with melena, 24% have no diagnosis by upper endoscopy.

Colonoscopy

Colonoscopy is the most frequently used diagnostic tool for evaluating LGIB. Successful colonoscopy requires timing the procedure to completion of adequate bowel preparation. It is important that the patient is adequately volume resuscitated and hemodynamically stable before the bowel preparation is initiated. The overall diagnostic yield of colonoscopy is 70% to 80%. Because of increased risk of perforation as the endoscope passes through poorly visualized areas, extreme care must be taken in patients with massive bleeding or suboptimal preparation. In these cases, other procedures may be used alternatively.

Capsule Endoscopy

Although upper endoscopy and colonoscopy are the standard tools utilized to evaluate acute GIB, visualization of the entire small bowel is not possible. In cases when findings in those two tests are negative, capsule endoscopy can be used for further visualization of the small bowel. The diagnostic yield has been shown to be as high as 92% in obscure GIB cases.

Tagged Red Blood Cell Scan

The technetium-99m–labeled red blood (RBC) cell scan can be used as a bedside evaluation of active lower GIB. Bleeding must exceed a rate of 0.1 mL/minute to be detected. The procedure is of very low risk; however, the test is positive <50% of the time. One use of this procedure is as a screening test before angiography. A patient with a negative tagged RBC

TABLE 6-1	ULCER REBLEEDING RISK BASED ON ENDOSCOPIC APPEARANCE

Endoscopic Finding	Risk of Rebleeding (%)
Arterial spurting	90
Visible vessel	50
Adherent clot	25
Oozing without visible vessel	10–20
Pigment spot	7–10
Clean-based ulcer	3–5

scan is unlikely to have a positive angiogram. If the test finding is negative, a colonoscopy is usually warranted for further evaluation of possible bleeding sources in the colon.

Angiography

Angiography offers accurate diagnosis and therapy in the rapidly bleeding patient. Bleeding rates of 0.5 to 1 mL/minute are required to detect extravasation into the bowel from a bleeding site. The overall diagnostic yield from arteriography ranges from 40% to 78%. If a bleeding source is identified, therapeutic modalities, such as infusion of vasopressin or selective embolization, can be used to stop bleeding. Complications of this procedure include contrast allergy, bleeding from arterial puncture, and embolism from dislodged thrombus. Arteriography should be reserved for those patients with massive, ongoing bleeding for which colonoscopy is not feasible.

Treatment

Again, resuscitation is the initial step in treatment of a patient with an acute GI bleed. Most patients in whom bleeding ceases require elective treatment of the source of bleeding, depending on diagnosis. Urgent therapeutic maneuvers are indicated for patients requiring transfusion of more than 3 U of red cells.

Peptic Ulcer Disease

- Appropriate therapy for PUD is dictated by findings at endoscopy. Table 6-1 gives the rebleeding rates after medical therapy of various endoscopic stigmata of hemorrhage. IV H_2-antagonists have not been shown to reduce surgery or mortality rates in patients with UGI hemorrhage. One randomized, controlled study demonstrated significant reduction in rebleeding, surgery, and mortality when patients at high risk for rebleeding were given high-dose proton pump inhibitors (PPI) (e.g., omeprazole, 40 mg PO BID for 5 days). The study did not include patients with visible arterial spurting, nor was endoscopic therapy performed. Other trials have studied omeprazole by intermittent IV bolus in patients with bleeding ulcers and most of them have shown no significant reduction in rebleeding, surgery, or mortality.
- Prognostic information can be obtained from the upper endoscopy report, which should document any stigmata of recent bleeding, such as active bleeding, a nonbleeding visible vessel, adherent clot, or flat pigment spots. Signs of active bleeding or the lack thereof (e.g., visualization of a clean-based ulcer) can be used to predict rebleeding and the need for therapeutic intervention.
- Ulcers that demonstrate arterial spurting or a visible vessel generally should be treated endoscopically. Thermal therapy (heater probe, electrocoagulation, laser) and injection therapy with epinephrine have both been shown to achieve hemostasis and decrease

rebleeding rates, shorten hospital stay, decrease transfusions and emergency surgery, and lower costs. Combination therapy appears to further reduce rebleeding. Some endoscopists attempt to dislodge adherent clots, so that an underlying vessel can be treated endoscopically. Patients with low-risk ulcers (i.e., clean base) may be discharged and followed on an outpatient basis. IV PPI have recently been shown to decrease rebleeding rates in patients who have already undergone endoscopic therapy; however, they may be unnecessary and expensive in patients who can tolerate oral PPI.

- Surgery is reserved for patients with intractable hemorrhage, recurrent bleeding despite repeated attempts at endoscopic therapy, or blood types that are difficult to crossmatch. Arterial embolization by selective arterial catheterization is an alternative for patients too unstable to undergo surgery.

Variceal Bleeding

- Initial management of variceal bleeding should be directed toward hemodynamic stabilization and airway protection because patients with variceal bleeding are at a high risk for decompensation. Octreotide acetate is a long-acting somatostatin analog that reduces splanchnic blood flow and portal pressure, thus improving hemostasis when used in conjunction with endoscopic therapy. It should be started immediately in any patient with suspected variceal hemorrhage. It is given as a 25- to 100-μg IV bolus followed by an infusion at 25- to 50 μg/hour for 48 to 120 hours. Vasopressin was formerly used as medical treatment of variceal hemorrhage but has been replaced by octreotide because of the cardiovascular side effects (systemic vasoconstriction that can cause arterial hypertension and myocardial ischemia) of vasopressin.

- Sclerotherapy, which involves injection of a variety of sclerosing agents (ethanolamine oleate, sodium tetradecyl sulfate, polidocanol, morrhuate sodium, or ethanol) directly into the varix, achieves hemostasis in >90% of cases. Recurrent bleeding within 10 days occurs in up to 50% of patients, however, and side effects of therapy include fever, ulceration, strictures, perforation, acute respiratory distress syndrome (ARDS), and sepsis. Endoscopic variceal ligation, which involves banding of the base of the varix, has largely replaced injection sclerotherapy in acute variceal hemorrhage, although some studies show that this may not be superior to sclerotherapy in terms of rebleeding and mortality. Regardless, with ligation the esophageal mucosa and submucosa strangulate, slough, fibrose and are eventually obliterated. Endoscopic variceal ligation is easier to perform and has been shown to reduce rebleeding, complications, and mortality. There are still some complications from ligation, however, which include treatment-induced ulceration, strictures, perforation, and hastening of portal hypertensive gastropathy. Patients who are stabilized from the acute episode of variceal bleeding often require scheduled intermittent endoscopic therapy for complete obliteration of the varices, which has been shown to prevent rebleeding and improve survival.

- Transjugular intrahepatic portosystemic shunt (TIPS) is reserved for patients with intractable variceal bleeding or if bleeding recurs after two or more endoscopic attempts at preventing rebleeding from esophageal varices. It creates a direct portosystemic shunt, thereby decreasing pressure within the portal vein. Technical success is achieved >90% of the time, but complications include hepatic encephalopathy in up to 25% of patients, shunt stenosis or thrombosis, and rebleeding. When TIPS is used in emergency situations, in-hospital mortality is around 10% and 30-day mortality as high as 40%. Of note, contraindications to TIPS include portal vein thrombosis, inferior vena cava obstruction, and polycystic liver disease. Surgical shunts are rarely used because of the availability of TIPS procedures. Portacaval and distal splenorenal shunts achieve hemostasis 95% of the time, but are associated with a high rate of postprocedure encephalopathy and mortality rates of 50% to 80%, largely because of severe underlying liver disease. They are often considered in patients with noncirrhotic portal hypertension and patients with Child's A cirrhosis.

- Balloon tamponade should only be used when hemorrhage is uncontrollable or when urgent endoscopy is not available. The Sengstaken-Blakemore tube and the Minnesota tube, both of which have gastric and esophageal balloons, are commonly used. The Linton-Nachlas tube has only a large gastric balloon. Hemostasis is achieved 70% to 90% of the time. Complications can be severe and include esophageal perforation, aspiration, chest pain, erosion, agitation, and death from asphyxiation from balloon migration with airway occlusion.
- Other complications can accompany variceal bleeding and should be promptly addressed. They include aspiration, infection, hypophosphatemia, and alcohol withdrawal. Patients with a history of alcohol use should be monitored for withdrawal and given thiamine. Infection occurs in 25% to 50% of patients with GIB and cirrhosis. Therefore, it has become common to give prophylactic antibiotics in patients with variceal bleeding.

Mallory-Weiss Tear
Endoscopic treatment is only used when tears involve active and ongoing bleeding. Epinephrine injection and thermal coagulation are both efficacious in controlling hemorrhage. Sclerosants should be avoided because of the risk of further tearing or perforation. PPI can promote healing after the acute episode.

Gastric Erosions
Management of gastric erosions is directed at primary prevention. In the intensive care unit (ICU), IV H_2-receptor blockers or oral PPI are used to prevent stress ulceration. PPI have replaced misoprostol for use in patients who require continued NSAID therapy.

Therapeutic Colonoscopy
Endoscopic therapy involves the uses of thermal coagulation (heater probe, bipolar or multipolar coagulation, laser therapy), and injection of vasoconstrictors and sclerosants. Placement of metallic hemoclips has also been successful in the treatment of diverticular bleeding. Approximately 25% of patients with lower GIB have lesions that are amenable to endoscopic therapy (angiodysplasia, diverticular bleeding with visible vessels, bleeding polypectomy sites, some colonic ulcers).

Intraarterial Vasopressin
Intraarterial vasopressin is effective in controlling hemorrhage from diverticula and angiodysplasia. In patients with persistent bleeding, vasopressin should be infused after selective catheterization of the bleeding vessels. Repeat contrast injection at 15 to 30 minutes should confirm cessation of the hemorrhage. The complication rate of vasopressin infusion is 5% to 15% and includes cardiovascular toxicity and problems associated with an indwelling catheter. Patients who do not respond to vasopressin therapy may require surgery or embolization. Patients receiving embolotherapy are at risk of developing the serious complication of bowel infarction. Lesser degrees of ischemia are more common. For these reasons, embolization techniques should be used as a last resort in patients who are poor surgical candidates. Older patients who develop lower GIB may be at greater risk for ischemic complications from embolic therapy because of diffuse arteriosclerosis.

Surgical Therapy
As with UGIB, surgery should not be postponed excessively in the patient with persistent LGIB and hemodynamic instability because morbidity and mortality increase with delay. Prior surgical practice included left hemicolectomy for LGIB and was associated with high rebleeding rates. Better preoperative localization reduces postoperative rebleeding rates. The surgical mortality rates for recent series are 5% to 10%. For the difficult situation of

recurrent massive bleeding without demonstration of a bleeding site, a subtotal colectomy may be indicated in patients with a good overall prognosis. When the patient is a high-risk surgical candidate, angiotherapy or a percutaneously or surgically placed portal-hepatic shunt for variceal bleeding can be considered as alternatives.

KEY POINTS TO REMEMBER

- Initiate resuscitative measures and appropriate level of monitoring before starting diagnostic testing and therapeutic intervention. Intensive care monitoring is appropriate for patients with unstable vital signs (not responding to resuscitative therapy) and those with comorbid conditions.
- GI bleeding is self-limited in almost 80% of cases.
- PUD accounts for nearly half of all UGIB episodes.
- A negative NG aspirate does not preclude UGIB.
- Ulcers with a clean base are at low risk for rebleeding; therefore, patients may be safely discharged with outpatient follow-up.
- Ulcers with active arterial spurting or a visible vessel are at high risk for rebleeding and should be treated endoscopically.
- Mortality from a single episode of variceal bleeding is 30%, with 60% to 70% of patients dying within 1 year.
- The portosystemic gradient must exceed 12 mm Hg for varices to form, but no correlation exists between portal pressure and risk of rupture.
- Whereas one-third of patients with cirrhosis have at least one variceal bleed, up to 50% of cirrhotics who present with UGIB have a source other than varices.
- Variceal band ligation has replaced sclerotherapy in acute variceal hemorrhage.
- Endoscopy (colonoscopy or sigmoidoscopy) is the test of choice for structural evaluation of LGIB.
- Arteriography should be reserved for patients with massive, ongoing bleeding that makes endoscopy unfeasible or when colonoscopy does not reveal a source of bleeding.
- Patients with persistent or recurrent LGIB may require surgical intervention. The accurate localization of bleeding before surgery decreases morbidity and mortality.
- In cases of LGIB in which no colonic cause is found and a UGIB source has been ruled out, evaluation of the small bowel may be necessary.

REFERENCES AND SUGGESTED READINGS

Brunner G, Chang J. Intravenous therapy with high doses of ranitidine and omeprazole in critically ill patients with bleeding peptic ulcerations of the upper intestinal tract: an open randomized controlled trial. *Digestion* 1990;45:217.

Cook D, Guyatt G, Salena B, et al. Endoscopic therapy for acute nonvariceal upper gastrointestinal hemorrhage: a meta-analysis. *Gastroenterology* 1992;102:139–148.

Edelman, DA, Sugawa C. Lower gastrointestinal bleeding: a review. *Surg Endosc* 2007;21:514–520.

Elmunzer BJ, Inadomi JM, Elta GH. Risk stratification in upper gastrointestinal bleeding. *J Clin Gastroenterology* 2007;41:559–563.

Freeman M, Cass O, Peine C, et al. The non-bleeding visible vessel versus the sentinel clot: natural history and risk of rebleeding. *Gastrointest Endosc* 1993;39:359–366.

Gostout GJ, Zuccaro G. A practical approach to acute lower gastrointestinal bleed. *Patient Care* 2000;29:23–31.

Lau JYW, Sung JJY, Lee KKC, et al. Effect of intravenous omeprazole on recurrent bleeding after endoscopic treatment of bleeding peptic ulcers. *N Engl J Med* 2000;343:310.

Lebrec D, Vinel JP, Dupas JL. Complications of portal hypertension in adults: a French consensus. *Eur J Gastroenterol Hepatol* 2005;17:403–410.

Morales GF, Pereira Lima JC, Hornos AP, et al. Octreotide for esophageal variceal bleeding treated with endoscopic sclerotherapy: a randomized, placebo-controlled trial. *Hepatogastroenterology* 2007;54:195–200.

Morrissey JF, Reichelderfer M. Gastrointestinal endoscopy. *N Engl J Med* 1991;325:1142–1149; 1214–1222.

Peter DJ, Daugherty JM. Evaluation of the patient with gastrointestinal bleeding: an evidence based approach. *Emerg Med Clin North Am* 1999;17:239–261.

Peura DA, Lanza FL, Gostout CJ, et al. and contributing America College of Gastroenterology members and fellows. The American College of Gastroenterology bleeding registry: preliminary findings. *Am J Gastroenterol* 1998;92:924.

Rockey DC, Auslander A, Greenberg PD. Detection of upper gastrointestinal blood with fecal occult blood tests. *Am J Gastroenterol* 1999;94:344–350.

Rollhauser C, Fleischer D. Nonvariceal upper gastrointestinal bleeding: an update. *Endoscopy* 1997;29:91–105.

Sanyal AJ, Freedman AM, Luketic VA, et al. Transjugular intrahepatic portosystemic shunts for patients with active variceal hemorrhage unresponsive to sclerotherapy. *Gastroenterology* 1996;111(1):138.

Silverstein F, Gilbert D, Tedesco F, et al. The national ASGE survey on upper gastrointestinal bleeding. *Gastrointest Endosc* 1981;27:73–79.

Yamada T. *Textbook and Atlas of Gastroenterology on CD-ROM*. Philadelphia: Lippincott Williams & Wilkins; 1999.

Zuccaro G Jr. Management of the adult patient with acute lower gastrointestinal bleeding. *Am J Gastroenterol* 1998;93:1202–1208.

Zuccaro G. Bleeding peptic ulcer: pathogenesis and endoscopic therapy. *Gastroenterol Clin North Am* 1993;22:737–750.

Zuckerman GR, Prakash C. Acute lower intestinal bleeding. Part I: Clinical presentation and diagnosis. *Gastrointest Endosc* 1998;48:606–616.

Zuckerman GR, Prakash C. Acute lower intestinal bleeding. Part II: Etiology, therapy, and outcomes. *Gastrointest Endosc* 1999;49:228–238.

Occult and Obscure Gastrointestinal Bleeding

Walter W. Chan

7

INTRODUCTION

Occult and obscure gastrointestinal (GI) bleeding rank among the most common reasons for referral to a gastroenterologist. They can often present significant diagnostic and therapeutic challenges, causing much frustration to both patients and their physicians. In this chapter, the causes, diagnostic approaches, and treatment options for both occult and obscure GI bleeding will be discussed. **Occult bleeding** is defined as either a positive fecal occult blood test (FOBT) or iron-deficiency anemia (IDA) without other evidence of visible blood in the stool. GI bleeding is the most common cause of IDA, especially in men and postmenopausal women. **Obscure bleeding** refers to GI bleeding that persists or recurs, with no identifiable origin after initial endoscopic evaluation. It can present in both the obscure-occult or obscure-overt forms depending on the presence of visible blood.

OCCULT BLEEDING

Causes

Pathophysiology
Bleeding can occur in any portion of the GI tract, and the excreted hemoglobin may be absorbed, degraded, or excreted with feces depending on the location of the bleeding. During transit through the GI tract, the globin chains of hemoglobin are degraded by proteases, which cleave the heme moiety from the globin. The free heme moiety may be resorbed in the small intestine or modified by bacteria in the colon. FOBT measure the presence of occult blood based on these properties of hemoglobin breakdown in the GI tract.

Iron loss from occult bleeding can deplete body iron stores and result in IDA. The time taken to develop IDA depends on the body stores of iron, rate of blood loss, and degree of compensatory increase in iron absorption. Daily losses of approximately 10 mL of blood are required to develop IDA. Iron deficiency can be associated with fatigue, pica, achlorhydria, and a spruelike, small intestinal lesion causing malabsorption of fat and fat-soluble vitamins.

Differential Diagnosis
An extensive list of disorders can cause occult GI bleeding, with or without IDA. Table 7-1 lists the common causes of occult blood loss.

Presentation

History and Physical Examination
Although, by definition, no known symptoms exist for occult GI bleed, the association with any abdominal symptoms, changes in bowel movements, dietary alterations, or constitutional symptoms remains important. In particular, careful attention must be paid to

TABLE 7-1	SOURCES OF OCCULT GASTROINTESTINAL BLEEDING
Source	Incidence (%)
Colorectal	25
Colorectal cancer	7
Polyps	9
Angiodysplasia	4
Colitis	1
Upper GI tract	41
Duodenal ulcer	5
Gastric ulcer	5
Esophagitis	11
Gastritis	8
Angiodysplasia	4
Gastric cancer	2
Celiac disease	1
No source found	41

medication history, especially over-the-counter nonsteroidal anti-inflammatory drugs (NSAIDs). Symptoms, such as fatigue, exertional dyspnea, tachycardia, and pica, suggest possible IDA. Physical findings of IDA are rare in developed countries, but may include brittle nails with longitudinal furrows or spooning (koilonychia), glossitis, cheilitis, and atrophic rhinitis. The Patterson-Kelly or Plummer-Vinson syndromes of postcricoid esophageal webs and IDA may occur. In the evaluation of IDA without menorrhagia, gross hematuria, or an obvious etiology, a GI source must be assumed.

Management

Fecal Occult Blood Tests

Although useful for initial screening, a positive FOBT does not always indicate true disease. False–positive results can occur because of diet, medications, or trauma while obtaining a sample. In fact, physiologic bleeding of up to 1.5mL/day can occur in healthy patients. The four basic types of FOBT are as follows.

- **Guaiac (hemoccult) test** is widely available, simple, and inexpensive, and thus most commonly used. It is a qualitative test, and provides little quantitative information. A colorless compound from tree bark that turns blue with peroxidase-like substances, such as heme and hydrogen peroxide, guaiac detects free heme or heme bound to its apoprotein (e.g., globin, myoglobin, and certain cytochromes). Heme degradation products that may form with more proximal (upper GI) bleeding are not detected. Because guaiac reacts with any peroxidase substance, the test can produce false–positive results with red meats or blood-containing foods, as well as plant peroxidases such as that found in radish. Iron, however, does not cause false–positive results. Vitamin C can cause a false–negative result.
- The **radiochromium-labeled erythrocyte test** remains the accepted gold standard for quantifying GI blood loss. It has limited clinical utility, however, because of cost, complexity, and requirement of 3 or more days of stool collection.

- **Immunochemical tests** use antibodies against human hemoglobin. They do not react with free heme and thus require no dietary restrictions before the test. Some of these tests may also provide quantitative information. Because these antibodies interact with the globin chain, they are only useful for colorectal bleeding, because globin from gastric bleeding is degraded.
- **Heme porphyrin assay (HemoQuant)** is a quantitative fluorometric assay of both heme and its degradation products. Although it has the advantage of detecting proximal bleeds, it is a complex test that requires confirmation in a reference laboratory.

Diagnostic Evaluation

Endoscopic evaluation remains the primary means of investigation in occult GI bleeding, because it allows direct visualization of the mucosa, tissue sampling, and therapeutic intervention. Both colonoscopy and esophagogastroduodenoscopy (EGD) can be performed during the same endoscopic session for a complete evaluation to eliminate the need for repeat sedation. Colonoscopy is typically performed first, especially in patients older than 50 years of age, because current colon cancer screening guidelines recommend evaluation of the colon after positive FOBT in this group of patients. Current data support proceeding with EGD after a negative colonoscopy result, because the upper GI tract has been shown to be a significant source for occult bleeding. If comorbid conditions, procedural risks, or patient preference preclude endoscopic evaluation, barium studies may serve as alternative to EGD, although they are limited by the inability to sample tissue or intervene. Often, endoscopy is required after an abnormal radiographic study. Therefore, it is preferable to perform endoscopy as the initial test whenever possible. Because most cases of occult bleeding with no clear source do not evolve into obscure bleeding, further testing beyond initial endoscopy is generally not indicated even if no cause is identified. In these cases, the patients should receive iron supplementation and be closely monitored for a response. If IDA persists despite oral iron supplementation, or if FOBT recurs or remains positive, further evaluation should proceed per the obscure bleeding algorithm (see Obscure Bleeding below).

Treatment

Treatment is directed at the underlying problem. For patients in whom no lesion can be identified, nonspecific therapy, such as iron supplementation and correction of coagulopathy or platelet disorders, is important.

OBSCURE BLEEDING

Differential Diagnosis

Obscure bleeding can present as both overt and occult bleeding, and it can originate from one or more lesions anywhere in the GI tract. As a result, the list of disorders that can cause obscure bleeding is exhaustive, encompassing those of both overt and occult bleeding. The incidence of these disorders varies, depending on the patient's age, gender, comorbid conditions, and presenting symptoms.

Presentation

Patients presenting with obscure bleeding have symptoms similar to those of acute overt and occult bleeding. Careful history and physical examination may help delineate the possible source of the bleeding.

Diagnostic Evaluation

Repeat EGD and colonoscopy remain the initial step in the evaluation of obscure bleeding. Previous studies have shown that repeat EGD and colonoscopy can identify initially missed lesions in 35% to 75% of patients. If repeat endoscopic studies remain negative, several other diagnostic modalities exist to help determine the source of bleeding.

- **Enteroscopy** allows direct visual examination of portions of the small bowel using a longer endoscope. Different methods of enteroscopy exist, including push enteroscopy and double-balloon enteroscopy.
  - **Push enteroscopy** involves advancing a longer endoscope manually into the small bowel. During repeat endoscopic evaluations of patients with obscure bleeding, the upper EGD is generally substituted by enteroscopy for a more thorough evaluation. This technique allows visualization of up to 50 cm of the small bowel beyond the ligament of Treitz.
  - **Double-balloon enteroscopy (DBE)** utilizes a modified enteroscope with two balloons attached toward the distal end. These balloons serve as anchors by gripping on to the intestinal wall to allow further advancement of the endoscope without loop formation. DBE can reach up to 300 cm beyond the ligament of Treitz. By approaching both orally and anally, DBE may allow evaluation of the entire small bowel. In addition to its expanded diagnostic capacity, DBE also contains intervention capabilities, including hemostasis, biopsy, polypectomy, and dilation.
- **Capsule endoscopy** has become available in recent years for the examination of the small bowel. This involves ingestion of a capsule containing a small camera that sends images to a recorder worn on the patient's belt at a rate of two pictures per second. Relying on normal intestinal peristalsis for the advancement of the capsule, this test is virtually painfree and noninvasive. It is limited, however, by the inability to either biopsy or intervene and the high incidence of incomplete studies because of long transit time. Without air insufflation, rinsing, or control of direction, parts of the mucosal surface might also be missed as the capsule gets pushed along by peristalsis. Capsule entrapment or retention, particularly in patients with stricture or diverticuli, remains the major risk, which occurs in <1% of cases. If within reach, retained capsules can be retrieved using an enteroscope; if beyond the reach of endoscopic instruments, surgery may be necessary.
- **Small bowel series** and **enteroclysis** use oral contrast to identify mucosal lesions in the GI tract radiographically. With a low sensitivity, they are generally reserved for cases in which more invasive testing cannot be performed or for ruling out endoluminal narrowing before capsule endoscopy.
- **Technetium-99m–labeled erythrocyte scans** can help identify the origin of obscure bleeding when other modalities fail to reveal a source. The test, however, must be performed during episodes of active bleeding at a rate exceeding 0.1 to 0.4 mL/minute. Results of the scan should be confirmed by an alternative test, such as angiography, because of significant false localization rate.
- **Angiography** usually follows a tagged erythrocyte scan and allows visualization of bleeding of at least 0.5 mL/minute. Sites not actively bleeding can sometimes be identified during angiography by demonstrating vascular patterns typically seen in certain lesions. Embolization can be performed during angiography for intervention. Caution should be taken and pretreatment might be needed in patients with suspected contrast allergy or renal insufficiency.
- **Intraoperative enteroscopy** may allow better and more complete visualization of the entire small bowel. It is usually reserved for transfusion-dependent bleeding without a source despite extensive diagnostic evaluation. The risks of continued bleeding should also be carefully evaluated and must outweigh the surgical risks of laparotomy.

Treatment

Treatment of obscure bleeding should be directed at the primary disorder leading to the bleeding. The treatment modalities generally fall into five main categories: endoscopic, pharmacologic, angiographic, surgical, and nonspecific. If all evaluations remain negative, nonspecific therapy, including iron supplementation, correction of coagulopathy or platelet disorders, or intermittent transfusion, should be continued.

KEY POINTS TO REMEMBER

- GI blood loss is the most common cause of IDA worldwide, especially in men and post-menopausal women.
- Guaiac tests are the most commonly used FOBT. Given the intermittent bleeding of tumors and the sensitivity of the screening tests, any positive result requires investigation.
- Red meat, blood-containing products, or plant peroxidases, such as radish, can lead to false-positive results on the guaiac test. Iron does not lead to false-positive test findings.
- Endoscopy is the primary mode of investigation.
- Evaluation of obscure bleeding should begin with repeat endoscopy.
- Treatment should aim at the primary disorder leading to the bleeding.
- If no bleeding source can be identified despite exhaustive evaluation, supportive therapy, such as iron supplement, correction of coagulopathy or platelet disorders, or intermittent transfusion, remains important.

REFERENCES AND SUGGESTED READINGS

Concha R, Amaro R, Barkin JS. Obscure gastrointestinal bleeding: diagnostic and therapeutic approach. *J Clin Gastroenterol* 2007;41(3):242–251.

Richter JM. Occult gastrointestinal bleeding. *Gastroenterol Clin North Am* 1994;23:53–66.

Rockey DC, Cello JP. Evaluation of the gastrointestinal tract in patients with iron deficiency anemia. *N Engl J Med* 1993;329:1691–1695.

Rockey DC, Koch J, Cello JP, et al. Relative frequency of upper gastrointestinal and colonic lesions in patients with positive fecal occult blood tests. *N Engl J Med* 1998;339:153–159.

Zuckerman G, Prakash C, Askin M, et al. AGA medical position statement: evaluation and management of occult and obscure gastrointestinal bleeding. *Gastroenterology* 2000;118:197–200.

Zuckerman G, Prakash C, Askin M, et al. AGA technical review on the evaluation and management of occult and obscure gastrointestinal bleeding. *Gastroenterology* 2000;118:201–221.

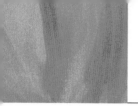

Jaundice

8

Brian B. Borg

INTRODUCTION

Jaundice is a common condition encountered in both inpatient and outpatient settings, with a broad spectrum of causes, ranging from benign to life-threatening. An in-depth understanding of the presentation and pathophysiology of jaundice is essential for appropriate investigation and accurate diagnosis.

Definition

Jaundice is defined as a yellow discoloration of skin, sclera, and mucous membranes caused by accumulation of bilirubin, a by-product of heme metabolism. It should be differentiated from yellow discoloration induced by ingestion of foods with a high content of lycopene, carotene (carotenemia), or drugs (quinacrine and busulfan). Upper limit of normal for total serum bilirubin is 1.0 to 1.5 mg/dL, of which direct bilirubin constitutes <0.2 mg/dL. Hyperbilirubinemia (serum bilirubin >1.5 mg/dL) may be present without overt jaundice, but it nevertheless represents an abnormal condition. Jaundice typically becomes apparent when the serum total bilirubin concentration reaches 2.5 to 3.0 mg/dL. Increased bilirubin levels may be caused by a defect at any site along the bilirubin metabolic pathway, from increased bilirubin production, decreased bilirubin clearance, or a combination of factors.

CAUSES

Pathophysiology

- Bilirubin is the end product of degradation of the heme moiety of hemoproteins, including hemoglobin (Fig. 8-1). Hemoglobin from senescent red blood cells (RBCs) accounts for 80% to 90% of the daily bilirubin production, the remainder coming from ineffective erythropoiesis and degradation of heme-containing proteins (cytochrome P450, peroxidase, and catalase). Normal daily bilirubin production averages 4 mg/kg of body weight (~300 mg). The reticuloendothelial system has the capacity to metabolize up to 1500 mg daily, so hemolysis rarely causes jaundice by itself, unless this ceiling is exceeded or unless hemolysis is associated with liver disease.
- Unconjugated or indirect hyperbilirubinemia is present when >80% to 85% of the total bilirubin is unconjugated. Defects proximal to, and including, the conjugation step result in primarily unconjugated hyperbilirubinemia. Defects after the glucuronidation step within the hepatocyte result in primarily conjugated hyperbilirubinemia. Conjugated or direct hyperbilirubinemia is present when >30% of the total bilirubin is in the conjugated form. Overlap between the two conditions can occur.

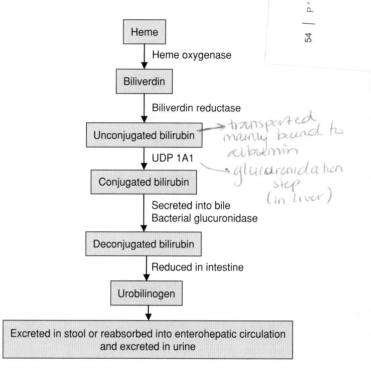

Handwritten annotations: "→ transported mainly bound to albumin", "→ glucaronidation step (in liver)"

FIGURE 8-1. Bilirubin metabolism. Heme oxygenase catalyzes the rate-limiting step within the reticuloendothelial system. Unconjugated bilirubin is transported bound primarily to albumin, at which point it is taken up by the hepatocyte and undergoes glucuronidation by uridine diphosphate glucuronyl transferase (UGT-1A1). It is then secreted in the water-soluble conjugated form into the canaliculi (70%–90% diglucoronide and 5%–25% monoglucoronide). Within the intestine, it is deconjugated and reduced by bacterial β-glucoronidases to urobilinogen, which is either excreted in stool or reabsorbed into the enterohepatic circulation. A defect at or before glucuronidation results in primarily unconjugated hyperbilirubinemia, whereas problems after this step cause conjugated hyperbilirubinemia.

Differential Diagnosis

Hyperbilirubinemia can be classified into unconjugated, conjugated, and mixed.

Unconjugated Hyperbilirubinemia ✗ know

- Hemolysis and ineffective erythropoiesis is seen with sickle cell anemia, thalassemia, G6PD deficiency, pyruvate kinase deficiency, malaria, ABO mismatch and lead toxicity. Bilirubin is usually <3 to 5 mg/dL, and overt jaundice is uncommon in the absence of severe hemolysis or concomitant liver disease.
- Neonatal jaundice
- Uridine diphosphate glucuronyl transferase deficiencies
  - Gilbert's syndrome affects 3% to 10% of the population (predominantly men) and presents with intermittent jaundice often precipitated by illness, stress, fatigue, or fasting. It is the most common cause of hyperbilirubinemia in outpatients, and is benign with no deleterious long-term consequences.

- Crigler-Najjar syndrome can be of two types: type I with complete deficiency of uridine diphosphate glucuronyl transferase 1A1, and type II with partial inactivation of the enzyme.
- Miscellaneous
  - Drugs: β-lactams, isoniazide, quinine, quinidine, rifampin, sulfonamides, sulfonylureas, thiazides, (α-methyldopa, ribavirin, nonsteroidal anti-inflammatory drugs (NSAIDs)
  - Decreased hepatic blood flow and bilirubin clearance: cirrhosis, portocaval shunt, congestive heart failure
  - Other: resolving hematoma, hypothyroidism, thyrotoxicosis, fasting, sepsis

Conjugated Hyperbilirubinemia
- Congenital forms: Rotor syndrome, Dubin-Johnson syndrome
- Familial forms: progressive familial intrahepatic cholestasis: PIFC-1 (Byler disease), PIFC-2 (BSEP mutation) and PIFC-3 (MDR-3 mutation), benign recurrent intrahepatic cholestasis (BRIC), cholestasis of pregnancy
- Choledochal cystic disorders: Caroli's disease and choledochal cysts
- Drugs:
  - Predominantly cholestatic (elevated alkaline phosphatase and total bilirubin): amoxicillin-clavulanic acid, anabolic steroids, chlorpromazine, clopidogrel, oral contraceptives, erythromycin, estrogens, irbesartan, mirtazapine, phenothiazines, terbinafine, tricyclics
- Extrahepatic cholestasis
  - Gallstones
  - Strictures: postsurgical
  - Sclerosing cholangitis: primary and secondary
  - Malignancies: hepatocellular carcinoma (intraluminal [tumor thrombus or fragments], extraluminal, hemobilia), cholangiocarcinoma, pancreatic cancer, ampullary tumors
  - Infection: acquired immunodeficiency syndrome (AIDS) cholangiopathy
  - Pancreatitis: chronic, autoimmune
  - Vascular enlargements (aneurysm, portal cavernoma)

Mixed Conjugated and Unconjugated Hyperbilirubinemia
A mixed pattern may be seen in hepatocellular disorders. A combination of unconjugated hyperbilirubinemia and parenchymal liver disease can also result in a mixed pattern of hyperbilirubinemia.
- Hepatocellular disorders:
  - Viral hepatitis, alcoholic liver disease, Wilson's disease, Reye's syndrome, hemochromatosis, autoimmune hepatitis, $α_1$-antitrypsin deficiency, celiac sprue, nonalcoholic steatohepatitis, pregnancy related (acute fatty liver of pregnancy and preeclampsia)
  - Drugs: acetaminophen, amiodarone, clindamycin, colchicine, ketoconazole, niacin, NSAID, salicylates, calcium channel blockers
- Intrahepatic cholestasis
  - Infiltrative disorders: granulomatous disease (sarcoidosis, lymphoma, mycobacterial infection, Wegener's granulomatosis), amyloidosis, malignancy (paraneoplastic syndrome: renal cell carcinoma)
  - Primary biliary cirrhosis
  - Infections: bacterial, sepsis, fungal, parasitic
  - Postoperative cholestatis and total parenteral nutrition (TPN)
  - Stem cell transplant-related: sinusoidal obstruction syndrome (veno-occlusive disease), graft-versus-host disease, chemotherapy-induced hepatitis

- Drugs: mixed cholestatic and hepatocellular picture (elevated alanine aminotransferase [ALT] and alkaline phosphatase and total bilirubin) can be seen with: azathioprine, allopurinol, captopril, clindamycin, carbamazepine, griseofulvin, haloperidol, hydralazine, H_2-receptor antagonists, nitrofurantoin, phenytoin, sulfonamides.
- Alcoholic hepatitis
- Vascular causes: hepatic vein thrombosis (Budd-Chiari syndrome), shock liver

Evaluation

The history, physical examination, and initial laboratory evaluation should be directed at answering the following questions:

- Is the hyperbilirubinemia unconjugated, conjugated, or mixed?
- If unconjugated hyperbilirubinemia, is it caused by increased production, decreased uptake, or impaired conjugation?
- If conjugated hyperbilirubinemia, is it caused by intrahepatic or extrahepatic cholestasis?
- Is the process acute or chronic?

History and Physical Examination

- Acute versus chronic jaundice can be differentiated by a thorough history, physical examination, and laboratory tests. Xanthelasma, spider angioma, presence of ascites, and hepatosplenomegaly are indicative of a chronic process. Similarly, hypoalbuminemia, thrombocytopenia, and prolonged prothrombin time (PT) are mostly seen in the setting of chronic jaundice. Fever, chills, right upper quadrant abdominal pain, leukocytosis, and hypotension are not only indicative of an acute cause but suggest ascending cholangitis and require urgent intervention. Asterixis, confusion, or stupor could represent fulminant hepatic failure and require immediate therapy.
- Patients with viral hepatitis often give a history of a viral prodrome, including anorexia, malaise, and myalgias. Infectious sexual exposures, intravenous drug use, and prior blood transfusions also support a diagnosis of viral hepatitis. Essential are a careful travel history and human immunodeficiency virus (HIV) status, as well as alcohol and drug history, including over-the-counter and herbal remedies, because a multitude of drugs can cause jaundice by diverse mechanisms, including hemolysis, hepatocellular damage, and cholestasis.
- Pruritus suggests a longer duration of disease and can be seen in both intrahepatic cholestasis and biliary obstruction. Increased urine urobilinogen may represent increased bilirubin production and subsequent enterohepatic circulation or decreased hepatic clearance of urobilinogen and, therefore, does not distinguish between hemolysis and liver disease. In the presence of cholestasis, however, conjugated bilirubin is filtered in the urine and urine bilirubin is an absolute indication of conjugated hyperbilirubinemia. Abdominal pain with radiation to the back can suggest pancreatic disease, whereas a right upper quadrant aching pain is frequently seen in patients with viral hepatitis.
- The **physical examination** should focus on evaluation for evidence of chronic liver disease, including muscle wasting, cachexia, palmar erythema, Dupuytren contracture, parotid enlargement, leuconychia, gynecomastia, and testicular atrophy. The findings of spider angiomata, palmar erythema, and caput medusae (or dilated veins) suggest cirrhosis. Liver size and consistency should also be evaluated. A shrunken and nodular liver would suggest cirrhosis, whereas a palpable mass can be indicative of a malignancy or an abscess. An enlarged liver with a span of >15 cm may be seen in nonalcoholic fatty liver disease (NAFLD), infiltrative disease, or congestive hepatopathy. Ascites is typically seen in advanced cirrhosis, but may also be seen with

severe viral and alcoholic hepatitis. Other useful findings include hyperpigmentation (hemochromatosis), xanthomas (primary biliary cirrhosis), and Kayser-Fleisher rings (Wilson's disease). Asterixis is indicative of end-stage liver disease and hepatic failure.

Aside from a thorough history and examination, the following specific points may help to identify the cause of the patient's jaundice.

- **Age:** Patients younger than 30 years of age are more likely to have acute parenchymal disease, including acute viral hepatitis, biliary tract disease, alcoholic liver disease, and autoimmune hepatitis, whereas those older than 65 years are more likely to have gallstones, malignancy, or drug-induced hepatotoxicity in the setting of polypharmacy. Autoimmune disease can have a second peak in the elderly.
- **Gender:** In male patients, consider alcohol, pancreatic cancer, hepatocellular carcinoma, and hemochromatosis. In female patients, gallstones, primary biliary cirrhosis, and autoimmune hepatitis are more common.
- **Pregnancy:** In pregnant patients, jaundice could be caused by disorders that are unique to pregnancy or coincident with, or exacerbated by, pregnancy (hepatitis E, herpes simplex, Budd-Chiari syndrome, choledocholithiasis). Low serum albumin level and high alkaline phosphatase (up to two to four times normal from placenta), fibrinogen, transferrin, and cholesterol levels can be considered part of expected pregnancy-related changes. Levels of transaminases, bilirubin, and gamma-glutamyl transferase (GGT) do not change with pregnancy, however, and abnormal levels need to be further investigated.
- Liver diseases associated with pregnancy occur at special time points. Mild elevations of alkaline phosphatase, bilirubin, and transaminases are seen in patients with hyperemesis gravidarum during the first trimester. **Intrahepatic cholestasis of pregnancy** normally presents with intense itching in the third trimester (up to 100 times increase in total serum bile acids). In **Dubin-Johnson syndrome** exacerbated by pregnancy, jaundice develops in the second or third trimester. Chronic hepatitis, autoimmune disease, Wilson's disease, and primary biliary cirrhosis may be exacerbated during pregnancy as well. Gallstone disease can occur at anytime. **Acute fatty liver of pregnancy** (with marked elevations of transaminases), preeclampsia or eclampsia and HELLP (hemolysis, elevated liver enzymes, and low platelet count) syndrome could present with jaundice, usually late in the pregnancy. When jaundice occurs late in the course of these hepatocellular diseases, it indicates severe hepatic dysfunction.
- **Critically ill patients:** Up to 40% of patients in the intensive care unit (ICU) and after major surgery may present with jaundice. Bilirubin overproduction caused by hemolysis of transfused blood (10% of RBC in a transfused unit are hemolyzed within 24 hours), drug-induced hemolysis, and prosthetic valves are most common explanation of this finding. Hepatocellular dysfunction secondary to ischemia (shock liver), right-sided heart failure, anesthetic agents, sepsis with multisystem organ failure, viral hepatitis, and TPN should also be considered in the differential diagnosis of nonobstructive jaundice. Choledocholithiasis, cholangitis, cholangiocarcinoma, pancreatic duct stricture, and pancreatic head mass are the most common causes of obstructive jaundice in patients in the ICU. Acalculous cholecystitis causes jaundice, especially after vascular surgeries, trauma, and burns. Injuries of the biliary tract are commonly seen in patients who have recently undergone a related operation (e.g. cholecystectomy).
- **Liver transplantation:** Cholestasis after liver transplantation can be related to early or late complications (an approximate cut-off of a 6-month period). Early complications include acute rejection, preservation injury (cold and rewarming ischemia), bacterial or viral infections, and drug-induced cholestasis. Late complications are predominantly related to chronic rejection and recurrence of the original disease.

MANAGEMENT

Diagnostic Tests

- Essential initial laboratory tests should include levels of direct and indirect bilirubin, transaminases (aspartate aminotransferase [AST] and ALT), alkaline phosphatase, total protein, albumin, and PT. If available, results of prior liver biochemical test results are essential to evaluate the trend of changes.
- If laboratory results are consistent with **unconjugated hyperbilirubinemia**, a hemolysis workup should be initiated (reticulocyte count, lactate dehydrogenase, haptoglobin, Coomb's test, and peripheral smear). In the absence of hemolysis, most asymptomatic healthy patients with isolated unconjugated hyperbilirubinemia have Gilbert's disease and require no further evaluation.
- If laboratory results demonstrate **conjugated hyperbilirubinemia** or are indeterminate, then additional workup is required. Patients with transaminases elevated out of proportion to the alkaline phosphatase most likely have a hepatocellular disorder. Levels of transaminases <300 IU/mL are seen in alcoholic hepatitis, drug-induced injury, and chronic liver disease and obstruction. Levels >1000 IU/mL are indicative of acute hepatitis, drug-induced hepatotoxicity (acetaminophen toxicity), and shock liver. If the alkaline phosphatase is elevated (usually more than three times upper limit of normal) out of proportion to the transaminases, this suggests intrahepatic cholestasis or extrahepatic obstruction. An increased GGT, 5'-nucleotidase, or leucine aminopeptidase confirms the hepatic origin of an elevated alkaline phosphatase. Disproportionate elevation of alkaline phosphatase compared with bilirubin could be seen in partial biliary obstruction or in early intrahepatic cholestasis (primary biliary cirrhosis and primary sclerosing cholangitis). High levels of alkaline phosphatase and bilirubin may, however, indicate presence of a common bile duct stone. High levels of GGT could be seen in many other medical conditions other than biliary disease, including congestive heart failure, alcohol intake, pancreatitis, chronic lung disease, renal failure, and diabetes, and as a result of use of many drugs.
- The presence of low albumin or prolonged prothrombin time suggests chronic liver disease with impaired synthetic function. In cirrhotic patients, high levels of globulins and low albumin levels are frequently seen. Prolonged PT may, however, also be seen in obstructive jaundice. Of note, parenteral administration of vitamin K corrects the coagulopathy in patients with obstructive jaundice but not hepatocellular disease. Testing for urinary bilirubin or urobilinogen may be of some use, because clinical jaundice may lag behind bilirubinuria. High cholesterol levels are seen in patients with cholestasis.
- If the initial evaluation does not reveal an obvious etiology (alcohol, drugs, infections), then specific biochemical studies should be ordered, including viral hepatitis serologies, antinuclear antibody, antimitochondrial antibody, antismooth muscle antibody, serum quantitative immunoglobulins, iron studies, ceruloplasmin, and α_1-antitrypsin levels. If the cause still remains unclear, then liver biopsy should be considered. Figure 8-2 is helpful in planning the evaluation of the patient with jaundice.
- The evaluation of **conjugated hyperbilirubinemia** requires careful selection of the appropriate imaging procedure, because many of these studies are expensive or invasive. If the initial evaluation suggests a possible vascular cause (Budd-Chiari syndrome or shock liver), then ultrasound with Doppler should be the initial study to evaluate patency of the hepatic and portal veins and hepatic artery. Increased transaminases should prompt a search for hepatocellular disorders. If the history and examination cause concern for malignancy, then an abdominal computed tomography (CT) scan and α-fetoprotein levels should be ordered, followed by ultrasound- or CT-guided liver biopsy, if appropriate.

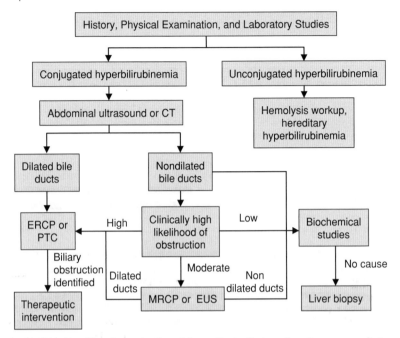

FIGURE 8-2. Algorithm for evaluation of the patient with jaundice. See comments in text regarding selection of appropriate imaging study when given a choice in the algorithm. ERCP, endoscopic retrograde cholangiopancreatography; PTC, percutaneous transhepatic cholangiography; EUS, endoscopic ultrasound; MRCP, magnetic resonance cholangiopancreatography.

- Patients with increased alkaline phosphatase should be evaluated for causes of cholestatic jaundice. Ultrasound should be the initial study to evaluate for evidence of biliary ductal dilatation. Abdominal CT can also be used to evaluate for ductal dilatation, but it has specific limitations. If ductal dilatation is present, or if the suspicion for obstruction remains high despite a normal study finding, then endoscopic retrograde cholangiopancreatography (ERCP) or percutaneous transhepatic cholangiography (PTC) should be performed. Of note, patients who have had prior cholecystectomy normally have a dilated common bile duct. If ductal dilatation is not seen and the suspicion for obstruction is low, then biochemical studies should be ordered as above to look for parenchymal disease. Again, liver biopsy should be considered if no etiology can be identified.

IMAGING PROCEDURES

Noninvasive Tests

Ultrasound
Ultrasound is the best initial study for detection of biliary obstruction as evidenced by ductal dilatation. It has a sensitivity of 77% and specificity of 83% to 95% for identification of bile duct dilation. Nondilated ducts, especially in the setting of acute or intermittent

obstructions, cannot definitively rule out biliary obstruction, however. Therefore, additional studies are required if a high suspicion of obstruction remains. Ultrasound can also identify hepatic parenchymal lesions, gallbladder disease, cholelithiasis, and choledocholithiasis. Its advantages are portability, noninvasiveness, and relatively low cost. Disadvantages include operator-dependent nature and decreased image quality in obese patients or in those with overlying bowel gas and poor visualization of distal ducts in 30% to 50% of patients.

Abdominal CT
Abdominal CT is a first-line study for evaluation of hepatic parenchymal lesions; it is also an alternative to ultrasound for identifying biliary obstruction. Its advantages are a less operator-dependent nature and improved images in obese patients. Limitations include higher cost, lack of portability, inability to detect noncalcified gallstones, and requirement of radiocontrast dye.

Magnetic Resonance Imaging
Magnetic resonance imaging (MRI) is a useful test for assessing liver parenchyma, specifically focal and malignant lesions. It is also sensitive in assessment of liver fat and iron. Magnetic resonance cholangiopancreatography (MRCP) is a special technique used to visualize the biliary tract. Advantages include its noninvasive nature and ability to accurately identify various liver lesions. Unlike ERCP, it does not have therapeutic capabilities.

Hepatic Iminodiacetic Acid Scan
The test of choice if acute cholecystitis with cystic duct obstruction or biliary leakage is suspected, is hepatic iminodiacetic acid (HIDA) scan. False-negative results should be expected, however, in the setting of TPN use or with fasting serum bilirubin concentrations >5 mg/dL.

Invasive Tests

Endoscopic Retrograde Cholangiopancreatography
Endoscopic retrograde cholangiopancreatography provides direct visualization of the biliary and pancreatic ducts and identifies the site of obstruction in >90% of patients. Advantages include high accuracy in locating the site of obstruction, as well as the ability to perform therapeutic interventions (sphincterotomy, stone extraction, stent placement, cytology, and brushing and direct visualization using SpyGlass). Disadvantages include expense, invasiveness, difficulty after certain surgeries (Roux-en-Y), and morbidity. Complications of perforation, bleeding, cholangitis, and pancreatitis are uncommon but can be serious (2%–3% overall morbidity rate).

Endoscopic Ultrasound
Endoscopic ultrasound (EUS) can detect small common bile duct stones with similar accuracy to ERCP and no risk of post-ERCP pancreatitis. It can detect small (<3 cm) pancreatic tumors that are usually not discovered by CT scans. Bile duct stones cannot be removed by EUS, which is a major disadvantage to ERCP.

Percutaneous Transhepatic Cholangiography
Percutaneous transhepatic cholangiography is also an excellent test for evaluating biliary obstruction, with accuracy similar to ERCP (up to 90%–100%) in identifying the site of biliary obstruction if the ducts are dilated. It is less accurate than ERCP, however, if there are nondilated ducts, and several passes into the liver may be required to access the biliary tree. Advantages include lower cost and therapeutic capabilities (decompression of biliary system). Aside from limited usefulness with nondilated ducts,

other problems include inability to perform the test in the presence of coagulopathy (PT >16 seconds and platelets <50,000) and ascites, as well as complication risks (bleeding, arteriovenous fistulas, sepsis, pneumothorax, peritonitis). The decision of whether to perform ERCP or PTC should be based partially on local expertise of the gastroenterologists and radiologists.

Liver Biopsy

If imaging studies are inconclusive and a hepatocellular process is suspected, a liver biopsy may be useful. It is an invasive procedure, however, and a complication rate of 0.1% to 3% is expected. Complications include pain, hemobilia, hemoperitoneum, arteriovenous (AV) fistula, pneumothorax, or hemothorax. In patients with thrombocytopenia, coagulopathy, and ascites, a transjugular approach is recommended. Ultrasound guidance may decrease some of the risks.

COMPLICATIONS

Complications of jaundice will depend on the primary cause and severity of the jaundice. Kernicterus caused by deposition of bilirubin in the brain can result in irreversible motor and cortical impairment. This is seen in infants when levels of total bilirubin are >20 mg/dL. Mechanical obstruction of the extrahepatic ducts can predispose to life-threatening complications, including cholangitis, secondary biliary cirrhosis, and hepatic abscess formation. Other long-term complications include: hepatic osteodystrophy, malabsorption of fat and fat soluble vitamins, and pruritus.

Treatment

Management of jaundice should be directed at the underlying cause. The goal of treating a patient with bile duct obstruction is to drain the bile to decrease the risk of complications and to provide symptom relief. In patients with choledocholithiasis, a laparoscopic cholecystectomy with common bile duct (CBD) exploration using intraoperative or postoperative ERCP is recommended. In many cases of CBD stones, an ERCP with sphincterotomy and stone extraction would be the appropriate therapeutic procedure. In old or frail patients who cannot undergo surgeries, externally inserted drains into the gall bladder or main hepatic ducts would be suggested to overcome malignant strictures or for temporary relief of symptoms.

KEY POINTS TO REMEMBER

- Jaundice is termed unconjugated or indirect hyperbilirubinemia when >80% to 85% of the total bilirubin is in the unconjugated form. It is termed conjugated or direct to hyperbilirubinemia when >30% of the total bilirubin is in the conjugated form.
- Hemolysis usually presents with bilirubin levels <3 to 5 mg/dL, and overt jaundice is uncommon unless there is severe hemolysis or concomitant liver disease. In the absence of hemolysis, isolated unconjugated hyperbilirubinemia is frequently caused by Gilbert's syndrome, a benign disorder that requires no further evaluation.
- In patients with conjugated hyperbilirubinemia, if transaminases are elevated out of proportion to the alkaline phosphatase, a hepatocellular disorder is likely; if the alkaline phosphatase is elevated out of proportion to the transaminases, intrahepatic cholestasis or extrahepatic obstruction is frequently to blame.

REFERENCES AND SUGGESTED READINGS

Bacon BR, DiBisceglie AM. *Liver Disease: Diagnosis and Management*. New York: Churchill Livingstone; 2000:36–46.

Bansal V, Schuchert VD. Jaundice in the intensive care unit. *Surg Clin North Am* 2006;86:1495–1502.

Faust TW, Reddy KR. Post operative jaundice. *Clin Liver Dis* 2004;8:151–166.

Feldman M, Friedman L, Brandt L. *Sleisenger and Fordtrans's Gastrointestinal and Liver Disease: Pathophysiology, Diagnosis, Management*. 8th ed. Philadelphia: Saunders Elsevier; 2006:301–316.

Green RM, Flamm S. AGA technical review on the evaluation of liver chemistry tests. *Gastroenterology* 2002:123;1367–1384.

Knox T, Olans L. Liver diseases in pregnancy. *N Engl J Med* 1996;335:569–576.

Lai ECH, Lau WY. Hepatocellular carcinoma presenting with obstructive jaundice. *ANZ J Surg* 2006;76:631–636.

Navarro V, Senior J. Drug-related hepatotoxicity. *N Engl J Med* 2006;354:731–739.

Trauner M, Meier P, Boyer J. Molecular pathogenesis of cholestasis. *N Engl J Med* 1998;339:1217–1227.

Yamada T, Alpers DH, Laine L, et al. *Textbook of Gastroenterology*. Lippincott Williams & Wilkins; 2003:911–928.

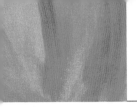

Abnormal Liver Chemistries

9

Manreet Kaur

INTRODUCTION

The evaluation of a patient with suspected hepatic or biliary disease can be aided by the measurement of various serum markers of liver function or injury. A thorough understanding of these markers of hepatic disease is essential for proper interpretation and accurate diagnosis. Whereas a single laboratory value rarely leads to a diagnosis in patients with hepatic disease, the pattern of liver enzyme abnormalities together with a thorough history and physical examination can help to direct additional workup to arrive at a diagnosis.

SERUM ENZYMES

Aminotransferases

Aspartate aminotransferase (AST, previously called SGOT) and alanine aminotransferase (ALT, previously called SGPT) are sensitive markers of hepatocellular injury or necrosis. ALT is the more specific indicator of liver injury because it is found primarily in the liver, whereas AST can be found in liver, cardiac and skeletal muscle, kidney, brain, pancreas, and other sites. A nonhepatic source should be considered in isolated elevations of AST. Marked elevations in AST and ALT (often >1000 U/L) are seen in acute viral, toxin-induced, and ischemic hepatitis. Small to moderate elevations in the transaminases are seen in a number of conditions, including chronic viral hepatitis, alcohol abuse, autoimmune hepatitis, nonalcoholic fatty liver disease, biliary obstruction, hemochromatosis, Wilson's disease, and α_1-antitrypsin deficiency, and as a side effect of various medicines (Table 9-1). The pattern of elevation can offer clues to the etiology. An AST:ALT ratio of $\geq$2 is highly suggestive of alcohol-induced injury, whereas a ratio of <1 is usually seen in patients with acute or chronic viral hepatitis or extrahepatic biliary obstruction.

Alkaline Phosphatase

Elevated alkaline phosphatase (AP) levels arise from two main sources—liver and bone—but the enzyme is also found in other tissues, including placenta, intestines, and leukocytes. Elevations in AP are seen in a variety of hepatobiliary conditions. Marked elevations in AP are typically seen in cholestatic syndromes (e.g., biliary obstruction, primary biliary cirrhosis, primary sclerosing cholangitis, and drug-induced cholestasis). Lesser elevations in AP are seen with infiltrative processes (sarcoidosis, other granulomatous diseases), liver metastasis, and other forms of liver disease. Elevations in AP can be confirmed as hepatic in origin by measuring either gamma-glutamyltransferase (GGT) or 5'-nucleotidase.

Gamma-Glutamyltransferase

GGT is found in bile duct epithelial cells, hepatocytes, and other tissues, including kidney, pancreas, and intestine. In the evaluation of hepatobiliary disease, it has two main

TABLE 9-1 DRUGS COMMONLY ASSOCIATED WITH ELEVATED LIVER ENZYMES

Antiarrhythmics	**Analgesics**
Amiodarone	Acetaminophen
Antibiotics	Nonsteroidal anti-inflammatory drugs (NSAIDs)
Synthetic penicillins	Sulfonylureas
Ciprofloxacin	Glipizide
Nitrofurantoin	Homeopathic substances
Ketoconazole	Ephedra
Fluconazole	Jin bu huan
Isoniazid	Senna
Erythromycin	Chaparral
Antihypertensives	Drugs of abuse
Methyldopa	Anabolic steroids
Captopril	Cocaine
Enalapril	3,4-Methylelenedioxy-
Antiepileptics	methamphetamine ("ecstasy")
Phenytoin	Phencyclidine
Carbamazepine	Toluene-containing glues
Hydroxymethylglutaryl	Chloroform
coenzyme A reductase inhibitors	Trichloroethylene
Atorvastatin	
Pravastatin	
Lovastatin	
Simvastatin	

uses. An elevated level helps confirm hepatobiliary origin of elevated AP. GGT also serves as a useful tool in diagnosing chronic alcohol abuse. A GGT that is twice the normal level in a patient with an AST:ALT ratio >2 is highly suggestive of alcohol abuse. The utility of GGT is somewhat limited by its lack of specificity. Elevations in GGT can be seen in a number of disorders, including pancreatic diseases, myocardial infarction, chronic obstructive pulmonary disease (COPD), renal failure, diabetes, and rheumatoid arthritis, as well as with the use of phenytoin, warfarin, barbiturates, and other drugs that induce microsomal enzymes.

5′-Nucleotidase

As with GGT, 5′-nucleotidase can be used to confirm hepatic origin of elevated AP.

EXCRETORY PRODUCTS

Bilirubin

Bilirubin is a degradation product of hemoglobin and hemoproteins composed of conjugated (direct) and unconjugated (indirect) fractions. Unconjugated hyperbilirubinemia results from excessive production, reduced hepatic uptake, or impaired conjugation of bilirubin. Conjugated hyperbilirubinemia occurs as a result of impaired intrahepatic secretion of bilirubin or extrahepatic biliary obstruction. Both forms of hyperbilirubinemia manifest clinically as jaundice. Usually a serum bilirubin concentration of >3 mg/dL is required for clinical detection of jaundice. A complete discussion of the pathophysiology and differential diagnosis of jaundice can be found in Chapter 8, Jaundice.

Serum Bile Acids

Cholic acid and chenodeoxycholic acid are synthesized from cholesterol in the liver and converted by bacteria in the intestine to deoxycholic and lithocholic acid, the secondary bile acids. Elevated levels of serum bile acids are specific markers of liver disease; however, the sensitivity is low, especially in mild disease, which limits their clinical utility.

MEASURES OF SYNTHETIC FUNCTION

Clotting Factors

Many of the proteins involved in hemostasis, including the coagulation factors, are synthesized in the liver. Normal activity of clotting factors II, VII, IX, and X depends on normal hepatic synthetic function, as well as the presence of vitamin K. As a result, two forms of hepatobiliary dysfunction can lead to coagulopathy manifested by prolongation of prothrombin time (PT).

- Significant hepatocellular injury or necrosis can impair hepatic synthetic function of clotting factors and leads to PT prolongation.
- Cholestatic syndromes may also prolong PT by interfering with intestinal absorption of vitamin K via impaired lipid absorption. This form should respond to parenteral administration of vitamin K, whereas coagulopathy purely from impaired hepatic synthesis should not.

Albumin

Serum albumin concentration, which is often decreased in chronic liver disease, reflects decreased synthesis. Other disease states as well as plasma volume expansion can also decrease albumin concentration. Levels may be normal in acute liver disease because of a half-life of approximately 20 days. The shorter half-life of prealbumin (1.9 days) makes it a sensitive marker of liver function in patients with acetaminophen overdose.

DIAGNOSTIC EVALUATION

A series of laboratory tests alone rarely leads to a diagnosis in a patient suspected of having hepatobiliary disease. Instead, the clinical context must be considered, and carefully chosen, disease-specific laboratory tests and other appropriate studies are necessary to arrive at a diagnosis. A thorough and accurate history is essential in the approach to a patient with abnormal liver chemistries; it should include the following:

- Symptoms of liver disease (e.g., weight loss, anorexia, fever, nausea, vomiting, abdominal pain, pruritus, jaundice)
- Medical and surgical history, including details of other medical illnesses, such as cardiac disease, inflammatory bowel disease, diabetes, arthritis, thyroid diseases, and so on
- Pregnancy can predispose to intrahepatic cholestasis of pregnancy, toxemia, and acute fatty liver of pregnancy. Isolated alkaline phosphatase elevation in the third trimester can be from a placental source of the enzyme.
- Careful review of prescription and over-the-counter medications

- Thorough social history, including history of alcohol consumption, illicit drug use, use of herbal remedies, sick contacts and exposure history, well water consumption, tattoos, recent travel, dietary history including an unusual diet (e.g., raw oyster, mushroom), sexual and menstrual history, occupational and environmental history, and transfusion history
- Family history of jaundice may be present in Gilbert syndrome, Dubin-Johnson syndrome, and hereditary hemolytic syndromes. Hemochromatosis, Wilson's disease, and α_1-antitrypsin deficiency are autosomal-recessive disorders. Other hepatobiliary disorders, including primary sclerosing cholangitis, primary biliary cirrhosis, and autoimmune hepatitis, may also have a genetic component.

The physical examination should focus on stigmata of liver disease as well as signs suggestive of systemic diseases that commonly affect the liver, including jaundice, palmar erythema, spider nevi, parotid enlargement, ascites, hepatosplenomegaly, encephalopathy, abdominal tenderness, and the Kayser-Fleischer rings of Wilson's disease.

A nonhepatic source must be considered in any patient with abnormal liver chemistries. When a hepatic source is suspected, it is helpful to divide the pattern of abnormality into one of three broad categories: *hepatocellular injury, cholestasis,* and *infiltrative processes.*

Hepatocellular Injury

Hepatocellular injury typically manifests with modest to profound elevations in serum aminotransferases. AP and bilirubin may or may not be elevated, depending on the nature and severity of the injury. As a general rule, the highest elevations in transaminases are seen with ischemic and acute viral hepatitis. In ischemic hepatitis or herpes simplex hepatitis, transaminase levels >10,000 can be noted (see also Chapter 18, Acute Liver Disease). Toxic injury is also typically associated with marked elevations in AST and ALT. Less-marked elevations in transaminases are seen with chronic viral hepatitis and cirrhosis. PT can be prolonged with hepatocellular injury, depending on the extent of hepatocellular necrosis and subsequent hepatic synthetic dysfunction. Albumin is normal in acute injury, but can decrease in chronic disorders when synthetic function is significantly impaired. Table 9-2 lists the common causes of hepatocellular injuries. The initial evaluation should

TABLE 9-2	CAUSES OF HEPATOCELLULAR INJURY PATTERN OF LIVER CHEMISTRIES

Viral hepatitis (A, B, C, D, E; cytomegalovirus [CMV], Epstein-Barr virus, herpes simplex virus, varicella zoster virus [VZV])

Cirrhosis

Alcoholic liver disease

Nonalcoholic fatty liver disease

Wilson's disease

Hemochromatosis

Shock liver (hypotension)

Budd-Chiari syndrome

Veno-occlusive disease

Acute fatty liver of pregnancy

Autoimmune hepatitis

α_1-Antitrypin deficiency

Medications

TABLE 9-3	SCREENING FOR ALT AND AST ELEVATIONS

Less than fives times the upper limit, screen for:

1. Alcohol abuse: Elevation of AST > ALT, especially a ratio >2:1 (AST rarely exceeds 300) with a twofold elevation of GGT.
2. Hepatotoxic medications or herbal supplements
3. Hepatitis B: Initial screening tests include Hep B surface Ag and Ab, Hep B core Ab.
3. Hepatitis C: Check Hep C Ab.
4. Hereditary hemochromatosis: Serum iron and TIBC to calculate iron saturation (serum iron/TIBC), if saturation is >45%, check ferritin; a ferritin level >400 in men and >300 in women supports the diagnosis. Liver biopsy to assess severity of liver injury and genetic testing should follow.
5. NASH: More common in women, associated with obesity and diabetes mellitus type 2. Ratio of AST:ALT is <1. Obtain imaging studies (ultrasound/computed tomography/magnetic resonance imaging).
6. Rarer nonhepatic etiologies include celiac disease, muscle disorders (e.g., rhabdomyolysis or polymyositis), thyroid disorders, adrenal insufficiency, and anorexia nervosa.

AST and ALT elevations >15 times the upper limit, screen for:

1. Drug-induced hepatotoxicity: Acetaminophen overdose is the most common cause of drug-induced fulminant hepatic failure.
2. Acute viral hepatitis (A-E, Herpes simplex)
3. Ischemic hepatitis
4. Autoimmune hepatitis: More common in young women. Screen with SPEP (80% of patients have hypergammaglobulinemia) followed by antinuclear (ANA) and antismooth muscle Ab (SMA). Liver biopsy is required to confirm the diagnosis.
5. Wilson's disease: Serum ceruloplasmin, ophthalmologic examination for Kayser-Fleischer rings, occasionally a 24-hour urine for copper excretion
6. Acute bile duct obstruction
7. Acute Budd-Chiari syndrome

ALT, alanine aminotransferase; AST, aspartate aminotransferase; GGT, gamma-glutamyl transpeptidase; NASH, nonalcoholic steatohepatis; SPEP, serum protein electrophoresis; TIBC, total iron binding capacity.

---

include specific testing of the most likely causes. Specific biochemical testing often reveals the etiology. Imaging with ultrasound or abdominal CT may be useful in identifying structural causes. For patients with unexplained abnormal transaminases, liver biopsy should be considered, especially if the levels remain elevated for >6 months (Table 9-3).

Cholestasis

Cholestatic injury typically produces moderate to profound elevations in AP, often with hyperbilirubinemia (elevations in bilirubin may be absent in certain clinical situations, such as with partial biliary obstruction). PT may be prolonged but responds to parenteral vitamin K administration. Depending on the nature of the cholestasis, serum transaminases may or may not be elevated. In early total common bile duct obstruction, AST and ALT may rise before AP. Evaluating a patient with cholestatic injury by routine liver chemistries can be particularly challenging. Once a nonhepatic source of elevated AP has been excluded, selection of other studies is directed by the degree of AP elevation. Table 9-4 lists

TABLE 9-4	CAUSES OF CHOLESTATIC INJURY PATTERN OF LIVER CHEMISTRIES

Malignancy (intrahepatic or extrahepatic)
Biliary stricture
Choledocholithiasis
Primary sclerosing cholangitis
Primary biliary cirrhosis
Sepsis
Rotor's or Dubin-Johnson syndrome
Medications

the common causes of cholestasis. Ultrasound is the best initial study, because it allows visualization of the liver parenchyma and biliary tree (Fig. 9-1). Depending on the ultrasound findings, further evaluation may include abdominal CT, endoscopic retrograde cholangiopancreatography, or liver biopsy.

Infiltrative Process

Infiltrative liver injury is seen most commonly with granulomatous diseases, including sarcoidosis and metastatic disease to the liver. The predominant feature is an elevation in AP and, to a lesser extent, elevated bilirubin. Unlike with cholestatic liver injury, PT prolongation would not be expected in infiltrative injury because intestinal absorption of vitamin K is not affected. Table 9-5 lists the common causes of infiltrative liver disease. Imaging with either ultrasound or abdominal CT, often followed by liver biopsy, forms the basis for evaluating infiltrative processes.

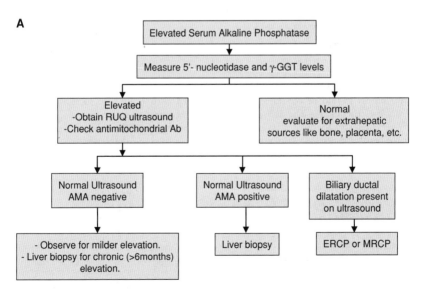

A

Elevated Serum Alkaline Phosphatase

Measure 5'- nucleotidase and γ-GGT levels

Elevated
-Obtain RUQ ultrasound
-Check antimitochondrial Ab

Normal
evaluate for extrahepatic
sources like bone, placenta, etc.

Normal Ultrasound
AMA negative

Normal Ultrasound
AMA positive

Biliary ductal
dilatation present
on ultrasound

- Observe for milder elevation.
- Liver biopsy for chronic (>6months)
elevation.

Liver biopsy

ERCP or MRCP

FIGURE 9-1. (A) Diagram for elevated serum alkaline phosphatase. *(continued)*

B

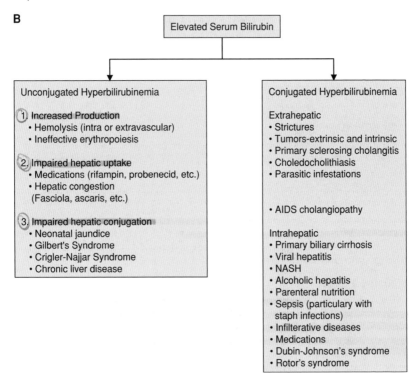

Elevated Serum Bilirubin

Unconjugated Hyperbilirubinemia

1. Increased Production
   • Hemolysis (intra or extravascular)
   • Ineffective erythropoiesis

2. Impaired hepatic uptake
   • Medications (rifampin, probenecid, etc.)
   • Hepatic congestion
     (Fasciola, ascaris, etc.)

3. Impaired hepatic conjugation
   • Neonatal jaundice
   • Gilbert's Syndrome
   • Crigler-Najjar Syndrome
   • Chronic liver disease

Conjugated Hyperbilirubinemia

Extrahepatic
• Strictures
• Tumors-extrinsic and intrinsic
• Primary sclerosing cholangitis
• Choledocholithiasis
• Parasitic infestations

• AIDS cholangiopathy

Intrahepatic
• Primary biliary cirrhosis
• Viral hepatitis
• NASH
• Alcoholic hepatitis
• Parenteral nutrition
• Sepsis (particulary with
  staph infections)
• Infilterative diseases
• Medications
• Dubin-Johnson's syndrome
• Rotor's syndrome

FIGURE 9-1. (Continued) (B) Diagram for elevated serum bilirubin. Abbreviations: AMA, antimitochondrial antibody; ERCP, endoscopic retrograde cholangiopancreatography; γ-GGT, gamma-glutamyl transpeptidase; MRCP, magnetic resonance cholangiopancreatography; NASH, nonalcoholic steatohepatitis; RUQ, right upper quadrant.

Clinical Indication for Performing a Liver Biopsy

Liver biopsy should be considered in patients with chronically (>6 months) elevated serum liver chemistries. The decision must be individualized to each patient's age, pattern of liver chemistry abnormalities. and associated comorbid conditions. Biopsies performed in patients with negative serologic markers are most likely to demonstrate a pattern of steatosis or steatohepatitis, occasionally associated with fibrosis.

TABLE 9-5	CAUSES OF INFILTRATIVE INJURY PATTERN OF LIVER CHEMISTRIES	
Metastatic cancer		Tuberculosis
Lymphoma		Sarcoidosis
Leukemia		Histoplasmosis
Primary hepatic tumors		Medications

- Alanine aminotransferase is the more specific indicator of liver injury because it is found primarily in the liver, whereas AST can be found in liver, cardiac and skeletal muscle, kidney, brain, pancreas, and other sites.
- Marked elevations in AST and ALT (often >1000 U/L) are seen in acute viral, toxin-induced, and ischemic hepatitis.
- Elevations in AP can be confirmed as hepatic in origin by measuring either GGT or 5'-nucleotidase.
- In choledocholithiasis, an AST increase is the earliest abnormality detected, and is usually less than five times the upper limit of normal. The AST increase is typically transient and returns to normal within 72 hours.
- In cholangitis, the AST can increase up to 10 times.
- Cholestatic syndromes may prolong PT by interfering with intestinal absorption of vitamin K via impaired lipid absorption. This form of PT prolongation should respond to parenteral administration of vitamin K, whereas coagulopathy purely from impaired hepatic synthesis should not.
- For patients with unexplained abnormal chemistries, liver biopsy should be considered, especially if the levels remain elevated for >6 months.
- Imaging with either ultrasound or abdominal CT, often followed by liver biopsy, forms the basis for evaluating infiltrative processes.

REFERENCES AND SUGGESTED READINGS

Green RM, Flamm S. AGA technical review on the evaluation of liver chemistry tests. *Gastroenterology* 2002;123:1367–1384.

Moselely R. Approach to the patient with abnormal liver chemistries. In: Yamada T, Alpers DH, Lane L, et al. ed. *Textbook of Gastroenterology*. Philadelphia: Lippincott Williams & Wilkins; 2003.

Moseley R. Evaluation of abnormal liver chemistry tests. *Med Clin North Am* 1996;80:887–906.

Pratt D, Kaplan M. Evaluation of abnormal liver-enzyme results in asymptomatic patients. *N Engl J Med* 2000;342(17):1266–1271.

Pratt D, Kaplan M. Laboratory tests. In: Schiff E, Sorrell M, Maddrey W, eds. *Schiff's Diseases of the Liver*. 8th ed. Vol. 1. Philadelphia: Lippincott–Raven; 1999:205–244.

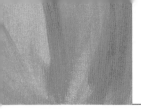

Ascites

Yume P. Nguyen

INTRODUCTION

Ascites is the abnormal accumulation of fluid in the peritoneal cavity. The etiologies of ascites are myriad, but the most common cause by far is portal hypertension due to cirrhosis of the liver. Once ascites develops in a patient with end-stage liver disease, the 1-year survival drops by as much as 50%. The presence of ascites can also lead to spontaneous bacterial peritonitis (SBP), hepatorenal syndrome, and hepatic hydrothorax. Development of ascites is one criterion used in determining the need for liver transplantation.

CAUSES

Liver Disease

Liver disease accounts for approximately 80% of ascites. Within 10 years of a diagnosis of cirrhosis, 50% of patients will have developed ascites. As a result of altered hepatic architecture, sinusoidal pressure increases in the fibrotic liver. This leads to increased hydrostatic pressure in the liver and splanchnic bed and accumulation of fluid in the peritoneum. The portal pressure usually has to exceed 12 mm Hg for ascites to develop. Cirrhosis also causes peripheral vasodilation from increased levels of arterial nitric oxide. This vasodilatory effect results in an effectively reduced plasma volume, initiating renal protective mechanisms and the renin-angiotensin-aldosterone system. The kidney avidly retains sodium and water, furthering fluid accumulation in a vicious cycle.

Malignancy

Tumors can lead to ascites by several pathways. In peritoneal carcinomatosis, proteinaceous material exuded into the peritoneal cavity produces an osmotic gradient with movement of fluid from the intravascular space. Hepatocellular carcinoma can cause portal hypertension from replacement of normal liver parenchyma. Carcinoma-induced hypercoagulable states can cause hepatic or portal venous thrombosis with subsequent ascites.

Cardiac Disease

Ascites caused by right-sided heart failure is fairly uncommon. Chronic, passive liver congestion results from increased central venous pressures which can lead to hepatocellular damage and fibrosis if sustained. Fluid accumulation is further exacerbated by the circulatory compromise and activation of the antinatriuretic, renin-angiotensin, and sympathetic nervous systems.

Infections

Peritoneal tuberculosis is a rare extrapulmonary manifestation that leads to proteinaceous exudate and subsequent movement of fluid into the peritoneal cavity.

Acute Pancreatitis

Pancreatic ascites can result from a pancreatic enzyme leak into the peritoneal cavity in severe acute pancreatitis. This can lead to intraperitoneal irritation or inflammation, further potentiating fluid accumulation.

Chylous Ascites

Obstruction of the thoracic duct seen with lymphoma or surgical trauma can lead to accumulation of chyle in the peritoneal cavity.

Nephrotic Syndrome

Patients with nephrotic syndrome have anasarca from hypoproteinemia, which can be associated with ascites. Ascites is further exacerbated by activation of renal protective mechanisms.

Connective Tissue Disorders

Serositis may yield an inflammatory ascites in connective tissue disorders including systemic lupus erythematosus.

PRESENTATION

History and Physical Examination

A thorough history and physical examination are essential to an accurate diagnosis in new-onset ascites. In the 20% of patients with a nonhepatic cause of ascites, the history should focus on uncovering conditions such as malignancy, heart failure, tuberculosis, or renal disease. The patient with ascites usually develops increased abdominal girth, often manifested as weight gain or increase in belt size. Ascites is usually not painful except when complicated by peritonitis, but tense ascites may be very uncomfortable or cause shortness of breath. Physical examination may reveal bulging flanks, shifting dullness, or the presence of a fluid wave if ≥500 mL of fluid is present. Ultrasound examination of the abdomen is extremely sensitive in identifying even small amounts of ascites. Other physical signs helpful in identifying specific causes of ascites include peripheral manifestations of chronic liver disease (palmar erythema, spider angiomata or jaundice); jugular venous distention and an audible S_3 in congestive heart failure; and Sister Mary Joseph nodule in malignant ascites.

Diagnostic Evaluation

- The two main purposes of performing diagnostic evaluation are (a) to identify the etiology of new-onset ascites, and (b) to evaluate for SBP in patients with known ascites presenting with abdominal or nonspecific systemic symptoms. A diagnostic paracentesis should be performed in new-onset ascites or in any patient with known ascites with any abdominal or systemic symptom bringing them to medical attention, because manifestations of spontaneous bacterial peritonitis may be subtle and nonspecific. Very few contraindications exist to performing a diagnostic paracentesis. No data support the administration of blood products to correct thrombocytopenia or coagulopathy before performing the procedure. Fluid should be obtained in a sterile fashion and evaluated for automated cell count and differential, albumin, protein, and culture. The sensitivity of ascites fluid culture is increased if blood culture bottles are inoculated at the bedside. If the clinical situation suggests other less common causes, fluid may also be sent for lactate dehydrogenase (LDH), glucose, amylase and triglyceride levels, cytology, flow cytometry, or mycobacterial smear and culture.
- The most important parameter in stratifying the diagnostic workup is the **serum-ascites albumin gradient (SAAG)**. The SAAG is simply the number obtained by

subtracting the ascites albumin level from the serum albumin level in grams per deciliter. The values for albumin from serum and ascites fluid should be obtained within a relatively close interval, preferably the same day. A SAAG of ≥1.1 g/dL is indicative of ascites related to portal hypertension with a specificity of 97%.

- Ascitic fluid **cell count and differential** help determine if the ascitic fluid is infected. An ascitic fluid neutrophil count of >250 cells/μL or total WBC count of >500 cells/μL indicates the presence of SBP, and warrants initiation of empiric antibiotic therapy.
- Ascitic fluid **protein** level of <1.0 g/dL places a patient in a high-risk group for SBP. In peritonitis from secondarily infected ascites (e.g., from gastrointestinal tract perforation), ascitic protein and LDH are high, and the glucose level is low. Surgical intervention is often required for secondarily infected ascites.
- **Amylase** levels are helpful in detecting pancreatic ascites, and **triglyceride** levels help identify chylous ascites. **Cytology** is useful when peritoneal carcinomatosis is suspected, but findings are less likely to be abnormal in hepatocellular carcinoma. If the cell count is remarkable for a high number of lymphocytes, tuberculosis or lymphoma is suggested. Acid-fast bacillus (AFB) stain and culture or flow cytometry can confirm the diagnosis.

Complications

Diagnostic evaluation of ascites is very rarely associated with complications. Only 1% of patients undergoing diagnostic paracentesis develop a procedure-related complication, such as hemoperitoneum or an abdominal wall hematoma. Entry of the paracentesis needle into the bowel occurs in fewer than 1 of 1000 cases.

MANAGEMENT

Management of ascites depends on the etiology, especially when it is caused by a process other than chronic liver disease. If a specific etiology is identified, management can be directed toward the causative lesion (e.g. antituberculous medications, chemotherapy for lymphoma or cancer). Management of ascites in cirrhosis is initiated in a stepwise fashion as discussed below.

Abstinence

In alcohol-related cirrhosis it is important to convince patients to stop drinking to prevent further injury to the liver. Abstaining from alcohol can significantly improve outcomes over time and result in better response to medical therapy. Alcohol-related liver injury has been shown to have a more reversible component than nonalcohol related liver injury.

Sodium Restriction

Management should begin with sodium restriction to 2 g/day. Although this may be insufficient in many cases, it is nearly impossible for patients to adhere to a stricter regimen in a nonhospital setting. Patients should be cautioned to avoid salt supplements containing potassium chloride, because use of these products can lead to life-threatening hyperkalemia, especially in association with aldosterone antagonists. Fluid restriction is usually not necessary but should be initiated in patients with dilutional hyponatremia (serum sodium <125 mmol/L).

Diuretic Therapy

Diuretic therapy is a necessary addition to dietary sodium restriction in most cases. The goal of diuretic therapy should be a weight loss of 1 kg/day in patients with edema and 0.5 kg/day without edema until ascites is adequately controlled. Dual therapy with furosemide and spironolactone simultaneously is initiated to prevent potassium derangements and to achieve desired diuresis efficiently. Spironolactone, 100 mg/day and furosemide 40 mg/day in a single oral dose are recommended for initiation. The dose can be increased every 3 to 5 days if necessary until a maximum of 400 mg/day of spironolactone and 160 mg/day of furosemide is reached or significant side effects occur. If ascites is minimal, use of spirono-lactone as a single agent can be useful, but furosemide alone is not adequate therapy in cir-rhotic ascites. If spironolactone in therapeutic doses results in intolerable gynecomastia, amiloride or triamterene can be substituted, although these agents are less effective in con-trolling ascites. Oral furosemide has good bioavailability and is preferred over the intravenous route, which has the undesired effect of lowering glomerular filtration rate. Patients must be carefully monitored for signs of intravascular volume depletion, renal insufficiency, and decompensation of liver disease. Diuretic therapy should not be initiated when the serum creatinine is unstable because of the risk of precipitating the hepatorenal syndrome.

Large Volume Paracentesis

Large volume paracentesis (LVP) remains an excellent technique to provide relief from the discomfort of tense ascites. Rare but important complications of LVP are cardiovascular collapse and renal failure. Infusion of albumin (5–8 g albumin/L ascites removed) may minimize the likelihood of these complications and should be considered in high-risk patients or when >5 L of fluid is expected to be removed.

Transjugular Intrahepatic Portosystemic Shunt

Less than 10% of cirrhotic ascites is refractory to medical therapy. Transjugular intrahepatic portosystemic shunt (TIPS) is currently the most effective method of managing ascites refractory to diuretics and LVP. The goal of this procedure is to lower portal pressures by making a shunt through the liver from the portal vein directly to the hepatic vein. This is achieved by accessing the hepatic vein through a jugular approach, puncturing liver tissue to access an intrahepatic portal vein radical, and establishing a conduit using an expandable stent. Complications include hepatic encephalopathy and decompensation of cirrhosis. These complications are more likely to occur in Child-Turcotte-Pugh class C liver disease.

Liver Transplantation

If worsening ascites is part of progressive decompensation of chronic liver disease, a workup for assessing candidacy for liver transplantation may be warranted.

KEY POINTS TO REMEMBER

- Ascites formation in cirrhosis is related to both a hydrostatic pressure gradient and to decreased effective plasma volume from peripheral vasodilation and subsequent sodium and water retention by the kidney in response to the renin-angiotensin-aldos-terone system.
- Diagnostic paracentesis should be performed on all patients with new-onset ascites and in those with established ascites and any abdominal or systemic symptom bringing them to medical care (to look for evidence of SBP).
- The SAAG is the most important determinant in the diagnostic evaluation of new-onset ascites. A SAAG of ≥1.1 g/dL is very specific for portal hypertension-related ascites.
- Ascitic neutrophil count of >250 cells/µL or ascitic total WBC count of >500 cells/µL is indicative of SBP and should prompt initiation of empiric antibiotic therapy.
- Management of ascites in cirrhosis should advance in a stepwise fashion with dietary sodium restriction, implementation of spironolactone and loop diuretics, and LVP in cases of tense ascites.
- Transjugular intrahepatic portosystemic shunting is currently the most effective therapy for refractory ascites, but it carries a significant risk of precipitating encephalopathy or liver decompensation.
- Liver transplantation should be considered in advanced cirrhosis and ascites.

REFERENCES AND SUGGESTED READINGS

Garcia-Tsao G. Current management of the complications of cirrhosis and portal hypertension. *Gastroenterology* 2001;120:726–748.

Lake J. The role of transjugular portosystemic shunting in patients with ascites. *N Engl J Med* 2000;342:1745–1747.

Runyon B. AASLD guideline: management of adult patient with ascites due to cirrhosis. *Hepatology* 2004;39:841.

Runyon B. Approach to the patient with ascites. In: Yamada T, ed. *Textbook and Atlas of Gastroenterology on CD-ROM.* Philadelphia: Lippincott Williams & Wilkins; 1999.

Runyon B. Care of patients with ascites. *N Engl J Med* 1994;330:337–342.

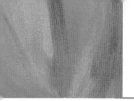

Nutrition

Vladimir Kushnir and Shelby A. Sullivan

INTRODUCTION

Background

Assessment of nutritional status is an important aspect in the care of all patients. The nutritional status represents the effectiveness of nutrient intake in maintaining body composition and meeting metabolic demands. The best overall approach to evaluating nutritional status involves a thorough clinical and physical examination, a nutritional history, and appropriate laboratory studies. To effectively manage a patient's nutritional status, it is imperative to be familiar with the basic principles of clinical nutrition.

Definitions

A state of over- or undernutrition can be called **malnutrition.** For the purposes of this chapter, malnutrition will refer to the state of undernutrition, where nutrient intake is not adequate to meet the body's metabolic demands.

Epidemiology

Undernutrition is prevalent in hospitalized patients, occurring in 20% to 70% of patients at admission or during the hospital course. In the outpatient setting, unintentional weight loss is encountered in up to 13% of the elderly and 50% to 60% of nursing home residents. In addition, malnutrition is frequently underdiagnosed by both practitioners and trainees. Studies have found only 40% of malnourished patients have documentation of their nutritional status and that trainees recorded measurements of nutritional status in <33% of malnourished patients. It is important for health care providers to understand the fundamentals of identifying, preventing, and treating malnutrition.

Natural History

Multiple consequences occur as the result of malnutrition in hospitalized patients. These include increased length of hospital stay, mortality, and susceptibility to infection; poor wound healing, increased frequency of decubitus ulcers; and impaired cardiopulmonary function. As little as 5% unintentional weight loss in 1 month can be clinically significant and a weight loss of 20% or more can impair most physiologic body functions.

CAUSES

Pathophysiology

- In terms of nutritional status, the body is made up of **lean body mass** (LBM) and **fat mass.** The LBM is the body's total mass minus the fat mass and includes muscle, organs, fluid, bones, and minerals. Fat, in the form of adipose tissue triglyceride, is the body's major fuel reserve. In times of stress, the body tries to preserve LBM; however, as fat stores run out, visceral protein mass is mobilized to meet metabolic needs, which include acting as gluconeogenic precursors and wound healing.

- Multiple changes occur in the body as a result of negative energy balance. Initially, there is a decrease in resting energy expenditure (REE). There is also a decrease in protein synthesis, particularly in persons with disease compared with healthy controls. This impaired protein synthesis can lead to a decrease in intestinal cell mass and, consequently, atrophy of the mucosa. Studies have shown variable degrees of mucosal atrophy associated with malnutrition, but these changes can normalize after refeeding.

- In most cases, malnutrition is multifactorial. Nutritional disturbance in hospitalized patients typically results from reduced food intake (prescribed by physicians, critical illness, dysphagia) and increased metabolic demands (burns, inflammatory states, fluids lost through drains). Unintentional weight loss is also commonly caused by malignancy, and gastrointestinal, endocrine, cardiovascular, and pulmonary disorders.

EVALUATION

Nutritional Assessment

No gold standard exists for evaluating the nutritional status of a hospitalized patient. Multiple tools have been developed to assist in nutritional assessment, including the Subjective Global Assessment, Mini Nutritional Assessment, Nutrition Risk Score, Nutrition Risk Index, and Geriatric Risk Index. Studies have been done to validate these tools in assessing for malnutrition, but no gold standard exists. The best overall approach involves a thorough nutritional history and physical examination.

Nutritional History

Nutritional assessment includes identification of preexisting malnutrition before acute presentation, relevant medical and surgical history, medications, social habits, and a focused dietary history. The presence of mild (<5%), moderate (5%–10%), or severe (>10%) unintentional weight loss in the last 6 months should be determined. Unintentional weight loss of >10% is associated with a poor clinical outcome. A thorough dietary history should assess changes in diet and, if present, the reasons for the changes.

Physical Examination

The physical examination should include careful inspection of hair, skin, eyes, mouth (including dentition), extremities, and fluid status as stigmata for protein calorie malnutrition or vitamin and mineral deficiencies. Temporal muscle wasting, sunken supraclavicular fossae, and decreased adipose stores are easily recognized signs of malnutrition. Body Mass Index (BMI = weight in kilograms/height in meters^2) should also be calculated as part of the physical examination with a weight obtained in the hospital (Table 11-1).

Laboratory Assessment

Historically, concentrations of several plasma proteins (e.g., albumin, transferrin, prealbumin) and total lymphocyte count have been used to determine the degree of protein malnutrition, and to predict clinical outcomes. It has been shown, however, that in many cases inflammation and injury, not malnutrition, are responsible for low levels of these markers and for the increased incidence of morbidity and mortality. As such, these parameters have poor sensitivity and specificity and will not be discussed further in this chapter.

TABLE 11-1	BODY MASS INDEX (BMI)-BASED ENERGY REQUIREMENTS FOR HOSPITALIZED PATIENTS	
BMI (kg/m^2)	Energy Requirements (kcal/kg/day)	
<15	36–45	
15–19	31–35	
20–29	26–30	
>30	15–25	

Adapted from Klein S. A primer of nutritional support for gastroenterologists. *Gastroenterology* 2002:122(6);1677–1687, with permission.

MANAGEMENT

Calculating the Nutrient Requirement

- Nutritional requirements are determined by the body's energy demands or total energy expenditure (TEE). The TEE is composed of the resting energy expenditure (70% TEE), thermal effect of food (digestion, 20% TEE), and physical activity (10% TEE). At times of illness or trauma, the resting energy requirement can increase by as much as 50%. Although it is often not feasible to measure energy expenditure directly in hospitalized patients, a number of predictive equations have been devised to estimate macronutrient requirements.

- The simplest approach to estimating the caloric needs of a hospitalized patient is based on BMI (Table 11-1). The general rule is that caloric requirement is inversely proportional to BMI, because LBM (which includes organ mass) is the main determinant of energy expenditure. Because organs do not significantly hypertrophy with increasing adiposity, energy expenditure per kilogram body mass progressively declines with increasing adiposity, but increases with lower body weights. In critically ill, insulin-resistant patients, a lower energy dose should be used to avoid the deleterious effects of hyperglycemia. In overweight patients, an adjusted body weight (see formula below) should be used to avoid overfeeding.

$$\text{Adjusted body weight} = \text{ideal body weight} + 0.25$$
$$(\text{actual body weight} - \text{ideal body weight})$$

The recommended protein intake is 0.8g/kg/day in healthy adults. Individual protein requirement depends on multiple factors, including the overall nutritional state, energy requirement, and nonprotein caloric intake. Normal weight medically ill patients require 1.0 to 1.5 g/kg/day of protein; however, in patients experiencing large protein losses from burns, wounds, or fistulas 2 to 2.5 g/kg/day of protein may be required.

Nutritional Support

- Loss of lean body mass is tightly associated with mortality and, therefore, the goal of nutritional support is to prevent significant weight loss and preserve LBM until recovery from the underlying illness has been achieved. Patients most likely to benefit from nutritional support are those with baseline malnutrition in whom a protracted period of starvation would otherwise occur. No absolute indications exist for nutritional support. A careful assessment of the patient's clinical condition and expected outcome help to determine the need for nutritional support. Factors that must be accounted for include amount of intake, amount of available endogenous stores (adipose tissue), lean muscle mass, and the rate of catabolism. Individuals who are severely malnourished at the outset of an illness often require immediate nutritional support, whereas patients with adequate stores can tolerate longer periods without significant nutritional intake. In general, well-nourished hospitalized patients do not require nutritional support for 7 to 10 days, whereas malnourished and critically ill patients may need nutritional support initiated within 48 to 72 hours of admission. The decision to initiate nutritional support must be individualized and the type of support carefully chosen.

- Types of nutrition support include volitional nutritional support (VNS), enteral nutrition (EN), and parenteral nutrition (PN). VNS is any liquid formulation taken by mouth for either complete nutrition or as a supplement to *ad libitum* food intake. VNS can be used if the patient is able to swallow and is willing to consume a liquid formula as the sole source of calories or as a supplement to solid food. The remainder of this section on nutrition support focuses on enteral nutrition and parenteral nutrition.

Enteral Nutrition

- **Enteral nutrition** is defined as the infusion of a nutrient liquid formulation into the upper gastrointestinal (GI) tract that can provide complete nutritional requirements. EN is thought to preserve GI tract barrier function and should be used when possible. Mechanical obstruction, paralytic ileus, bowel ischemia, unstable GI bleeding, and high output enteric fistulas are relative contraindications to enteral feedings. EN can be used with caution and careful monitoring in the setting of severe pancreatitis, and may be associated with fewer complications than PN.
- For short-term support (<30 days), nasogastric (NG) or nasoenteric tubes are preferred over gastrostomy or jejunostomy tubes. Gastrostomy tubes are indicated if the duration of enteral feeding is expected to be >30 days. The underlying condition and local expertise should dictate percutaneous, radiologic, or surgically placed gastrostomy tubes. Tube feeds should be started at a low dose (150–200 mL) every 4 to 6 hours and increased by 50 to 100 mL each feeding until the feeding goal is reached. Each feeding should be followed by a water flush. The amount of water flush depends on the patient's volume status. With NG tube feeding, a single elevated residual volume is an indication to recheck the residual volume in 1 hour. The feeding should not automatically be stopped, however. Patients' upper bodies should remain upright or elevated by at least at 30 degrees during bolus tube feeds and for 2 hours after to avoid aspiration.
- If short term postpyloric or small bowel feeding is required, small caliber nasojejunal feeding tubes can be placed past the ligament of Treitz. They are associated with a decreased risk of aspiration, and are better tolerated by patients with impaired motility. They may also be associated with less pancreatic stimulation and are often used in the setting of severe acute pancreatitis. If long-term small bowel feeding is required, percutaneous, surgical, or radiographic jejunostomy tubes can be placed. Small bowel feeds are given as a continuous pump-controlled infusion, and typically start with 10 to 30 mL/hour and are increased in small increments (10 mL/hour every 8–12 hours) until the goal feeding is reached. Again, these tubes should be flushed with water every 4 hours to avoid tube occlusion. Bolus feeds should not be used with small bowel feeding tubes to prevent fluid shifts, abdominal distension, and diarrhea.

Choosing an Enteral Formula

Standard tube feeding formulas (Ensure, Osmolite, Isocal) are sufficient for most patients. They are free of gluten and lactose, and are isotonic. They contain 1.0 calorie/mL, and intake of 1500 to 2000 mL/day provides 100% of carbohydrates, protein, fat, vitamins, and minerals. Use of disease-specific and elemental formulas (monomeric and oligomeric) is controversial because these formulas are more expensive than standard formulas.

Complications of Tube Feedings

Tube feeding is a relatively safe procedure, and complications usually can be avoided or adequately managed. In addition to the complications of percutaneous tube placement (infection, bleeding, inadvertent colonic placement), patients may experience aspiration, diarrhea, and alterations in drug absorption and metabolism.

Aspiration: To limit the risk of aspiration, the head of the patient's bed should be raised ≥30 degrees during feeding and for 2 hours afterward. Intermittent or continuous feeding regimens, rather than the rapid bolus method, should be used. Gastric residuals should be checked regularly, and all patients should be observed for signs of feeding intolerance. Jejunal access is helpful in patients with recurrent tube feeding aspiration (not oropharyngeal) or in critically ill patients at risk for impaired gastric motility.

Diarrhea: To minimize the incidence of diarrhea, it is advisable to use an isosmotic, lactose-free formula and to advance tube feeds slowly. If diarrhea becomes a problem, helpful steps include decreasing the rate of the feeds, switching to continuous tube feeds, and adding fiber to the formula. It is important to remember to check for antibiotic-associated diarrhea in these high-risk patients and to look for sorbitol in other orally administered medications. If the above measures fail and infectious causes have been ruled out, an antidiarrheal agent may be appropriate.

Hyperglycemia: Adequate blood glucose monitoring is necessary when starting EN. Initially, sliding scale regular insulin can be used to control blood glucose concentrations. Once the feedings have reached 1000 kcal/day, intermediate duration insulin given every 12 hours can be used in conjunction with sliding scale regular insulin for blood glucose control.

Small Bowel Necrosis: Patients who require pressor support to maintain an adequate blood pressure are at risk for small bowel necrosis with small bowel feeds. The early signs of bowel ischemia are not specific and include bloating, loss of bowel sounds, abdominal pain, and ileus. If EN is necessary in a patient with hypotension, he or she should be carefully monitored for any signs of early bowel ischemia.

Parenteral Nutrition

Parenteral nutrition is the infusion of a nutritional liquid formulation through a central or peripheral venous catheter that can provide complete nutritional requirements. PN may be given if the GI tract is not accessible or functional, as occurs in patients with bowel obstruction, diffuse peritonitis, short gut syndrome, or malabsorption. In some cases, prolonged ileus or severe pancreatitis may also require PN. PN can be administered via a peripheral vein, but the nutrition formula cannot exceed 900 mOsm/kg (e.g., 10% dextrose, 2% amino acids, and electrolytes). This generally provides inadequate calories and, therefore, hyperosmolar solutions (which more adequately meet caloric goals) are used, which require central venous access. The optimal location of the tip of the central venous catheter is at the junction of the superior vena cava and the right atrium.

Composition and Administration of Parenteral Nutrition

- The PN solution can be purchased commercially or can be made by the hospital pharmacy. The total number of calories and amount of protein are determined using the guidelines described in the "Calculating the Nutrient Requirement" section seen above. The lipid content of the PN ideally provides 20% to 30% of the daily calories; a 20% lipid emulsion yields 2.0 kcal/mL. The carbohydrate component is dextrose, and provides the remainder of the calories; it contains 3.4 kcal/g.

- When initiating PN, most practitioners start at one half to two thirds of the total volume over the first 24 hours to avoid large fluid shifts and hyperglycemia. The volume is then advanced as tolerated. Once goal volume has been reached, the rate of infusion can be increased, and PN can be infused over 10 to 14 hours. Cyclic (rather than continuous) infusion of PN improves quality of life and decreases incidence of hepatobiliary complications. Shortened infusion time, however, can lead to periods of hyperglycemia. During initiation of nutrition support, close monitoring is indicated, with frequent measurement of vital signs, daily weights, intake and output, as well as blood sugar checks every 6 to 8 hours. A comprehensive metabolic panel should be checked daily until feeds are at goal, and then twice weekly. Complete blood count (CBC) may be checked once weekly. Electrolytes, minerals, trace elements, and a multivitamin preparation are generally added to the parenteral solution. Note that *iron* is not generally part of the standard additives.

Complications of Parenteral Nutrition

- Mechanical complications may occur during central line placement. These include pneumothorax, brachial plexus injury, subclavian or carotid artery puncture, hemothorax, and chylothorax.
- Metabolic complications include fluid overload, hypertriglyceridemia, hypercalcemia, hypoglycemia, hyperglycemia, and specific nutrient deficiencies.
- **Hyperglycemia** is defined as blood glucose >200 mg/dL. It should be managed by minimizing the dextrose to <200 g/day as well as adding 0.1 U of regular insulin for each gram of dextrose in PN. Blood sugars should be checked frequently and sliding scale insulin (SSI) used to control hyperglycemia. If blood sugars remain elevated despite SSI, additional insulin should be added to the PN solution, equal to 50% of the SSI from the previous 24 hours. If this fails, an intravenous (IV) insulin drip or further reduction in PN carbohydrate dose may be required.
- Hypertriglyceridemia can also be problematic. Triglyceride (TG) levels >1000 mg/dL can cause or exacerbate acute pancreatitis and have been associated with thrombocytopenia. TG levels should be checked at baseline and at least once during lipid emulsion infusion to assure adequate clearance. Most practitioners reduce or eliminate lipids in the emulsion with serum TG levels >400 mg/dL. Remember, the sedative propofol is administered in a 10% (1.1 kcal/mL) lipid emulsion, and should be counted as part of the lipid calories.
- Thrombosis or pulmonary embolism can occur secondary to central venous catheter use. Radiologically evident subclavian vein thrombosis occurs commonly (25%–50%), but clinically significant manifestations (e.g., upper extremity edema, superior vena cava syndrome, or pulmonary embolus) are rare. Inline filters should be used with all PN solutions.
- Infectious complications are most commonly caused by *Staphylococcus epidermidis* or *Staphylococcus aureus*. In immunocompromised patients, gram-negative rods and *Candidal* species are also a major concern.
- Hepatobiliary complications include elevated serum transaminases and alkaline phosphatase. In addition, steatosis, steatohepatitis, lipidosis, cholestasis, fibrosis, and cirrhosis can occur. Although these abnormalities are usually benign and transient, more serious and progressive disease can develop in a small subset of patients, usually after 16 weeks of PN. Biliary complications typically occur with PN administered for longer than 3 weeks and include acalculous cholecystitis, gallbladder sludge, and cholelithiasis.

- Metabolic bone disease, including osteomalacia or osteopenia, may be seen with long-term (>3 months) total PN.

Refeeding Syndrome

- Refeeding syndrome occurs when a severely malnourished patient is initiated on nutritional support; it results in massive fluid and electrolyte shifts, which can lead to volume overload, cardiovascular collapse, and death. Electrolyte depletion is the most dangerous complication of initial refeeding. With administration of a carbohydrate load, serum levels of phosphorous, potassium, and magnesium rapidly fall, because of insulin-mediated transcellular shifts in the face of whole body electrolyte depletion. The rapid fall in phosphate can lead to respiratory muscle paralysis and cardiovascular collapse. Additionally, the rapid fall in potassium and magnesium can lead to cardiac dysfunction and arrhythmias. Volume overload (secondary to fluid administered with the nutritional supplement and insulin-mediated sodium retention) is also characteristic of refeeding syndrome, and may progress quickly to congestive heart failure. Other cardiac abnormalities include prolongation of the QT interval which, combined with plasma electrolyte abnormalities seen in early refeeding, leads to an increased risk of ventricular arrhythmias and sudden cardiac death during the first week of refeeding. Thiamine deficiency can lead to acute beriberi, which in turn can lead to lactic acidosis, impaired sensory perception, edema, and heart failure.
- The best approach to refeeding syndrome is prevention by starting feeds slowly and aggressively supplementing potassium, magnesium, and phosphate in patients with normal renal function. Serum levels should be checked at least once a day. Thiamine should be supplemented at 50 to 100 mg/day for 3 days. To prevent fluid overload, initial fluid intake and sodium should be limited, and patient weight should be monitored daily. Weight gain in excess of 0.25 kg/day or 1.5 kg/wk should be treated as volume overload; fluid intake should be reduced and diuretics used as necessary. Initial feeding should start at 15 kcal/kg/day, and can advance slowly as tolerated. Finally, an electrocardiogram (ECG) should be obtained at baseline, and patients should be monitored on telemetry during early refeeding.

KEY POINTS TO REMEMBER

- No gold standard exists for evaluating the nutritional status of hospitalized patients. The best overall approach involves a thorough clinical and physical examination, as well as a nutritional history.
- BMI is a useful indicator of nutritional status.
- Individuals who are severely malnourished at the outset of an illness often need nutritional support early, whereas patients with adequate stores can tolerate longer periods without adequate nutritional intake (7–10 days).
- If the gut works, use it! Enteral feeding is preferred over parenteral feeding whenever possible.
- Parenteral nutrition should be given if the GI tract is not accessible or functional.
- Refeeding syndrome is a serious complication when artificial nutrition is given to profoundly malnourished patients. Start calorie intake and fluids below goal amounts to prevent refeeding complications. Close monitoring of volume status, heart rhythm, and serum electrolytes is essential during initiation of nutritional support.

REFERENCES AND SUGGESTED READINGS

Gramlich L, Kichian K, Pinilla J, et al. Does enteral nutrition compared to parenteral nutrition result in better outcomes in critically ill adult patients? A systematic review of the literature. *Nutrition* 2004;20(10):843–848.

Kirby DF, Delegge MH, Fleming CR. AGA technical review on tube feeding for enteral nutrition. *Gastroenterology* 1995;108:1282–1301.

Klein S. A primer of nutritional support for gastroenterologists. *Gastroenterology* 2002; 122(6):1677–1687.

Koretz RL, Lipman TO, Klein S. AGA technical review on parenteral nutrition. *Gastroenterology* 2001;121:970–1001.

Koretz RL., Avenell A, Lipman TO, et al. Does enteral nutrition affect clinical outcome? A systematic review of the randomized trials. *Am J Gastroenterol* 2007:102(2): 412–429.

MacFie J. Enteral versus parenteral nutrition. *Br J Surg* 2000;87(9):1121–1122.

Muskat PC. The benefits of early enteral nutrition. In: Shikora SA, Blackburn GL, eds. *Nutrition Support: Theory and Therapeutics*. New York: Chapman & Hall; 1997: 231–241.

Singh H, Watt K, Veitch R, et al. Malnutrition is prevalent in hospitalized medical patients: are housestaff identifying the malnourished patient? *Nutrition* 2006;22: 350–354.

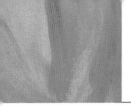

Esophageal Disorders

Julie A. Holinga

GASTROESOPHAGEAL REFLUX DISEASE

Introduction

- Gastroesophageal reflux disease (GERD) is extremely common and, if left untreated, can result in serious complications, including esophageal ulceration, stricture formation, hemorrhage, Barrett's esophagus, and adenocarcinoma. With the advent of proton pump inhibitors (PPI), most cases of GERD can be treated medically.
- **GERD** can be defined as symptoms or mucosal damage that occur secondary to the abnormal reflux of gastric contents into the esophagus. Although the symptoms classically associated with GERD include heartburn, regurgitation, and dysphagia, atypical symptoms such as chest pain, cough, or wheezing may occur. Complications from GERD can also arise in patients who are asymptomatic.
- Reflux of acidic gastric contents into the esophagus is a normal event that occurs in healthy people. Such physiologic reflux can result in transient symptoms directly after a meal. Prolonged exposure of the esophagus to gastric acid is abnormal, however, and may produce symptoms of GERD and mucosal injury.
- The prevalence of GERD is difficult to ascertain because it is based on the number of patients in the population with subjective complaints of regular episodes of heartburn, regurgitation, or dysphagia, which is thought to be secondary to esophageal reflux. Various studies have estimated the prevalence of patients in the Western world with GERD to be as low as 3% and as high as 20% of the population.

Causes

- Several mechanisms underlie abnormal reflux, all of which result in the failure of the gastroesophageal junction to prevent gastric contents from entering the esophagus. The gastroesophageal junction is composed of the lower esophageal sphincter (LES), the crural diaphragm, and the phrenoesophageal ligament. Most cases of GERD are related to transient, inappropriate LES relaxations and, less frequently, to decreased LES resting tone.
- Certain medications or endogenous chemicals can decrease LES tone. In addition, impaired peristalsis allows refluxed contents to remain in contact with the esophageal mucosa. Poor gastric emptying can contribute to the process. Hypersecretion of gastric acid, as seen with the Zollinger Ellison syndrome, increases physiologic reflux to cause pathologic esophageal acid exposure and severe reflux esophagitis.
- Regardless of the mechanism, the acid and enzymes present in gastric contents directly injure the squamous lining of the esophagus. Significant damage occurs when the esophagus is exposed to a pH <4 for a prolonged period of time. Reflux of duodenal contents, most notably bile, may also play an important role.

Presentation

The evaluation of GERD has three important aspects:

- Cardiac diseases should be excluded, especially when chest pain is a symptom.
- Any "alarm symptoms" (see below) should be elicited.
- Severity of GERD should be assessed.

Many lifestyle-related risk factors can worsen GERD symptoms, including alcohol and caffeine intake, smoking, obesity, some medications, and lying supine immediately following meals. *Helicobacter pylori* infection does not contribute to reflux disease and may actually be protective.

Clinical Presentation

- The duration, frequency, and severity of heartburn should be determined. Because many patients with ischemic heart disease describe symptoms that are similar to GERD, the relationship of symptoms to exercise should be ascertained.
- Patients with GERD commonly report "acidic" taste in mouth and nocturnal wheezing or coughing. Other symptoms that may suggest GERD include hoarseness, chronic sore throat, or apnea. Behaviors that increase reflux should be sought, including smoking, caffeine use, large meals, and recumbency after eating. The presence of "alarm symptoms" should be determined, including dysphagia, weight loss, occult or overt gastrointestinal (GI) bleeding, symptoms >5 years, age older than 45 years, and symptoms unresponsive to PPI.
- The physical examination should include an assessment of body habitus (obesity) and an evaluation of the stool for occult blood.

Management

Diagnosis

- Although the degree of esophageal irritation does not always correlate with patient symptoms, many clinicians advocate a trial of a PPI to confirm the diagnosis in patients with suspected GERD.
- In the presence of alarm symptoms, uncertainty of diagnosis, or inadequate response to PPI, further workup is necessary. Also, patients with long-standing GERD (>5–10 years) should have endoscopy performed to evaluate for Barrett's esophagus. Further workup often involves endoscopy, barium swallow, and 24-hour esophageal pH monitoring.
- **Endoscopy** may reveal esophagitis on gross examination, although many patients have evidence of GERD only on histologic examination. The main utility of esophagogastroduodenoscopy (EGD) is to evaluate for complications of GERD, such as stricture, hemorrhage, Barrett's esophagus, and adenocarcinoma.
- **Barium swallow** is often a low-yield examination, although hiatus hernias, and complications of GERD, such as strictures or neoplasia, can be detected.
- **Esophageal pH studies** involve placement of an esophageal luminal pH monitor with measurement over a 24- or 48-hour period. This study is most useful in two clinical scenarios. If the diagnosis of GERD is in doubt, then monitoring can be performed off acid suppression. Generally, an elevated acid exposure time is suggestive of GERD, if the esophageal pH is <4 for ≥5% of the time. Another use is in determining whether chest pain or other atypical symptoms correlate with acid reflux events. The pH study is also used to determine adequacy of acid suppression in a patient with known GERD, when performed on acid suppression. The patient is asked to record episodes of chest pain in a log. The correlation between chest pain and esophageal pH can then be determined.

- Laboratory information is of limited use in the evaluation of GERD. A complete blood count (CBC) may reveal a microcytic anemia if bleeding occurs from esophagitis, cancer, or an erosion.

Treatment
- The goal of treatment is to alleviate symptoms, heal the esophageal damage, and prevent the occurrence of complications of GERD. First-line therapy for moderate to severe GERD includes lifestyle modification and a PPI.
- **Lifestyle modifications** include weight loss, smoking cessation, avoidance of meals within 3 hours of bedtime, and elevation of the head of the patient's bed. Encourage patients to decrease consumption of alcohol, caffeine, and aggravating foods, such as onions and tomatoes. Patients should also avoid use of medications that lower LES tone, such as calcium channel blockers, beta-blockers, nitrates, and anticholinergic drugs. Lifestyle modification is not recommended in isolation, but rather in conjunction with pharmacologic therapy.
- **PPI** administered once daily can heal erosive esophagitis and relieve heartburn. In terms of efficacy, all of the PPI are more effective than H_2-blockers or motility agents in healing esophageal lesions. The PPI can be administered twice daily with improved therapeutic benefit if once-daily dosing is unsuccessful at relieving symptoms of GERD, or if patients have severe erosive esophagitis, strictures, ulcers, or Barrett's esophagus. If twice-daily PPI does not relieve nocturnal symptoms, an H_2-blocker may be added at night.
- **Surgical management** is reserved for patients with documented GERD who do not respond to maximal medical therapy or do not wish to be on lifelong PPI. Patients typically undergo preoperative esophageal physiologic testing, including motility studies and ambulatory pH monitoring. The surgical procedure most often used is laparoscopic Nissen fundoplication. Surgery is as effective as properly dosed PPI with less incidence of pulmonary aspiration. It entails more morbidity and mortality, however.
- GERD symptoms are relieved for most patients with pharmacologic treatment and lifestyle modifications.

Complications
Complications of long-standing or incompletely treated GERD include esophageal stricture, hemorrhage, Barrett's esophagus, and adenocarcinoma.

ESOPHAGEAL MALIGNANCIES

Introduction
- Squamous cell carcinoma and adenocarcinoma represent the two most common malignancies of the esophagus. Barrett's esophagus refers to a premalignant condition in which there is metaplasia of normal esophageal squamous epithelium into specialized intestinal-type epithelium.
- In the United States, squamous cell carcinoma is decreasing in incidence, but the risk remains elevated in black men. The incidence of adenocarcinoma has risen over the past 20 years. Both diseases have a strong male predilection and a high mortality rate. Most patients have regional and distant lymph node metastases at the time of diagnosis.

Causes
- Esophageal squamous cell carcinoma is believed to develop from carcinogenic exposure in susceptible individuals. The most common locations of disease are the proximal and distal esophagus, and the incidence increases with advancing age.

- Adenocarcinoma of the esophagus is believed to develop as a consequence of an accumulation of genetic mutations in the normal squamous epithelium. Most cases develop near the gastroesophageal junction and it is believed that predisposing factors include chronic, long-standing GERD. The continual reflux of gastric acid is thought to cause genetic damage to cells in the adjacent esophageal tissue, leading to eventual transformation into malignancy.
- Barrett's esophagus represents the metaplasia of normal esophageal stratified squamous epithelium in the distal esophagus to specialized intestinal-type epithelium. Patients with Barrett's esophagus have a risk of developing esophageal adenocarcinoma that is approximately 100 times that of patients without the disease.

Presentation

Risk Factors

- For squamous cell carcinoma of the esophagus, risk factors include chronic tobacco and alcohol use, chronic ingestion of hot liquids, history of mediastinal or breast irradiation, human papillomavirus (HPV) 16 or 18 infection, and achalasia. The heavy use of both alcohol and tobacco is a synergistic risk factor, increasing the risk of developing squamous cell carcinoma 100-fold.
- For adenocarcinoma of the esophagus, several risk factors have been identified including Barrett's esophagus, GERD, obesity, scleroderma, history of colon cancer, and medications (including chronic use of theophylline or beta-agonists). Infection with *H. pylori* may have a protective effect. Most cases occur near the gastroesophageal junction and mostly present in obese middle-class men.
- Barrett's esophagus is seen in the setting of long-term, untreated GERD, occurring in approximately 10% of patients with GERD. Most patients with GERD and Barrett's esophagus are symptomatic from GERD, but a significant portion of patients may be asymptomatic.

History and Physical Examination

A thorough history and physical examination should be performed. Key points to look for are a history of dysphagia and unintentional weight loss. Risk factors, especially country of origin, tobacco use, and alcohol consumption, are useful in the diagnosis.

Evaluation

Laboratory tests provide little information to aid in the diagnosis of esophageal malignancies. Basic laboratory tests may reveal a microcytic anemia if bleeding has occurred. A low albumin concentration may suggest malnutrition secondary to dysphagia.

Management

Workup

A barium swallow may reveal a mass in the esophageal lumen or compression from adjacent structures. EGD allows visualization of the esophageal lumen and biopsy of lesions and is the gold standard for diagnosis. Once the diagnosis of cancer has been established, the evaluation should focus on resectability, including endoscopic ultrasound and computed tomography (CT) scan of the chest and abdomen to assess for local and distant spread. Positron emission tomographic (PET) scanning is often useful to exclude distant metastases. Many patients, however, have local or distant spread at the time of diagnosis.

Follow-up of Barrett's Esophagus

Barrett's esophagus can progress from low-grade dysplasia to high-grade dysplasia and then adenocarcinoma, making treatment of it and the underlying GERD very important. Once Barrett's esophagus is diagnosed, repeat endoscopic biopsies should be performed at 1- to 2-year intervals. If low-grade dysplasia is found, follow-up is recommended in 6 to 12 months. If high-grade dysplasia is found, the patient should be referred for endoscopic ablation or esophagectomy. It is important to note that a large portion of patients referred to surgery with high-grade dysplasia may have undetected adenocarcinoma.

Treatment
- For squamous cell carcinoma of the esophagus, the standard of care is surgery alone or in combination with radiation and chemotherapy. Mounting evidence indicates that adjuvant chemoradiotherapy plus surgery may be effective therapy. Patients often present with severe dysphagia that can be relieved with external-beam radiation therapy, surgical resection, or endoscopic stent placement.
- Management of adenocarcinoma of the esophagus is similar to squamous cell carcinoma. Patients who are not surgical candidates should be offered palliative chemotherapy or radiation therapy.

Prognosis
Five-year survival rates for both squamous cell carcinoma and adenocarcinoma of the esophagus remain poor at 10% to 15%. In cases detected at an early stage, however, cure can be possible.

INFECTIOUS ESOPHAGITIS

Introduction
- With the advent of acquired immunodeficiency syndrome (AIDS), the incidence of infectious esophagitis has increased, and the causal organisms have shifted over the past 20 years. The diagnosis of these diseases often requires endoscopic evaluation. Many of these diseases, however, have typical presentations and findings that may obviate invasive diagnosis.
- Infectious esophagitis is most commonly seen in the immunosuppressed patient. Fungal and viral diseases are the most common agents, especially as the T-cell CD4 count falls.
- Approximately 30% of patients with human immunodeficiency virus (HIV) infection have symptoms of esophageal infection during the course of their disease. Almost all of these diseases are treatable, however, and their incidence is decreasing with use of highly active antiretroviral therapy.

Causes
Infectious esophagitis is most often associated with immunosuppression, and most often occurs as a secondary disease in the setting of AIDS. It also is seen in patients on immunosuppressant medications and in those having chemotherapy. There are instances, as discussed below, where infectious esophagitis is seen in immunocompetent hosts.

Differential Diagnosis
- **Immunosuppressed Hosts**
  - **Fungal Esophagitis:** Candidiasis is the most common infectious disease of the esophagus in patients infected with HIV, accounting for roughly 70% of all cases. The most common species is *Candida albicans*, but other species of *Candida* may be involved. Other fungi, such as *Histoplasma capsulatum*, can cause esophagitis, but these infections are rare. It is important to note that patients with AIDS may present with multiple esophageal infections at the same time. Almost all of these cases include *Candida* as one of the causal organisms.
  - **Viral Esophagitis:** The most common viral cause of esophagitis in patients infected with HIV is cytomegalovirus (CMV). The risk of infection is low with CD4

counts >100 cells/μL. Unlike in immunocompetent patients and in those with immunodeficiency from other causes (e.g., organ transplant), herpes simplex virus (HSV) esophagitis is uncommon in those with HIV. Varicella zoster virus (VZV) can cause a devastating esophagitis in severely immunocompromised hosts. Other viruses, such as Epstein-Barr virus and human papilloma virus, can infect the esophagus, but are very rare.

- **Bacterial Esophagitis**: Bacterial infection of the esophagus in patients infected with HIV is rare but can be seen. Pathogens involved are *Mycobacterium avium complex*, *Mycobacterium tuberculosis*, *Nocardia*, *Actinomyces*, and *Lactobacillus*.

Idiopathic esophageal ulceration (IEU) is common in patients with a CD4 count <50 cells/μL. The etiologic agent of this disease has not been determined, although HIV itself has been implicated. In those infected with HIV taking antiretroviral therapy, it is important to consider pill esophagitis as a cause of symptoms.

- **Immunocompetent Hosts.** HSV and VZV are the only common esophageal infections of the immunocompetent patient, although they are rare. HSV infection usually occurs in male patients and involves the mid-esophagus. VZV esophagitis often occurs in children with chickenpox or adults with herpes zoster.

Presentation

Clinical Presentation

- Risk factors for infectious esophagitis include HIV or AIDS, ongoing treatment with chemotherapy, and other causes of immunosuppression. A thorough history and physical examination should be performed, with emphasis on hydration and HIV status, and other key features listed below.
- **Candidiasis.** Dysphagia is the most common symptom of candidiasis. Odynophagia, fever, nausea, and vomiting are less common. Patients often have thrush. Up to one-half of patients with other esophageal infections and AIDS have concomitant esophageal candidiasis.
- **Cytomegalovirus.** Odynophagia and chest pain are the most common symptoms of CMV. Patients may also have a low-grade fever, nausea, and vomiting. Dysphagia is uncommon.
- **Herpes Simplex Virus.** Patients with HSV most commonly present with both odynophagia and dysphagia. Most patients also present with chest pain and fever.
- **Varicella Zoster Virus.** The typical skin lesions of chickenpox in children or herpes zoster in adults may be seen in VZV, otherwise, it presents similarly to HSV.
- **Idiopathic Esophageal Ulceration**

Almost all patients with IEU present with severe odynophagia and, as a result, are malnourished and dehydrated at presentation. The diagnosis is made when other causes have been ruled out.

Evaluation

An elevated white blood cell (WBC) count may suggest infection, although this finding is variable in patients with immunodeficiency. The CD4 count is useful in determining which pathogen is likely involved in patients with AIDS.

CD4 Count	Typical Organisms Involved
>200	HSV, VZV
100–200	Candida, HSV
<100	Candida, CMV, HSV
<50	IEU

Management

Diagnosis

Many clinicians recommend giving a patient with AIDS and dysphagia, but without other symptoms, an empiric course of fluconazole, because *Candida* is the most likely pathogen. If the patient does not improve in 7 days or has other symptoms (e.g., weight loss, dehydration, or fever), further evaluation is needed. EGD can distinguish between the types of esophageal infections by gross or histologic appearance of the lesions.

- **Candidiasis.** Multiple adherent, white or yellow, "cottage cheese" plaques are easily seen on endoscopy. Brushings or biopsies reveal yeast or budding hyphae. Culture is useful in patients with a history of esophageal candidiasis for determining species and susceptibilities.
- **Cytomegalovirus.** Few large, well-demarcated ulcers are seen in CMV. Immunohistochemistry (special CMV staining) of biopsy specimens aids in the diagnosis.
- **Varicella Zoster Virus.** Multiple vesicles and confluent ulcers are seen in VZV. The cytology is difficult to distinguish from HSV and often requires immunohistochemistry or culture.
- **Herpes Simplex Virus.** HSV appears as either small, superficial ulcers or a diffuse esophagitis in later stages. Cytology reveals giant cells and ground-glass nuclei. Immunohistochemistry or culture confirms the diagnosis.
- **Idiopathic Esophageal Ulceration.** A few well-circumscribed, often large, ulcers are seen in idiopathic esophageal ulceration. Multiple biopsies should be taken to exclude other processes.

Treatment

- **Candidiasis.** First-line treatment is fluconazole, 200-mg oral loading dose, followed by 100 mg/day for a total of 5 to 10 days. In patients with azole-resistant *Candida*, the oral dose of fluconazole may be increased, or treatment with intravenous (IV) amphotericin can be initiated. Severe, refractory cases may not improve until treatment of HIV is undertaken to raise the CD4 count.
- **Cytomegalovirus.** First-line therapy includes IV ganciclovir, 5 mg/kg q12h, if the patient is not pancytopenic. Alternate therapy includes IV foscarnet, 60 mg/kg q8h. Treatment continues until healing occurs, usually up to 1 month. Approximately 30% of patients relapse.
- **Herpes Simplex Virus.** First-line therapy includes acyclovir, 5mg/kg IV q8h for 7 to 14 days or 400 mg PO 5 times a day for 14 to 21 days. Other effective agents are famciclovir, valacyclovir, and ganciclovir. Foscarnet is reserved for resistant strains because of its adverse effects.
- **Varicella Zoster Virus.** Therapy includes acyclovir 5mg/kg IV q8h for 7 to 14 days. Higher dosing may be needed for refractory cases.
- **Idiopathic Esophageal Ulceration.** Treatment involves corticosteroids. Oral prednisone can be used; if the patient cannot tolerate PO intake, then IV formulations are used. The use of corticosteroids often predisposes to *Candida* infection, and many clinicians also give fluconazole twice weekly as long as prednisone is given. Thalidomide is effective in treating IEU as well.
- **Prophylaxis.** Many of these diseases have high recurrence rates and warrant prophylaxis. Primary prophylaxis of *Candida* is not recommended; however, secondary prophylaxis in patients with multiple recurrences is used. Often, once weekly oral fluconazole, 100 mg, is effective. Although primary prevention of CMV is recommended in patients with CD4 counts <100, no data support a decreased incidence of GI disease. Primary prophylaxis for HSV is not recommended. Secondary prophylaxis is recommended for patients with recurrent disease with acyclovir, 600 mg PO daily.

EOSINOPHILIC ESOPHAGITIS

Introduction

- Eosinophilic esophagitis, also referred to as *allergic esophagitis*, is a relatively new diagnosis that continues to be described with increasing frequency over the past few decades. The etiology, prevalence, and predisposing factors for eosinophilic esophagitis are incompletely understood and remain an area of continued research and investigation.
- Eosinophilic esophagitis is characterized by infiltration of the esophageal mucosa with eosinophils. Although eosinophilic infiltration of the esophagus can be seen secondarily in association with other conditions, such as GERD, eosinophilic esophagitis is now recognized as a primary diagnosis, presumably from an allergic or idiopathic cause.
- For unclear reasons, there seems to be an increasing incidence of eosinophilic esophagitis that is not solely accounted for by increasing recognition. Little epidemiologic data currently exist.

Causes

- The pathogenesis of eosinophilic esophagitis is unknown. Once eosinophils have infiltrated the esophageal mucosa, however, their presence appears to trigger a self-sustaining cascade of inflammatory mediators. This, in turn, is thought to perpetuate esophageal inflammation and sometimes leads to mechanical narrowing of the esophageal lumen. These physiologic changes then can result in symptoms of dysphagia, GERD, food impaction, and esophageal dysmotility.
- In addition to the primary diagnosis of eosinophilic esophagitis, recruitment of eosinophils to the esophagus is seen as a secondary response in many other inflammatory and infectious conditions, such as gastroesophageal reflux and inflammatory bowel disease.

Presentation

Risk Factors

There seems to be an increased incidence of eosinophilic esophagitis in pediatric patients with a history of asthma, allergic rhinitis, eczema, and food or environmental allergies. This association has not been fully studied in adult populations, however. There is also a reported association of eosinophilic esophagitis in adults with eosinophilic gastroenteritis and peripheral eosinophilia.

Clinical Presentation

A thorough history and physical examination should be performed. Questions regarding risk factors, including those listed above, should be elicited. The most common presenting symptoms of eosinophilic esophagitis are dysphagia and heartburn or chest pain. Less common presenting symptoms include a history of food impaction or symptoms consistent with esophageal dysmotility. No physical examination findings are specific to or indicative of this diagnosis.

Evaluation

The esophageal mucosa is abnormal by endoscopy in more than half of patients. It is notable, however, that even in those patients with grossly normal esophageal mucosa, significant eosinophilia is seen on histologic evaluation.

Management

Workup

- Currently, no established consensus exists on the diagnostic criteria for eosinophilic esophagitis. Generally speaking, the diagnosis is most often made based on the presence of characteristic clinical features, confirmation of large numbers of eosinophils on esophageal biopsy after a trial of acid suppression with a PPI, and exclusion of other possible diagnoses (e.g., GERD, parasitic and fungal infections, Crohn's disease, allergic vasculitis, and other connective tissue diseases).

- To evaluate for the presence of eosinophilic esophagitis, biopsies should be obtained along the length of the esophagus. Biopsies should also be obtained in the stomach and duodenum to determine whether the disorder is confined to the esophagus or is a manifestation of eosinophilic gastroenteritis. A CBC count can be done to evaluate for peripheral eosinophilia, although this phenomenon is more frequently seen in the pediatric population with eosinophilic esophagitis. A barium swallow and esophageal pH study may add further data regarding a patient's anatomy and assessing for pathologic reflux, but they are not required in the routine management and treatment of this disease. Allergen skin testing has been suggested by some to avoid potential precipitating foods or allergens.

Treatment

Currently, there is no universally accepted treatment regimen for this disease. Although many patients with eosinophilic esophagitis present with symptoms consistent with GERD, PPI often give minimal and inadequate relief. Systemic corticosteroids have been shown to give significant benefit in pediatric patients. Symptoms recur quickly on cessation, however, and given the multiple deleterious side effects of long-term *systemic* corticosteroid use, this remain a poor treatment option. Currently, the most commonly accepted course of treatment includes avoidance of known environmental and food allergens and treatment with *topical* corticosteroids. One of the primary studies supporting the use of topical steroids in this manner involved the use of fluticasone. Patients were instructed to swallow rather than inhale the medication. Relief of dysphagia was seen in all study participants within the initial week of treatment. Although a low incidence of esophageal candidiasis has been described with this treatment regimen, the systemic effects of topical corticosteroids are thought to be much decreased in comparison to systemic corticosteroids.

Prognosis

The prognosis of eosinophilic esophagitis is not well described. There is no known risk of associated dysplasia or malignancy. It is not yet established whether these patients should undergo surveillance endoscopy.

Complications

Various morphologic findings in the esophagus have been described in association with eosinophilic esophagitis, presumably in some way a result of the chronic inflammatory process which occurs. Proximal esophageal strictures have been observed as well as mucosal rings, esophageal ulceration, and esophageal polyps.

ESOPHAGEAL STRICTURES

Introduction

- Esophageal strictures often arise as complications of other disease processes. Any type of chronic inflammation can lead to esophageal strictures. Common causes include GERD, repetitive vomiting, caustic ingestion, infections, and pill esophagitis. Other less common causes include nasogastric (NG) tube injury, iron-deficiency anemia, and Crohn's disease.
- Peptic strictures are relatively common, occurring in approximately 10% of patients with GERD. Other strictures include lower esophageal (Schatzki's) ring, and less commonly, esophageal webs.

Presentation

- Patients do not often develop symptoms of dysphagia until a significant amount of the esophageal lumen is obliterated. Peptic strictures that are associated with GERD typically occur in the distal esophagus. Strictures as a result of esophageal infections, caustic ingestion, NG tube trauma, repetitive vomiting, or Crohn's disease often are more extensive. Lower esophageal (Schatzki's) rings often occur in the distal esophagus and are associated with GERD, pill esophagitis, and hiatal hernias. They are an extremely common cause of intermittent, solid food dysphagia. Plummer-Vinson syndrome, which includes iron deficiency, dysphagia, and upper esophageal webs, usually occurs in middle-aged women.
- A careful history is crucial in the assessment of dysphagia. In addition to helping rule out diseases other than stricture, the type of dysphagia and regurgitation can often localize the site and involvement of disease. Key points of the history should include onset and duration of symptoms, association of dysphagia with type of foods, description of regurgitated material if present, history of weight loss, and history of GERD.
- Physical signs of weight loss, dehydration, and malnutrition help to assess severity. (See Chapter 1, Dysphagia and Odynophagia, for a discussion of the evaluation of suspected dysphagia.)

Management

Workup

- A barium swallow test is a useful step in the workup of suspected stricture, ring, or web. Radiologic findings inconsistent with the patient's history warrant further evaluation with direct visualization with EGD. EGD is also useful for relieving identified areas of dysphagia with bougie or balloon dilation.
- Laboratory studies are generally not useful in the workup of stricture. Iron-deficiency anemia may support the diagnosis of Plummer-Vinson syndrome. A low albumin concentration may reflect nutritional deficiency.

Treatment

- **Peptic Stricture**. Aggressive acid control with high-dose PPI can cause regression of the stricture. Dilation is often required, however, and it is performed endoscopically. Limited data exist on the benefit of stent placement for benign strictures, and the obvious risk is stent migration. Occasionally, dysphagia is not relieved by maximal medical therapy, and surgery is required.
- **Schatzki's Ring**. Patients with Schatzki's ring describe intermittent dysphagia for solids, often when eating meats or bread or when eating too quickly. In mild disease, patients should be advised to masticate their food carefully. Patients with more severe disease are at increased risk for food bolus impaction and benefit from passage of an endoscopic dilator. Refractory cases may require pneumatic dilation, electrocautery incision, or surgical repair. Patients should be assessed for GERD and treated with a PPI as needed.
- **Plummer-Vinson Syndrome (Esophageal Web)**. Dysphagia associated with Plummer-Vinson syndrome is very responsive to iron repletion. Severe cases may require endoscopic dilation with bougienage. These patients have an increased risk of developing squamous cell carcinoma of the esophagus. It is unclear whether they should receive screening EGD.

ESOPHAGEAL MOTILITY DISORDERS

Introduction

Motility disorders of the esophagus can involve both the striated and smooth muscle of the esophagus. Often, dysfunction of one or multiple components of the esophageal neuromuscular system can be identified. These diseases can result in extreme morbidity for patients. Fortunately, new treatments are becoming available.

Causes

Swallowing involves two types of muscular activity. It is initiated by neural impulses from the central nervous system (CNS), controlling voluntary muscles of the oropharynx. It is completed by the involuntary contraction of the smooth muscle of the esophagus in a coordinated sequence. Dysfunction at any step can cause dysphagia.

- **Striated Muscle.** The striated muscles of the oropharynx can be affected by a number of conditions, including cerebrovascular accidents, myasthenia gravis, polymyositis, Parkinson's disease, and amyotrophic lateral sclerosis. Neuromuscular dysregulation results in the loss of a coordinated swallow and can lead to dysphagia, regurgitation, and pulmonary aspiration. An inappropriately contracting cricopharyngeus muscle can lead to dysphagia in some patients.
- **Smooth Muscle.** Esophageal smooth muscle dysfunction results from the loss of inhibitory neurons in the esophagus. The loss leads to dysregulation of peristalsis and an increased LES tone. This process, which leads to achalasia, can result from various causes. The differential diagnosis for esophageal dysmotility secondary to smooth muscle dysfunction is broad and includes infectious, malignant, autoimmune, and neurologic causes. Achalasia can be primary or secondary caused by invasive cancer or by *Trypanosoma cruzi* infection causing Chagas' disease. Diffuse esophageal spasm (DES) and nutcracker esophagus are similar disorders of abnormal inhibitory neuron function that are nonprogressive. Scleroderma causes the smooth muscles of the distal esophagus to atrophy and LES tone to decrease. In early stages, it causes solid food dysphagia but can progress to severe dysphagia when complications of severe GERD develop.

Presentation

- The history should focus on conditions that can cause motility disorders, such as cerebrovascular accident, amyotrophic lateral sclerosis, and myasthenia gravis. A history of travel to Central and South American countries may warrant workup for Chagas' disease. As with strictures, the type, duration, and severity of dysphagia are important to address. A description of regurgitated contents is useful as well. Complications of motility disorders, such as severe weight loss and aspiration pneumonia, should be assessed. The most common symptoms at presentation are dysphagia and chest pain.
- The physical examination should include a thorough neurologic examination as well as assessment of nutritional status.

Oropharyngeal Dysphagia

Patients with oropharyngeal dysphagia often present with drooling, regurgitation of food immediately after swallowing, and pulmonary aspiration.

Achalasia

Achalasia often presents as progressive dysphagia and chest pain. Severe disease can result in solid and liquid dysphagia with accompanying weight loss. Patients frequently report a history of regurgitated, undigested food, often while sleeping.

Nutcracker Esophagus and Diffuse Esophageal Spasm

Patients with nutcracker esophagus or diffuse esophageal spasm present with nonprogressive, intermittent chest pain and dysphagia, which can range in severity from mild to extremely severe, sometimes with radiation to other parts of the body. Hence, it is important to rule out myocardial ischemia or infarct in patients with this presentation. Patients often have solid and liquid dysphagia, especially with very hot or cold items.

Management
Workup
Barium swallow and esophageal manometry are very useful in diagnosing esophageal motility disorders.

- **Achalasia.** Barium swallow often reveals a characteristic "bird's beak" tapered distal esophagus with proximal dilation. This appearance can also occur with neoplastic compression of the lower esophagus (pseudoachalasia). Manometry reveals a lack of primary peristalsis and increased LES tone. If patients have simultaneous and repetitive contractions, the disease is termed *vigorous achalasia*. EGD should always be performed to exclude mass lesions as a cause of secondary achalasia or pseudoachalasia.
- **Diffuse Esophageal Spasm.** Barium swallow often reveals a typical "corkscrew" or "rosary-bead" appearance. Nutcracker esophagus often appears normal. Manometry in DES reveals simultaneous contractions of the entire esophageal body. Nutcracker esophagus is defined by an elevated distal esophageal peristaltic amplitude. EGD often appears normal, although patients often have evidence of GERD.

Treatment
- **Achalasia.** The only effective medical therapy is endoscopic botulinum toxin injection of the LES. Effectiveness requires repeated injections and development of resistance and scarring can occur. The standard nonsurgical treatment is endoscopic esophageal dilation. Most patients experience immediate relief. A risk of esophageal perforation exists, however. Laparoscopy with surgical myotomy of the LES is gaining popularity and has more long-term efficacy than other treatment modalities. Patients with achalasia have an increased risk of squamous cell esophageal carcinoma (develops in 2%–7%), and there is debate about whether regular surveillance EGD should be performed.
- **Diffuse Esophageal Spasm.** Patients with DES and GERD require reassurance that their disease is nonprogressive and not fatal. Psychiatric disorders should be considered because they are often comorbid with DES and nutcracker esophagus. Medications, such as nitrates and calcium channel blockers, are often used in treatment. PPI should also be included in the treatment regimen, given the strong link of GERD with these disorders. The use of dilation or pneumatic dilation is of limited value considering the episodic nature of these diseases. Laparoscopic surgical esophageal myotomy is indicated only in patients with severe refractory symptoms.
- **Scleroderma.** Treatment of scleroderma should involve aggressive acid control with high-dose PPI. The motor dysfunction is very refractory to treatment, however.

KEY POINTS TO REMEMBER

- During the evaluation of GERD, it is important to exclude other causes of chest pain—especially cardiac causes.
- A trial of standard-dose, once-daily PPI is often used to confirm the diagnosis of uncomplicated GERD. Presence of dysphagia, weight loss, anemia, occult blood in stools, lack of response to PPI, or age older than 50 years warrants further evaluation with EGD.
- Patients with squamous cell carcinoma often have a long history of tobacco and alcohol use, whereas patients with adenocarcinoma are often obese and have a long history of GERD.

(continued)

KEY POINTS TO REMEMBER (continued)

- Patients with Barrett's esophagus represent a high-risk group for the development of esophageal adenocarcinoma and should be treated with aggressive acid control and endoscopic surveillance.
- The most common causes of esophagitis in patients with AIDS are *Candida*, CMV, HSV, and IEU. Infections in an immunocompetent host are rare but can include HSV and VZV.
- Patients with suspected esophagitis who do not respond to an empiric trial of fluconazole or those with symptoms, such as severe odynophagia or fever, should have an upper endoscopy study.
- Eosinophilic esophagitis is an emerging disease entity characterized by infiltration of the esophageal mucosa with eosinophils in response to a primary allergic or immunologic mechanism.
- Peptic strictures are common complications of GERD. Schatzki's rings are the most common cause of intermittent solid food dysphagia.
- Striated muscle dysfunction often presents with difficulty swallowing in the context of known neuromuscular diseases. Treatment of underlying diseases and swallowing therapy are the most effective treatments.
- Achalasia typically presents as progressive dysphagia and chest pain. It can be treated with botulinum toxin injections, dilations, or surgery.

REFERENCES AND SUGGESTED READINGS

Adler DG, Romero Y. Primary esophageal motility disorders. *Mayo Clin Proc* 2001; 76(2):195–200.

Arora AS, Perrault J, Smyrk TC. Topical corticosteroid treatment of dysphagia due to eosinophilic esophagitis in adults. *Mayo Clin Proc* 2003;78:830.

Bonacini M, Young T, Laine L. The causes of esophageal symptoms in human immunodeficiency virus infection: a prospective study of 110 patients. *Arch Intern Med* 1991;151:1567–1572.

DiPalma JA. Management of severe gastroesophageal reflux disease. *J Clin Gastroenterol* 2001;32(1):19–26.

Falk GW. Gastroesophageal reflux disease and Barrett's esophagus. *Endoscopy* 2001;33(2):109–118.

Goyal RK. Diseases of the esophagus. In: Fauci AS, Braunwald E, Isselbacher KJ, et al., eds. *Harrison's Principles of Internal Medicine.* New York: McGraw-Hill; 1998: 1588–1596.

Gupta SK, Fitzgerald JF, Davis MM. Treatment of allergic eosinophilic esophagitis with oral prednisone and swallowed fluticasone: a randomized, prospective study in children [Abstract]. *Gastroenterology* 2003; Abstract ID 101884.

Heath EI, Forastiere AA, Limburg PJ, et al. Adenocarcinoma of the esophagus: risk factors and prevention. *Oncology* 2000;14(4):507–514.

Hetzel DJ, Dent J, Reed WD, et al. Healing and relapse of severe peptic esophagitis after treatment with omeprazole. *Gastroenterology* 1988;95:903–912.

Hoffman RM, Jaffee PE. Plummer-Vinson syndrome. *Arch Intern Med* 1995;155: 2008–2011.

Klinkenberg-Know EC, Nelis F, Dent J, et al. Long-term omeprazole treatment in resistant gastroesophageal reflux disease: efficacy, safety, and influence on gastric mucosa. *Gastroenterology* 2000;118:661–669.

Landres RT, Juster GG, Strum WB. Eosinophilic esophagitis in a patient with vigorous achalasia. *Gastroenterology* 1978;74:1298.

Liacouras CA, Wenner WJ, Brown K, et al. Primary eosinophilic esophagitis in children: successful treatment with oral corticosteroids. *J Pediatr Gastroenterol Nutr* 1998; 26:380.

Lundell L, Miettinen P, Myrvold HE, et al. Continued follow-up of a randomized clinical study comparing antireflux surgery and omeprazole in gastroesophageal reflux disease. *J Am Coll Surg* 2001;192:172–181.

Noel RJ, Putnam PE, Rothenberg ME. Eosinophilic esophagitis. *N Engl J Med* 2004; 351:940.

Shiflett DW, Gilliam JH, Wu WC, et al. Multiple esophageal webs. *Gastroenterology* 1979; 77;556.

Straumann A, Simon HU. Eosinophilic esophagitis: escalating epidemiology? *J Allergy Clin Immunol* 2005;115:418.

Streitz JM, Ellis FH, Gibb SP, et al. Achalasia and squamous cell carcinoma of the esophagus: analysis of 241 patients. *Ann Thorac Surg* 1995;59:1604–1609.

Wilcox CM, Monkemuller KE. Diagnosis and management of esophageal disease in the acquired immunodeficiency syndrome. *South Med J* 1998;91(11):1002–1007.

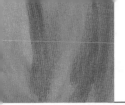

Gastric Disorders

Thomas A. Kerr

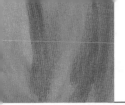

13

PEPTIC ULCER DISEASE

Background

Gastric disorders, in particular peptic ulcer disease (PUD), are among the most common problems encountered by internists and gastroenterologists. PUD accounts for a significant portion of health care expenditures and imposes significant morbidity on many individuals. PUD is characterized by denudation of mucosa exposed to gastric acid. By definition, this denudation extends into the muscularis propria layer. Lesions >5 mm are called *ulcers*, whereas those <5 mm are called *erosions*. PUD most commonly occurs in the gastric antrum or duodenal bulb. Duodenal ulcers are more common than gastric ulcers.

Epidemiology

Peptic ulcer disease is a worldwide problem. The lifetime risk of acquiring the disease is approximately 1 in 10. Each year, in the United States, approximately 500,000 new cases of PUD occur and 4 million cases recur. The annual mortality rate of PUD is low and is mostly owing to complications, which include hemorrhage, perforation, and obstruction. Duodenal ulcers are slightly more common in men than in women, but gastric ulcers occur with equal frequency in both genders. Duodenal ulcers present at a slightly younger age range than gastric ulcers: ages 25 to 55 years and ages 40 to 70 years, respectively. This difference is believed to be owing to increased use of nonsteroidal anti-inflammatory drugs (NSAID), which are associated primarily with gastric ulcers, in the elderly population. The incidence of PUD has declined since 1955, which partly has been attributed to increased sanitation and antibiotic use leading to decreased rates of *Helicobacter pylori* infection.

Pathophysiology

The development of PUD is not entirely understood. It is believed to result from an imbalance between gastric mucosal protective factors provided in part by prostaglandins and noxious influences such as *H. pylori*, pepsin, NSAIDs, bile salts, and acid. Gastric ulcers are typically associated with normal or reduced levels of acid secretion, whereas duodenal ulcers are generally characterized by increased levels of acid secretion. Both can occur in the setting of *H. pylori* infection. Other factors that may play a role in PUD are elevated serum gastrin levels, increased acid output, and rapid gastric emptying, all of which have been associated with idiopathic PUD. A list of risk factors associated with PUD is found in Table 13-1.

Differential Diagnosis

Forms of PUD are listed in Table 13-2. The most common forms of PUD are associated with *H. pylori* or the use of NSAID; these comprise 90% of cases of PUD. In patients in whom *H. pylori* infection, NSAID use, Crohn's disease, and Zollinger-Ellison syndrome have been ruled out, no apparent etiology is found in 50% of cases.

TABLE 13-1   RISK FACTORS FOR PEPTIC ULCER DISEASE

Infection with *Helicobacter pylori*	Having a first-degree relative with peptic ulcer disease
Nonsteroidal anti-inflammatory drug use	Emigration from a developing nation
Smoking	
African American or Hispanic ethnicity	

Natural History

The natural history of PUD varies from resolution without treatment to recurrence with or without complications. Before the discovery in the 1980s of *H. pylori* infection as the most common cause of PUD, this disease was believed to be caused by stress, dietary factors, or gastric acid, but it frequently recurred despite treatment with antacids and antisecretory medications. Surgery was often performed for recurrent disease. Now, *H. pylori*–associated PUD is treated with eradication of *H. pylori*. As a result, the recurrence rate of PUD has markedly decreased, and elective surgery for PUD is exceedingly rare. Vigorous efforts should be expended to avoid surgery for PUD induced by *H. pylori* or NSAID use.

Causes

Helicobacter pylori–Associated Peptic Ulcer Disease

- *Helicobacter pylori* infection has been associated with up to 90% of duodenal ulcers and 70% to 90% of gastric ulcers. It is also a risk factor for gastric adenocarcinoma and gastric mucosa–associated lymphoid tissue (MALT) lymphomas. The incidence of *H. pylori* in PUD appears to be decreasing, as more recent studies in the United States have demonstrated that 20% to 58% of ulcers are not associated with *H. pylori*. *H. pylori* infection is associated with lower socioeconomic status and is typically acquired in childhood.
- *Helicobacter pylori* is a gram-negative bacillus that lives in the mucous layer overlying gastric epithelium, leading to inflammation. It can also be found within epithelial cells and attached to mucous cells. In the case of duodenal ulcers, *H. pylori* is believed to infect the gastric antrum or ectopic gastric mucosa in the duodenum. This is associated with increased acid production and duodenal ulceration. The

TABLE 13-2   FORMS OF PEPTIC ULCER DISEASE

Most Common

Helicobacter pylori–associated
Nonsteroidal anti-inflammatory drug–associated

Other Forms

Stress ulcers
Zollinger-Ellison syndrome
Gastroduodenal Crohn's disease
Viral infection
Chemotherapy
Radiation therapy
Vascular insufficiency

corpus of the stomach is relatively spared of inflammation, parietal cell function is intact, and ulceration occurs in the area of greatest inflammation. Conversely, *H. pylori* infection that involves the acid-producing mucosa of the stomach can lead to hypochlorhydria or achlorhydria, and subsequent gastric ulceration.

- The ability of *H. pylori* to induce gastritis likely stems from a combination of qualities. The bacterium does not appear to have a predominant virulence factor. The bacterium secretes a urease enzyme that breaks down urea in the stomach to produce ammonia, which helps to neutralize the acidic gastric environment and thereby protect the organism. This urease activity provides the basis for many of the laboratory tests used to evaluate for *H. pylori* infection. In addition, *H. pylori* infection is believed to increase the permeability of the gastric mucous layer to pepsin and acid. Finally, the bacterium produces cytotoxins (CagA) that may also contribute to its pathogenicity.

Nonsteroidal Anti-inflammatory Drug-Associated Peptic Ulcer Disease

- The second most common cause of PUD after *H. pylori* is NSAID use. NSAID use has been associated with 30% to 75% of *H. pylori*-negative ulcers and 15% of *H. pylori*-positive ulcers. The rate of GI complications in patients taking long-term NSAID varies from 7.3 per 1000 patients per year for osteoarthritis to 13 of 1000 patients per year for rheumatoid arthritis. NSAID have a direct toxic effect because of their acidic nature and because they can decrease the hydrophobicity of gastric mucus, allowing injury of the epithelium by acid and pepsin. The predominant mechanism for NSAID-associated PUD is inhibition of endogenous prostaglandin synthesis. Therefore, enteric-coated, parenteral, or rectal NSAID or acetylsalicylic acid (ASA) use presents the same risk of ulcers as their oral counterparts. Moreover, administration of NSAID with food does not decrease ulcer risk. Suppression of prostaglandin synthesis is mediated through inhibition of the cyclooxygenase (COX)-1 enzyme, which acts as a "housekeeping" enzyme to maintain the integrity of the gastric mucosa, where it is constitutively expressed. Inhibition of prostaglandin synthesis decreases mucus production, bicarbonate secretion, mucosal perfusion, and epithelial proliferation. This impairs the integrity of the mucosa, allowing damage by harmful factors such as NSAIDs, pepsin, bile salts, and acid. Because the anti-inflammatory effects of NSAIDs are believed to be mediated through the COX-2 enzyme, which is not expressed in the gastric mucosa, COX-2–selective inhibitors may be less likely to cause GI complications.
- Risk factors for the development of NSAID-associated PUD include concomitant corticosteroid use, anticoagulants, and older age (Table 13-3). Corticosteroids alone are not a risk factor. The role of *H. pylori* infection in NSAID-associated PUD remains incompletely defined, with different studies showing conflicting results. It is

TABLE 13-3	RISK FACTORS FOR NSAID-ASSOCIATED PEPTIC ULCER DISEASE
Concomitant corticosteroid use	Prior peptic ulcer disease (associated with *Helicobacter pylori* or NSAIDs)
Concomitant bisphosphonate use	
Concomitant anticoagulant use	Increasing NSAID dose or prolonged use
Older age	Poor overall health
Female gender	

NSAID, nonsteroidal anti-inflammatory drugs.

generally believed, however, that *H. pylori* and NSAID may act synergistically to induce PUD.

- NSAID use can cause a spectrum of lesions that can affect any area of the stomach, although the gastric antrum is most frequently involved. The various types of lesions seen range from superficial lesions to ulcers that are complicated by hemorrhage or perforation. Superficial lesions include petechiae and erosions, and these are likely caused by the direct toxic effects of NSAID and may occur within hours of NSAID administration. These lesions are confined to the mucosa and, as such, do not cause complications. Ulcers extend to the submucosa and are larger than erosions. Endoscopic evidence of mucosal damage has been found in up to two-thirds of patients who use NSAID and frank ulceration is found in 10% to 25%.
- NSAID-associated ulcers are often complicated by hemorrhage and perforation. In fact, 60% or more of complicated gastroduodenal ulcers are associated with the use of NSAID or ASA. These complications occur with similar frequency among duodenal and gastric ulcers. Hemorrhage is the most common complication. Platelet dysfunction may contribute to the tendency toward hemorrhage, especially in the case of ASA. Hemorrhage can occur at any time during the course of NSAID treatment, and the risk of hemorrhage at any given time does not change over an extended period of NSAID use.

Zollinger-Ellison Syndrome

Uncontrolled acid hypersecretion in the setting of a gastrinoma, or the Zollinger-Ellison syndrome, accounts for only 0.1% of all peptic ulcers. The ulcers are caused by gastrin-producing endocrine tumors of the pancreas or duodenum. The increased gastrin levels cause histamine release from enterochromaffin-like cells in the gastric mucosa. The histamine then binds to histamine receptors on parietal cells, causing hypersecretion of hydrochloric acid. Peptic ulcers develop as the normal defense mechanisms against acid are overwhelmed by the high gastric acid output. Ulcers typically form in the duodenal bulb, but may also be seen in the distal duodenum and jejunum, and multiple ulcers are commonly seen. Diarrhea may also develop because of gastric acid-mediated damage to the small bowel mucosa resulting in a secretory pattern, and contributed to by the excessive volume of gastric secretion. The diagnosis should be suspected in any patient with multiple ulcers in unusual locations or in patients with a family history suggestive of possible multiple endocrine neoplasia type I. An elevated gastrin level suggests the diagnosis, and a secretin stimulation test or measurement of elevated fasting gastric acid output helps confirm the diagnosis.

Presentation

History

- History alone is unreliable in diagnosing PUD. Approximately 70% of patients who report dyspepsia have nonulcer dyspepsia, and up to 40% of patients with active PUD have no abdominal pain. The classic symptom complex of a patient with a gastric ulcer includes pain that occurs 5 to 15 minutes after oral intake, and is relieved with fasting. For this reason, patients may learn to avoid food and lose weight. Patients with duodenal ulceration, by contrast, may have pain that is temporarily relieved by eating, but returns 1 to 2 hours after eating. The pain from a duodenal ulcer may manifest at night. Because of the potential of duodenal ulcers to result in right upper quadrant abdominal pain, the pain may mimic that of acute cholecystitis. Perforation of a peptic ulcer may be heralded by an acute change in symptoms, peritoneal signs on physical examination, and decreased bowel sounds. Chronic PUD can lead to scarring and gastric outlet obstruction in which case nausea, vomiting, or weight loss may be the presenting complaint.

- Patients should be questioned carefully about NSAID and ASA use, including over-the-counter NSAIDs. Even if patients have discontinued NSAID use, they may still present with GI toxicity up to 1 year later. NSAID-associated ulcers are more likely than other forms of peptic ulcers to be painless and may present initially with bleeding rather than dyspepsia.

Physical Examination

In the absence of complicated PUD, the physical examination is not very helpful. Patients may have epigastric tenderness. The sensitivity, specificity, positive predictive value, and negative predictive value of epigastric tenderness on deep palpation are ≤50%, however. Patients with perforated peptic ulcers usually exhibit signs of peritonitis. Patients with bleeding ulcers may have fecal occult blood, melena, or hematemesis. If they are hemodynamically compromised, they may be tachycardic or hypotensive. Bleeding may be the presenting sign in 15% of cases of PUD.

Management

Diagnostic Evaluation

- Routine laboratory studies are usually unremarkable. CBC may show iron-deficiency anemia from chronic fecal occult blood loss or anemia from acute blood loss.
- Patients in whom PUD is suspected should be tested for *H. pylori* infection. Patients with a history of documented peptic ulcer or gastric MALT lymphoma should also be tested, although some would argue that the likelihood of *H. pylori* infection in individuals with no history of NSAID use and a history of documented PUD is so high that testing is unnecessary. As a corollary, patients should not be tested for *H. pylori* infection unless treatment is intended. Moreover, asymptomatic patients without a history of PUD and patients on long-term treatment with proton pump inhibitors (PPI) for GERD do not need to be tested.
- Several types of tests have been developed to detect the presence of *H. pylori*. These tests include *serology*, *urease assays*, and *histology*. Some of these tests are noninvasive, whereas others require endoscopy. The decision regarding which test to perform and whether to perform endoscopy depends on the individual patient. Culture is not generally performed because it is expensive, time consuming, and difficult. Culture should not be considered unless a patient does not respond to eradication treatment and there is concern about antibiotic resistance.
  - **Serology.** Serology tests for IgG antibodies to *H. pylori*. Serology diagnoses *H. pylori* infection rather than the presence of PUD *per se*. Because of their high sensitivity, serologic tests are more accurate in areas with a high prevalence of *H. pylori*. The most common serologic tests are laboratory-based enzyme-linked immunosorbent assay (ELISA) tests. Less commonly used serology tests are based on immunochromatography and western blotting. The accuracy of ELISA testing can extend up to 95%. Serologic testing is inexpensive, but antibodies may remain positive for >1 year after treatment of the infection, so it is difficult to evaluate *H. pylori* infection with serology after treatment.
  - **Urease Assays.** Urease assays test for the presence of the urease enzyme, which is produced in high amounts by *H. pylori*. These tests include noninvasive urea breath testing and biopsy urease tests. They can be used both to diagnose active infection and to confirm cure of *H. pylori* infection. False–negative results can occur in the setting of treatment with PPI, H_2-receptor blockers, antibiotics, or bismuth-containing medications. Therefore, PPI should be held for 7 to 14 days before testing. In addition, urease breath testing to confirm cure of *H. pylori* should be held until 4 weeks after completing treatment for *H. pylori* infection.

The urea breath test is the best noninvasive method of diagnosing *H. pylori* infection. The two forms of urea breath tests are (a) the ^{14}C-urea breath test and (b) ^{13}C-urea breath test. The two breath tests use urea that has been labeled with either a radioactive (^{14}C) or nonradioactive (^{13}C) isotope. Labeled urea is given orally to the patient; in the presence of urease, the urea is broken down into ammonia and labeled CO_2. After absorption of CO_2 into the circulation, it is expelled into the breath. $^{13}CO_2$ is detected by mass spectroscopy, whereas $^{14}CO_2$ is detected by scintillation counting. Radioactive urea breath testing is contraindicated in pregnant women and in children. The theoretic advantage of urea breath testing over biopsy urease tests is a decreased number of false-negative tests owing to sampling error.

Biopsy urease tests include the CLOtest, PyloriTek, and Hp-fast. Biopsy urease testing is the best endoscopic method of diagnosing *H. pylori*. Most of these tests involve a pH-sensitive dye that changes color because of an increase in pH secondary to the production of ammonia from urea. In addition to false-negative results in the setting of prior treatment with PPI, false-negative results can occur if blood from recent or active bleeding is present. If it is not possible to hold PPI before testing, biopsies should be taken from both the antrum and the fundus to increase the likelihood of a positive result.

- **Histology.** Histology is not usually necessary to diagnose *H. pylori* infection. Histology requires the performance of endoscopy. It is indicated in gastric ulcers because of the risk of malignancy or in cases of PUD in which urease testing might be falsely negative (e.g., in the setting of use of PPI before endoscopy). In the case of gastric ulcers, biopsies should be obtained from around the ulcer crater and edges to rule out malignancy, but they should be obtained from other areas of the stomach to test for *H. pylori*. Biopsy may be less sensitive in the setting of bleeding ulcers, so other sampling-independent testing, such as serology, should be performed. Patients with a gastric ulcer should undergo follow-up endoscopy at 8 to 12 weeks to document ulcer healing and exclude malignancy. Duodenal ulcers do not require biopsy or repeat endoscopic evaluation because of the extremely low risk of malignancy.
- ***Helicobacter pylori* Testing in Complicated Peptic Ulcer Disease.** *H. pylori* testing is more likely to be negative in complicated PUD. Among patients with bleeding duodenal ulcers, only 70% are infected with *H. pylori*. Moreover, in one study among patients with perforated peptic ulcers, only 50% were infected. The lower rate of *H. pylori* in complicated PUD may be at least partially owing to a higher false-negative rate for biopsy urease tests. Therefore, a negative biopsy urease test in the case of a complicated peptic ulcer warrants additional testing for *H. pylori*. If the patient has never had treatment for *H. pylori*, serology is the test of choice in the setting of PUD complicated by hemorrhage.
- **Endoscopy.** Decisions regarding endoscopy in patients with symptoms of PUD should be made based on a patient's symptoms and the risk of gastric cancer. With a high suspicion of PUD based on the history and physical examination, consideration may be given to performing noninvasive testing, such as serology and urease breath testing without endoscopy, especially if the patient is relatively young and otherwise healthy. These tests are more cost-effective than esophagogastroduodenoscopy. Endoscopy should be performed, however, in patients who have signs or symptoms worrisome for gastric cancer. These include anorexia, dysphagia, epigastric mass, severe vomiting, weight loss, anemia, advanced age, and family history of upper GI cancer. Patients with significant dyspepsia, acute GI bleeding, fecal occult blood, or abdominal pain of unclear etiology should also undergo endoscopy. Gastric ulcers should be biopsied to rule out gastric cancer.

Treatment

Medications used to treat PUD include antisecretory drugs and mucosal protectants such as sucralfate. Antisecretory drugs include histamine₂ (H₂)-receptor antagonists, PPI, and prostaglandin analogues. H₂-receptor antagonists inhibit acid secretion by blocking the binding of histamine to its receptor on the parietal cell. They inhibit both basal and food-induced acid secretion. The H₂-receptor blockers available in the United States include cimetidine, famotidine, nizatidine, and ranitidine. This class of drugs is well tolerated, although doses should be adjusted in patients with renal insufficiency. In general, when used in the treatment of gastroduodenal ulcer disease, H₂-blockers are most effective when administered between dinner and bedtime. PPI are prodrugs that, when activated by acid, bind to and inhibit the parietal cell H^+/K^+-adenosine triphosphatase (ATPase). Because they require acid for activation, they are most effectively taken before or with a meal and in the absence of other antisecretory drugs. PPI pose a theoretic risk of inducing enterochromaffinlike cell hyperplasia and carcinoid tumors, but these drugs have been used safely in the United States for the past decade without a notable increase in the incidence of carcinoid tumors. Misoprostol is a prostaglandin analog that inhibits acid secretion. It is the only drug that has been approved by the U.S. Food and Drug Administration (FDA) for prophylaxis of NSAID-induced peptic ulcers. Because of its mechanism of action, misoprostol might cause diarrhea or spontaneous abortion.

- **Helicobacter pylori–Associated Peptic Ulcer Disease.** Patients with documented *H. pylori* infection should be treated with antibiotics and antisecretory therapy. Treatment of *H. pylori* infection with antibiotics significantly lowers the recurrence rate. Patients treated with antisecretory therapy alone have a recurrence rate of 60% to 100%, compared to <15% in patients treated with *H. pylori* eradication.

  A number of regimens have been developed for *H. pylori* eradication, mostly through trial and error. Because *H. pylori* is difficult to eradicate, effective *H. pylori* regimens usually involve more than one antibiotic and ≥10 days of therapy. Some regimens are relatively inexpensive but require four times daily dosing, which may decrease compliance. Because most regimens involve two or more antibiotics, they can also be associated with unpleasant side effects. Accepted treatment regimens for *H. pylori* eradication are listed in Table 13-4.

  Current therapy standards recommend triple therapy with clarithromycin, amoxicillin, and a PPI for 10 to 14 days as an accepted primary regimen (Table 13-4). Of

TABLE 13-4	**TREATMENT REGIMENS FOR *Helicobacter pylori* ERADICATION**

PPI PO BID; amoxicillin, 1000 mg PO bid; clarithromycin, 500 mg PO BID

PPI PO BID; amoxicillin, 1000 mg; metronidazole 500 mg PO BID

PPI PO BID; bismuth subsalicylate, 525 mg PO QID; metronidazole, 500 mg PO QID; tetracycline, 250 mg PO QID

PPI PO BID; metronidazole 500 mg PO TID; bismuth subsalicylate 2 tablets TID or QID; tetracycline 500 mg PO TID

Ranitidine bismuth citrate, 400 mg PO BID for 28 days; clarithromycin, 500 mg PO BID for 14 days

Note: With the exception of ranitidine bismuth citrate, treatment duration is 14 days.

PPI, proton pump inhibitor.

note, amoxicillin and clarithromycin are pH-dependent antibiotics that work more effectively in combination with antisecretory drugs. Regimens include multiple antibiotics to maximize the likelihood of eradication and to prevent the spread of antimicrobial resistance. Monotherapy is inadequate. Even so, none of these regimens eradicates *H. pylori* in all patients. In general, the eradication rate is 70% to 90%. *H. pylori* therapy may be unsuccessful because of noncompliance or antibiotic resistance. In the United States, resistance most commonly occurs with metronidazole and rarely clarithromycin. A four-drug regimen that includes bismuth subsalicylate, tetracycline, metronidazole, and a PPI can be used as a salvage regimen and in patients allergic to penicillin; alternate salvage regimens incorporate levofloxacin (Levaquin).

In addition to antibiotics, patients should also be treated with antisecretory therapy. Debate exist to whether antisecretory medications accelerate the rate of healing; however, they do allow faster resolution of symptoms. The course of antisecretory treatment depends on the location of the ulcer. Duodenal ulcers should be treated for 4 weeks, and gastric ulcers should be treated for 8 weeks. In general, with ulcers >1 cm, it is reasonable to treat with a longer course of antisecretory therapy.

- **Confirmation of *Helicobacter pylori* Eradication.** In patients with uncomplicated PUD, confirmation of cure is not required because recurrence would most likely also be uncomplicated. Testing for *H. pylori* eradication should be performed, however, in patients with recurrent symptoms, complicated PUD, gastric MALT lymphoma, or early gastric cancer. Because of the high rate of bleeding recurrence in untreated *H. pylori*-positive bleeding ulcers, testing for eradication is critical. Confirmation of cure can be performed by urea breath testing. In the case of *H. pylori*-positive, complicated PUD, testing for cure of *H. pylori* should be done after treatment to minimize recurrence. To avoid false–negative results, urea breath testing should be performed ≥4 weeks after the end of *H. pylori* therapy and 2 weeks after finishing treatment with PPI. Serology testing to document eradication is less useful, because the antibody may remain positive for up to 1 year after successful eradication.

- **NSAID-Associated Peptic Ulcer Disease.** For patients with NSAID-associated PUD, consideration should be given to stopping the offending drug, because continuation of NSAID use delays ulcer healing. Discontinuing NSAID is not always practical, however. In patients who must continue to take NSAID, GI toxicity may be reduced by decreasing the dose or switching to a less gastrotoxic medication, such as a COX-2 inhibitor. Concomitant corticosteroid, anticoagulant, or bisphosphonate therapy should be discontinued if possible.

  Direct treatment of NSAID-induced ulcers is acid suppression with an H_2-receptor antagonist or a PPI. Studies have shown that even with continued NSAID use, approximately 75% of gastric ulcers and 87% of duodenal ulcers heal after 6 to 12 weeks of treatment with conventional doses of H_2-receptor antagonists. Continuation of NSAID use does result in delayed healing, and larger ulcers also take longer to heal. A number of trials comparing PPI to H_2-receptor antagonists in patients with NSAID-induced ulcer disease who continue to take NSAID have demonstrated higher rates of ulcer healing with PPI than with H_2-receptor antagonists. The current recommendation, therefore, is to treat NSAID-associated ulcers with PPI if the patient is to continue to take NSAID. PPI therapy should continue as long as the patient is being treated with NSAID to reduce the risk of ulcer recurrence.

- **Recurrent Peptic Ulcer Disease.** The most important risk factors for ulcer recurrence are *H. pylori* infection and NSAID use. Among untreated, bleeding *H. pylori*-positive peptic ulcers, approximately one-third present with recurrent bleeding within 1 year. Treatment of *H. pylori* dramatically reduces the rate of recurrent disease. The incidence of *H. pylori* reinfection after eradication is very low in developed countries.

TABLE 13-5	RISK FACTORS FOR GASTRIC ADENOCARCINOMA
Helicobacter pylori infection	Prior gastrectomy
Chronic atrophic gastritis	Blood type A
Pernicious anemia	Family history of gastric cancer
Gastric adenoma	Low socioeconomic status

- **Maintenance Antisecretory Therapy.** Maintenance antisecretory therapy after treatment of *H. pylori* infection is not cost-effective and is generally unnecessary in the treatment of PUD. It may be considered in high-risk cases, such as patients with complicated PUD, patients with *H. pylori*-negative ulcer disease, and patients in whom *H. pylori* eradication is unsuccessful.

GASTRIC ADENOCARCINOMA

In the early 1900s, stomach cancer was the most common cancer in the United States. Over the last 80 years, the incidence has decreased dramatically for unclear reasons. In 2000, in the United States, approximately 33,800 new cases of gastric cancer and 25,100 deaths were recorded. Gastric cancer, however, remains a major cause of death in other parts of the world, necessitating routine screening in Japan, for example. Multiple risk factors for gastric cancer have been identified (Table 13-5).

Presentation

Many patients with gastric cancer are asymptomatic or have nonspecific symptoms, including indigestion, epigastric discomfort, anorexia, early satiety, and weight loss. By the time symptoms have been investigated, many gastric cancers are advanced. The physical examination may reveal an epigastric mass, ascites, occult blood in the stool, or lymphadenopathy. An enlarged left supraclavicular node (Virchow's node) or periumbilical lymph node (Sister Mary Joseph's node) represents a metastatic site.

Management

Diagnostic Evaluation

Laboratory evaluation is of limited use but may demonstrate iron-deficiency anemia from chronic blood loss from the cancer. Diagnosis is best made with upper endoscopy, because this allows direct visualization as well as tissue sampling. Most gastric cancers are exophytic or fungating masses, but some manifest as nonhealing ulcers or with perforation of the gastric wall. All gastric ulcers should be aggressively biopsied to exclude malignancy. Repeat esophagogastroduodenoscopy should be performed at 8 to 12 weeks to document healing in any patient with a gastric ulcer. Once the diagnosis of gastric adenocarcinoma is established, staging should be performed with endoscopic ultrasound or abdominal computed tomography (CT) scans to determine whether surgical resection is an option.

Treatment

Surgical resection offers the only chance for cure. Approximately 60% of gastric cancers are deemed unresectable, however, because of local or metastatic spread at the time of diagnosis. Depending on location, partial or total gastrectomy may be performed. Even with complete resection, 5-year survival is only approximately 20%. Palliative chemotherapy can be given to patients who are not surgical candidates, but the median survival is only 6 to 9 months.

GASTROINTESTINAL STROMAL TUMORS

Background

Gastrointestinal stromal tumors (GIST) represent 1% to 2% of all malignant GI tumors. Before the molecular definition of GIST in 1998, GIST were commonly unrecognized and unreported. Since that time, despite the increasing recognition by gastroenterologists of this condition, the true incidence remains unknown, although it has been estimated to be approximately 15 cases per million or approximately 5000 new cases per year in the United States. The median occurrence is in the fifth decade of life and GIST are found more commonly in women than in men.

Pathophysiology

The term gastrointestinal stromal tumor was coined in 1983 to encompass noncarcinomatous intra-abdominal tumors. In 1998, the pathophysiology was discovered to involve mutations in KIT signaling pathways leading to tumor proliferation. The definition of GIST has subsequently been narrowed to include a subset of tumors arising from the interstitial cells of Cajal, over 90% of which exhibit KIT mutations. Approximately 5% of GIST tumors do not express KIT mutations. These have been found to have mutations in other pathways including platelet-derived growth factor signaling.

Clinical Presentation

GISTs can be found throughout the GI tract, although 60% to 70% arise in the stomach. They may be discovered incidentally on endoscopy or imaging. If not discovered incidentally, they often present after achieving a large size, thus causing mass effect or obstruction. Patients may complain of nonspecific symptoms, such as nausea, vomiting, or early satiety. Approximately 40% of GIST lesions may present with acute upper GI hemorrhage.

Treatment

Surgical resection is the treatment of choice for localized tumors. If, however, the tumor has metastasized, chemotherapy is an option. GIST demonstrates striking resistance to traditional cytotoxic chemotherapeutics; however, imatinib mesylate (a tyrosine kinase inhibitor) has yielded in striking results, with clinical benefits seen in >80% of patients.

GASTRIC LYMPHOMA

Background

The stomach is the most common location of GI lymphoma in developed countries. Gastric lymphomas can be of the diffuse large B-cell type, or MALT type. Approximately 40% are the MALT type, and they are thought to arise from transformation of B cells in the marginal zone of the stomach in response to *H. pylori* infection (>90%).

Clinical Presentation

The most common presenting symptoms are abdominal pain and dyspepsia with B-type symptoms being rare. Although *H. pylori* infection is a risk factor, the incidence in *H. pylori* infected individuals is between 1 in 30,000 to 80,000.

Treatment

Reports are that MALT lymphoma completely regresses after eradication of *H. pylori* in up to 75% of patients with stage I disease. In patients who do not respond to antibiotic therapy for *H. Pylori*, radiation, chemotherapy, and surgery may be considered and they are effective.

KEY POINTS TO REMEMBER

- The most common forms of PUD are associated with *H. pylori* or the use of NSAIDs. These comprise 90% of PUD cases.
- Gastric ulcers should be biopsied to rule out malignancy. Most patients should have repeat endoscopy at 8 to 12 weeks to document ulcer healing.
- Treatment of *H. pylori* dramatically reduces recurrence of PUD.
- In patients with uncomplicated PUD, confirmation of cure is not required because recurrence would most likely also be uncomplicated. Testing for *H. pylori* eradication should be performed, however, in patients with recurrent symptoms, complicated PUD, gastric MALT lymphoma, or early gastric cancer.
- The current recommendation is to treat NSAID-associated ulcers with PPIs if the patient is to continue to take NSAIDs. PPI therapy should continue as long as the patient is being treated with NSAIDs to reduce the risk of ulcer recurrence.
- Many patients with gastric cancer are asymptomatic or have nonspecific symptoms, including indigestion, epigastric discomfort, anorexia, early satiety, and weight loss.
- Palliative chemotherapy can be given to patients with gastric cancer who are not surgical candidates, but the median survival is only 6 to 9 months.

REFERENCES AND SUGGESTED READINGS

Cappell MS, Schein JR. Diagnosis and treatment of nonsteroidal anti-inflammatory drug-associated upper gastrointestinal toxicity. *Gastroenterol Clin North Am* 2000;29:97–124, vi.

Cecil RL, Goldman L, Bennett JC. *Cecil Textbook of Medicine.* 21st ed. Philadelphia: WB Saunders; 2000.

Chey WD, Wong BC; Practice Parameters Committee of the American College of Gastroenterology. American College of Gastroenterology guideline on the management of Helicobacter pylori infection. *Am J Gastroenterol* 2007;102:1808–1825.

Cohen H. Peptic ulcer and Helicobacter pylori. *Gastroenterol Clin North Am* 2000; 29:775–789.

Friedman SL, McQuaid KR, Grendell JH. *Current Diagnosis & Treatment in Gastroenterology.* 2nd ed. New York: Lange Medical Books/McGraw-Hill, Medical Publishing Division; 2003.

Graham DY. Therapy of Helicobacter pylori: current status and issues. *Gastroenterology* 2000;118:S2–S8.

Howden CW, Hunt RH. Guidelines for the management of *Helicobacter pylori* infection. Ad hoc committee on practice parameters of the American College of Gastroenterology. *Am J Gastroenterol* 1998;93:2330–2338.

McColl KE. *Helicobacter pylori*-negative ulcer disease. *J Gastroenterol* 2000;35(Suppl 12): 47–50.

Sleisenger MH, Feldman M, Friedman LS, et al. *Sleisenger & Fordtran's Gastrointestinal and Liver Disease: Pathophysiology, Diagnosis, Management.* 8th ed. Philadelphia: Saunders Elsevier; 2006.

Walsh JH, Peterson WL. The treatment of *Helicobacter pylori* infection in the management of peptic ulcer disease. *N Engl J Med* 1995;333:984–991.

Wolfe MM, Lichtenstein DR, Singh G. Gastrointestinal toxicity of nonsteroidal antiinflammatory drugs. *N Engl J Med* 1999;340:1888–1899.

Wolfe MM, Sachs G. Acid suppression: optimizing therapy for gastroduodenal ulcer healing, gastroesophageal reflux disease, and stress-related erosive syndrome. *Gastroenterology* 2000;118:S9–S31.

Small Bowel Disorders

Anisa Shaker and Deborah C. Rubin

INTRODUCTION

- The small bowel is approximately 600 cm in length, with a functional surface area >600 times that of a hollow tube. Three features unique to the gut enhance the surface area of the small intestine: the plicae circulares, the villi, and the microvilli. The plicae circulares, or circular folds, are visible mucosal and submucosal invaginations located predominantly in the duodenum and jejunum. Villi are fingerlike projections, consisting of a layer of epithelial cells overlying the lamina propria, approximately 0.5 to 1.5 mm long, which protrude into the intestinal lumen and cover the mucosal surface. Microvilli, tubular projections visualized by electron microscopy, are extensions of the apical cell membrane and compose the brush border. These unique mucosal features create an enormous area for digestion, absorption, and secretion.

- Diseases of the small intestine often result in malabsorption, an interruption of normal digestion, absorption, and transport of a number of nutrients and minerals. Malnutrition, diarrhea, steatorrhea, and weight loss are frequent consequences. Clinical manifestations of small bowel disorders often reflect deficiencies of various macro- and micronutrients.

MALABSORPTION

Causes

Small bowel disorders, pancreatic exocrine insufficiency, and cholestatic liver disease account for most causes of malabsorption. Table 14-1 lists the most common causes of malabsorption. Cholestatic liver diseases are discussed in Chapter 19, Chronic Liver Disease. Pancreatic disorders are discussed in Chapter 21.

Presentation

Many patients with malabsorption present with weight loss despite a good appetite and adequate oral intake. In addition, most patients have an increased number of foul-smelling stools with an oily character. Malabsorption of specific fat-soluble vitamins leads to various clinical findings, including night blindness (vitamin A), osteopenia (vitamin D), bleeding diathesis (vitamin K), or neurologic symptoms (vitamin E). Iron deficiency may develop, because the duodenum is the site for most iron absorption. Patients with an abnormal ileum or ileal resection may develop malabsorption of vitamin B_{12} and bile salts. Abdominal distention, flatulence, and abdominal cramps are common with carbohydrate malabsorption. Other common nonspecific findings include fatigue, muscle wasting, edema, amenorrhea, and orthostatic hypotension. Other, more specific clinical findings are discussed with the respective diseases below.

TABLE 14-1   CAUSES OF MALABSORPTION

Small Intestine Disorders	Pancreatic Exocrine Insufficiency
Celiac sprue	Chronic pancreatitis
Ileal resection	Cystic fibrosis
Short bowel syndrome	Pancreatic cancer
Radiation enteritis	Cholestatic liver disease
Small bowel lymphoma	Extrahepatic biliary obstruction
Bacterial Overgrowth	Intrahepatic biliary obstruction
Crohn's disease	Cirrhosis
Tropical sprue	
Whipple disease	
Acquired immunodeficiency syndrome	
Abetalipoproteinemia	
Diabetes mellitus	
Amyloidosis	

Evaluation

A number of tests may be useful in the evaluation of the patient with suspected small bowel disease.

Fecal Fat Analysis

Fecal fat analysis may be useful in patients with suspected malabsorption. Qualitative analysis using Sudan staining is a simple, rapid, inexpensive screening test for fat malabsorption. A positive result should be confirmed with quantitative analysis, which involves measurement of fecal fat content for 48 to 72 hours while the patient is on a 100 g per 24-hour fat diet. Normal fat absorption is >95% efficient, so >5 g/day of fecal fat is abnormal and suggests the presence of abnormal fat absorption. This test does not distinguish mucosal causes of malabsorption from hepatobiliary and pancreatic causes.

Xylose Absorption Test

If a patient has an abnormal quantitative fat analysis, the D-xylose absorption test is useful to determine whether a small bowel disorder is present. Although not often used, it is important to understand the principle on which it is based. D-xylose is a 5-carbon sugar that is absorbed in the small intestine, but does not require intraluminal digestion. Therefore, abnormal xylose absorption can distinguish between mucosal disease (absorption will be decreased) and pancreatic disease (absorption will be normal). Of note, bacterial overgrowth (discussed below) can also result in decreased absorption because some enteric bacteria can metabolize D-xylose. The patient is given 25 g of xylose orally, and urinary excretion, hydrogen breath testing (discussed below), or serum concentration of xylose is then measured. A 5-hour urine collection should contain at least 5 g of D-xylose.

Small Bowel Imaging Studies

- Traditional imaging of small bowel pathologic processes can be performed with barium small-bowel follow-through examinations, single- or double-contrast intubated enteroclysis, and computed tomography (CT) cross-sectional imaging. Capsule endoscopy, push endoscopy, and double-balloon endoscopy are newer techniques that have been developed to examine the small bowel in its entirety.

- Cross-sectional imaging techniques provide good visualization of both superimposed bowel loops and extraluminal findings and complications. In addition, the emergence of CT and magnetic resonance (MR) enterography have led to further improvements in the noninvasive evaluation of the small bowel. Advantages of MR enterography include the lack of ionizing radiation, improved soft tissue contrast, and the ability to provide real-time and functional evaluation. MR imaging (MRI) may prove especially useful in patients with polyposis syndromes, such as Peutz-Jeghers syndrome and familial adenomatous polyposis who must undergo routine surveillance and thus be exposed to a potentially significant cumulative radiation dose. Advances have also been made in CT cross-sectional imaging with the development of CT enterography. Advantages of this technique include superior temporal and spatial resolution compared with MR, more wide spread access, and decreased cost. Indications for cross-sectional imaging of the small bowel continue to evolve but include evaluation of obscure gastrointestinal (GI) bleeding, the presence and activity of Crohn's disease, and suspected neoplasia. Studies are ongoing comparing these new and evolving imaging techniques in evaluation of small bowel disease.

Endoscopic Biopsy

Biopsy of the small intestine is extremely useful in patients with suspected malabsorption. Specific histologic findings allow diagnosis of the more common causes of malabsorption, such as celiac sprue, as well as more infrequent causes, such as lymphoma and amyloidosis.

Hydrogen Breath Tests

- Hydrogen breath tests using glucose, lactose, or lactulose are commonly used for the diagnosis of small bowel bacterial overgrowth and lactase deficiency. Bacterial carbohydrate metabolism is the only source of exhaled hydrogen under normal conditions. In the setting of a disaccharidase deficiency, such as lactase deficiency, ingested carbohydrates are not absorbed in the small intestine and are instead metabolized by colonic bacteria. As a result, there is an increase in exhaled hydrogen. The hydrogen breath test can be used to diagnose lactase deficiency. Exhaled hydrogen is measured after the patient is given 25 to 50 g of oral lactose dissolved in water. Hydrogen (H_2) levels in end-expiratory breath samples are measured every 15 minutes for up to 3 hours. An increase >20 ppm over basal values indicates lactose malabsorption. A positive test usually peaks at 2 to 4 hours.
- More recently, hydrogen breath tests have been used to diagnose small bowel bacterial overgrowth (SBBO). In this setting, ingested carbohydrates are metabolized in small intestine, producing an earlier peak in hydrogen exhalation. An oral load of 10 g lactulose or glucose in a dose of 50 to 75 g dissolved in water can be used. An earlier than expected peak may be consistent with SBBO, but other conditions that should be considered include rapid small bowel transit or oral flora substrate fermentation. These tests, therefore, have a number of limitations and significant potential for false-negative and false-positive results. Interpretation of these tests is also not always uniform. The reported sensitivity and specificity of the lactulose hydrogen breath test in detecting SBBO is 68% and 44%, respectively, and for the glucose breath test 62% and 83%, respectively.

CELIAC SPRUE

Causes

- **Celiac disease** is defined as a permanent intolerance to the storage proteins or *gluten* found in wheat, rye, and barley. A consequence of complex adaptive and

innate immune responses to dietary gluten, it is characterized by chronic inflamm
tion of the proximal intestinal mucosa. The adaptive immune response is mediated
by gluten-reactive CD4$^+$ T cells. Gluten-derived peptides are presented to CD4$^+$ T
cells by HLA antigen class II molecules DQ2 and DQ8. Deamidation of these peptides by tissue transglutaminase allows higher affinity binding to the binding groove
of DQ2 or DQ8. Innate immune responses are mediated by intraepithelial lymphocytes, which are activated via interleukin-15 produced by enterocytes.

- The prevalence of celiac disease in the United States is approximately 1%, with a
range of 0.71% to 1.25%. HLA antigen class II DQ molecules DQ2 and DQ8 are
necessary but not sufficient for phenotypic expression of the disease. High risk populations include the following: first-degree relatives of patients with celiac disease
(prevalence 10%); patients with unexplained iron-deficiency anemia (prevalence
2%–5%); osteoporosis and bone demineralization (prevalence 1.5%–3%); type 1
diabetes mellitus (prevalence 2%–5% in adults, 3%–8% in children); patients with
liver disease, such as elevated transaminase levels of unknown cause (prevalence
1.5%–9.0%); autoimmune hepatitis (prevalence 2.9%–6.4%); primary biliary cirrhosis (prevalence 0%–6.0%); patients with genetic disorders (prevalence in patients
with Down syndrome ranges from 3%–12%); patients with autoimmune thyroid
disease (prevalence 1.5%–6.7%); and patients with reproductive disorders (prevalence 2.1%–4.1%).

Presentation

The spectrum of mucosal changes is wide, but classically there is atrophy of the small intestinal villi, deepening of the crypts, and infiltration of the lamina propria and intraepithelial compartments with chronic inflammatory cells, particularly affecting the proximal
small intestine. Consequences of chronic inflammation, such as ulceration or structuring,
may occur, although with less frequency. The spectrum of clinical presentations is broad
and includes predominantly GI symptoms, extraintestinal symptoms, or asymptomatic
disease discovered during serologic screening or endoscopy and biopsy for another reason.
Intestinal symptoms include those characteristic of malabsorption, including weight loss
and steatorrhea, along with fatigue and abdominal cramps. The most common presentation of celiac disease appears to be in those patients who present with nongastrointestinal
symptoms, such as unexplained iron-deficiency anemia, short stature, osteoporosis (calcium or vitamin D malabsorption), or infertility. Dermatitis herpetiformis is another
extraintestinal manifestation of celiac disease. It presents as a severely pruritic, blistering
rash that primarily affects extensor surfaces.

Management

Diagnostic Evaluation

Serologic testing with either **endomysial antibody (EMA IgA)** or **tissue transglutaminase
(tTG IgA)** is appropriate as an initial screening test in suspected cases of celiac disease. The
reported sensitivity and specificity of EMA are close to 90% and 99%, respectively. The
reported sensitivity and specificity for tTG IGA are 90% and >95%, respectively. A correlation has been shown between the sensitivities of these serologic tests and the degree of
histologic activity. Ideally, diagnostic evaluation should begin before the institution of
dietary modification because both serologic test results and histologic abnormalities may
resolve with a gluten-free diet. If serologic studies are negative, other causes of malabsorption have been evaluated, and suspicion for celiac disease remains, **measurement of serum
IgA levels** is appropriate because the prevalence of selective IgA deficiency in the celiac disease population is 1.7% to 3.0%, 10 to 15 times higher than in the general population.
Currently, the gold standard for establishing the diagnosis of celiac disease is with small
intestinal mucosal biopsy. It is the recommendation of the American Gastrointestinal

at a **small intestinal mucosal biopsy** confirm the diagnosis of celiac disease positive serologic test results before introduction of a lifelong dietary modifi- where the diagnosis remains unclear, analysis of the **HLA-DQ2/DQ8 alle-les** may be helpful because virtually all patients with celiac disease have these alleles and their absence has a negative predictive value close to 100%.

Treatment

- Treatment of celiac sprue involves strict lifelong adherence to a **gluten-free diet** (GFD). Dietary compliance often proves very difficult, because gluten is widespread in many different types of foods, especially those that are processed. Wheat, rye, and barley should be removed from the diet and food labels should be checked. The most common reason for resistant disease is inadvertent ingestion of gluten. Improved knowledge about the disease, as well as how to identify gluten-containing products, appears to correlate with increased compliance. Assistance from a dietitian is important and membership in a local celiac society may also be helpful.
- Evaluation at regular intervals by a physician and a dietician are appropriate. Optimal means to monitor adherence to a GFD have not been established, although monitoring of serologies (i.e., tTGA or EMA) may help to verify adherence. Serologic testing is sensitive for major but not minor dietary indiscretions and negative serologic test results do not necessarily mean improvement beyond severe or total villous atrophy. In addition to avoidance of gluten, specific nutrient deficiencies (e.g., iron, folate) should be evaluated and corrected. Bone mineral density should be performed to assess for osteoporosis. There is an increase in overall mortality in patients with celiac sprue, especially those presenting with malabsorption or not adhering to GFD. This may be due to the slightly increased incidence of small bowel lymphoma. The risk of lymphoma normalizes after a 5-year gluten-free period.
- Persistent symptoms despite complete removal of gluten should prompt evaluation for other diagnoses, such as pancreatic exocrine insufficiency, bacterial overgrowth, disaccharidase deficiency, intestinal lymphoma, and small bowel strictures. Once these conditions have been excluded, refractory sprue should be considered. Refractory celiac disease is characterized by severe villus atrophy associated with severe malabsorption that either does not or no longer responds to a GFD. The possibility remains that some of these cases of refractory sprue are not associated with gluten sensitivity. Therefore, other treatable forms of enteropathy, such as autoimmune enteropathy, common variable immunodeficiency syndrome, tropical sprue, and eosinophilic gastroenteritis, should be evaluated. Symptoms are consistent with those of an enteropathy and include frank malabsorption associated with hypoalbuminemia and malnutrition. It occurs most often in older patients and may be associated with carriage of a double dose of DQ2. A role may exist for corticosteroids or immunosuppression in confirmed cases.

SMALL BOWEL BACTERIAL OVERGROWTH

Causes and Presentation

- Small bowel bacterial overgrowth refers to an abnormal proliferation of bacteria within the small intestinal lumen. This bacterial overgrowth may impair nutrient digestion within the lumen and cause damage to the small bowel mucosa, leading to nutrient malabsorption. Conditions predisposing to SBBO include intestinal stasis, abnormal connections between the small and large intestines, reduced gastric acid barrier to ingested bacteria, and immunodeficiency. Common causes of intestinal stasis include strictures that occur in Crohn's disease, radiation enteritis, adhesions, malignancy, postsurgical blind loops, and motility disorders. Clinical manifestations may include diarrhea, weight loss, abdominal pain, and bloating. Symptoms likely are related to malabsorption of fat, carbohydrates, protein, and vitamins.

- Small bowel bacterial overgrowth is common in older adults and is an under recognized cause of malabsorption. In one series of adults ages 65 or older who suffered from malabsorption, SBBO was the most common cause (70.8%). Therefore, SBBO should be considered in the older patient who has chronic diarrhea, unexplained weight loss, or laboratory findings suggestive of malabsorption. The reported prevalence of SBBO in the asymptomatic elderly population is also high (14.5%–38%), although in the absence of symptoms, the significance of this finding is uncertain.

Diagnosis

The gold standard for diagnosis of SBBO is microbiological culture of small bowel aspirate. Typical small bowel intraluminal bacteria concentrations are $<10^4$ colony forming units per milliliter (CFU/mL), most which are gram-positive aerobes. SBBO is defined as bacterial count of $>10^5$ CFU/mL of colonic type bacteria from proximal small bowel aspirate. This approach, however, is invasive, time consuming, and expensive. The mainstay of diagnosis, therefore, has become hydrogen breath testing, using glucose or lactulose (as described above).

Treatment

Treatment options for SBBO include reversal of the underlying structural abnormality (surgical resection of strictures), broad-spectrum antibiotics, prokinetic agents, and probiotics. Quinolones and clavulanic acid or amoxicillin have both been shown to be effective. Repeat courses of antibiotics are often required, however. Probiotics may possibly maintain remission after antibiotic therapy, although they do not induce remission. The role of rifaximin, a non-absorbable antibiotic, for the treatment of SBBO is under investigation.

SHORT BOWEL SYNDROME

Causes

Short bowel syndrome (SBS) refers to the symptoms and disorders associated with malabsorption that are the result of removal of a significant portion of the small or large intestine. This generally occurs when <200 cm of small intestine remain. Congenital SBS occurs in infants with intestinal atresia and a variety of other intestinal anomalies. More commonly, SBS is an acquired condition that results from multiple resections for recurrent Crohn's disease, catastrophic vascular events, trauma, intestinal adhesions, and extensive aganglionosis.

Presentation

- Resection of small intestine reduces the absorptive surface area. Depending on the length of bowel resected, this may cause no symptoms or may result in severe malabsorption. The length of remaining small intestine and whether or not the colon is in continuity determine disease severity. Nutritional risk is greatest for those individuals with duodenostomy or jejunoileal anastomosis with <35 cm of residual small intestine, jejunocolic or ileocolic anastomosis with <60 cm residual small intestine, or end jejunostomy with <115 cm residual small intestine. Loss of the ileocecal valve also causes more significant disease. The intestinal adaptive response to resection or disease is a complex process that involves an increase in absorptive surface area that develops as a consequence of crypt cell hyperplasia and an increase in villus height. For nutrients normally absorbed in the proximal jejunum, residual ileum adapts and assumes the role of macronutrient absorption. The specialized terminal ileum cells where vitamin B_{12} intrinsic factor receptors are located and where bile salts are reabsorbed, however, cannot be replaced by jejunal hypertrophy. The specific nutrient deficiencies depend not only on the specific segment but also the extent of bowel resected. Extensive jejunal resection, for example, results in folate, calcium, and iron malabsorption despite hyperplasia of the ileum. Ileal resection causes depletion of bile salts and vitamin B_{12} owing to loss of specific receptors in the terminal ileum.

- Following small intestine resection, dysmotility may develop predisposing to SBBO and malabsorption. In addition, ileocecal valve resection allows colonic bacteria to populate the small intestine and also result in SBBO. Alterations in proteins and hormones (glucagonlike peptide-1, neurotensin) normally released from distal ileal and colon cells stimulated by fat or bile salts may occur after resection. These changes can lead to rapid gastric emptying, contributing to fluid losses.

Diagnosis

Diagnosis of SBS is usually relatively simple, because patients present with symptoms of malabsorption, volume depletion, or the above described specific nutrient deficiencies in the setting of prior bowel resection.

Treatment

Treatment of short bowel syndrome depends on the length of remaining intestine and the specific segments that have been resected. The goal of medical therapy is for the patient to resume work and as normal a lifestyle as possible. This can be more easily accomplished by decreasing, and ideally eliminating, the requirement for total parenteral nutrition (TPN). The objectives of medical management are to provide adequate nutrition to prevent energy malnutrition and specific nutrient deficiencies. It is also important to prevent dehydration and to correct and prevent acid-base disturbances. Attempts should always be made to maintain nutrition via enteral intake. This involves supplementation with minerals and vitamins. To increase absorptive time, diphenoxylate-atropine or loperamide can be used to slow GI tract motility. In the event that adequate nutrition and fluid intake cannot be maintained with oral intake, long-term TPN may be required.

SMALL BOWEL NEOPLASMS

Introduction

- The small intestine comprises 75% of the length of the entire GI tract and 90% of the mucosal surface; however, <2% of GI malignancies originate in the small bowel. The age-adjusted incidence of small bowel malignancies is 1 per 100,000, and the prevalence is 0.6%. Leiomyomas are the most frequent symptomatic benign tumors of the small bowel. Adenomas, lipomas, and hamartomas are other frequent benign tumors. Of the malignant tumors, approximately 30% to 50% are adenocarcinomas, 25% to 30% are carcinoids, and 15% to 20% are lymphomas. The duodenum is the site at highest risk for adenocarcinomas, whereas the ileum is the site for highest risk of carcinoids and lymphomas. The most common tumors are discussed in more detail below.
- Hereditary conditions that predispose to small intestinal tumors include Peutz-Jeghers syndrome (PJS) (hamartomatous polyps occurring primarily in the jejunum and ileum) and familial adenomatous polyposis (adenoma and adenocarcinoma). Small intestinal inflammatory disorders of the small bowel, such as Crohn's disease and celiac disease, can also increase the risk of adenocarcinoma and lymphoma, respectively.
- Small intestinal tumors can cause intermittent abdominal pain, anemia, bleeding, or obstruction, but their presentation is often insidious and nonspecific. As a result, the diagnosis is often delayed. In one large series, mean time to diagnosis was 7 months. Malignant tumors are most likely to produce symptoms, whereas benign tumors remain asymptomatic and are discovered incidentally or at autopsy. Tumors

are also commonly found unexpectedly during surgery in cases of small bowel obstruction.

Leiomyomas

Leiomyomas are the most common symptomatic, benign small bowel tumors. They most commonly occur in the sixth and seventh decade. The most frequent location is the jejunum, followed by the ileum and duodenum. Endoscopically, they appear as single, firm, grayish-white, well-defined masses. They often have central umbilication with ulceration and covered with normal epithelium. Because they are highly vascular tumors, GI bleeding is the most frequent presentation (65%), especially in the duodenum. Bleeding can be overt with severe hemorrhage or occult with chronic iron-deficiency anemia. Other common findings include obstruction or intussusception (25%).

Adenomas

- Adenomas are the most common asymptomatic benign small bowel tumor. Villus component, atypia, or large size increase the risk for malignancy. Because of their malignant potential, all adenomas should be removed or ablated endoscopically if possible. The type of resection depends on the location of the tumor. Duodenal polyps can generally be resected endoscopically, and local resection is adequate. Periampullary tumors can also be removed endoscopically, but often require surgical management because of the increased risk of malignancy.
- Prognosis is excellent for those tumors that lack malignant change or in which malignancy is confined to superficial layers. Patients who have had local tumor resection should undergo surveillance endoscopy to ensure complete ablation and to monitor for recurrence.

Adenocarcinoma

Only 1% of adenocarcinomas of the GI tract arise from the small bowel. Adenocarcinoma is the most common small bowel malignancy, accounting for 30% to 50%. The annual incidence is 3.9 cases per million, with a slight male predominance, most commonly presenting in the sixth or seventh decade. In most cases, adenocarcinomas are located in the proximal small bowel. The duodenum and, more specifically, the periampullary region are the most common location. Obstruction of the distal common bile duct outlet can result in obstructive jaundice. The clinical manifestations of small bowel adenocarcinoma are usually nonspecific and appear late in the course of disease. Unlike the general population, >75% of small bowel cancers in patients with Crohn's disease are located in the ileum. Surgery provides the only potential for cure, and pancreaticoduodenectomy (Whipple procedure) is often required for tumors of the first or second part of the duodenum. Some small bowel adenocarcinomas may be sensitive to chemotherapy and radiation therapy, although these interventions have not been shown to improve survival in patients with advanced disease. The prognosis of small bowel adenocarcinoma remains dismal, with an overall 5-year survival rate of 30%.

Lymphoma

Lymphoma is the third most common small bowel malignancy after adenocarcinoma and leiomyosarcoma, accounting for 15% to 20% of all small bowel cancers. Most are high-grade malignancy and require aggressive therapy. Depending on the series, non-Hodgkin's lymphoma comprises 18% to 24% of all small intestinal cancers. These patients often present with abdominal pain, weight loss, abdominal mass, perforation, or obstruction. The diagnosis can occasionally be made with small bowel biopsy, but exploratory laparotomy may be required to confirm the diagnosis. Most patients present with advanced disease and often require combined therapy with surgery, chemotherapy, or radiation therapy.

KEY POINTS TO REMEMBER

- Small bowel disorders, pancreatic exocrine insufficiency, and cholestatic liver disease account for most causes of malabsorption.
- Fecal fat analysis should be performed in all patients with suspected malabsorption.
- Treatment of celiac sprue involves strict adherence to a gluten-free diet.
- The length of remaining small intestine determines the severity of disease in short bowel syndrome. Generally, patients with <100 cm suffer from malabsorption.
- Ileal resection causes depletion of bile salts and vitamin B_{12} owing to loss of specific receptors in the terminal ileum.
- Although the small intestine comprises 75% of the length of the entire GI tract and 90% of the mucosal surface, only 1% of adenocarcinomas of the GI tract arise from the small bowel.

REFERENCES AND SUGGESTED READINGS

AGA Institute Medical Position Statement on the Diagnosis and Management of Celiac Disease. *Gastroenterology* 2006;131:1977.

Buchman AL, Scolapio J, Fryer J. AGA technical review on short bowel syndrome and intestinal transplantation. *Gastroenterology* 2003;124:1111.

Delaunoit T, Neczyporenko F, Limburg P, et al. Pathogenesis and risk factors of small bowel adenocarcinoma: a colorectal cancer sibling? *Am J Gastroenterol* 2005;100: 703–710.

Elpick HL, Elpick DA, Sanders DS. Small bowel bacterial overgrowth: an under-recognized cause of malnutrition in older adults. *Geriatrics* 2006;61:21–26.

Fidler J. MR imaging of the small bowel. *Radiol Clin N Am* 2007;45:317.

Gill S, Heuman D, Mihas A. Clinical reviews: the small intestine and nutrition. *J Clin Gastroenterol* 2001;33(4):267.

Macari M, Megibow A, Balthazar E. A pattern approach to the abnormal small bowel: observations at mdct and ct enterography. *AJR* 2007;188:1344.

Rostom A, Murray JA, Kagnoff MF. AGA institute technical review on diagnosis and management of celiac disease. *Gastroenterology* 2006;131:1981.

Rubin DC. Small intestine: anatomy and structural anomalies. In: Yamada Y, Alpers DH, Kaplowitz N, et al. (eds). *Textbook of Gastroenterology.* Philadelphia: Lippincott, Williams & Wilkins; 2003.

Simrén M, Stotzer PO. Use and abuse of hydrogen breath tests. *Gut* 2006;55;297–303.

Tabrez S, Roberts I. Malabsorption and malnutrition. *Primary Care: Clinics in Office Practice* 2001;28(3):505.

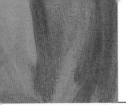

Colon Neoplasms

Anne K. Nagler and Dayna S. Early

INTRODUCTION

Background

More than 140,000 new cases and 55,000 deaths are attributed to **colorectal cancer (CRC)** in the United States each year. CRC is the second leading cause of cancer death and prognosis is closely linked to stage at diagnosis. The 5-year survival rate for localized cancers is >90%, whereas the 5-year survival for those with invasive cancer is <10%. Nearly all CRC develops from colorectal adenomas, with a progression that occurs over 5 to 15 years. Consequently, screening colonoscopy and polypectomy has been shown to reduce mortality from CRC. The high survival rate of patients with localized CRC and the ability to detect and resect precursor polyps makes screening a vital tool in the treatment and prevention of CRC.

Epidemiology

- The prevalence of adenomatous polyps in asymptomatic patients varies from 23% to 41%. Several factors predict the risk of developing colorectal adenomas and cancer. The most important risk factor, older age, is associated not only with a higher prevalence of polyps, but also with multiple polyps, severe dysplasia, and larger adenoma size. The lifetime incidence of CRC is roughly 5% for average risk individuals, with 90% of cases occurring after age 50 years. Distribution of polyps is fairly uniform throughout the colon. In patients older than 60 years and in women, adenomas tend to be more common in the proximal colon. In recent years, a gradual shift has occurred to greater incidence of proximal (ascending colon and cecal) CRC.
- Different ethnic populations carry varying risks for developing colorectal adenomas and cancer. For example, Hawaiian-Japanese have a prevalence of adenoma as high as 50% to 60%; in contrast, Japanese living in Japan have prevalence rates <12%. This disparity suggests lifestyle and environmental influences are additional risk factors in developing CRC. Developing countries have lower rates of CRC than North America, Australia, and Europe, which may be explained by diets high in red meat and fat, and low in fruits, vegetables, and fiber in developed countries.

Causes

Pathophysiology

Colorectal adenomas are precursors to CRC in nearly all instances, the exception being CRC that develops in patients with idiopathic inflammatory bowel disease manifesting as colitis. Adenomatous polyps are believed to develop in a stepwise fashion as a result of a series of genetic mutations. These arise in colonic crypts in which the proliferative component of the crypt, usually confined to the base, extends through the entire crypt. Histologically, the tubular adenoma is the most common subgroup, representing 80% to 86%

of all adenomatous polyps. These lesions tend to be small and exhibit only mild dysplasia, seen microscopically as a complex network of branching adenomatous glands. Villous adenomas tend to have a higher degree of dysplasia, with adenomatous glands extending through to the center of the polyps, thereby appearing grossly as fingerlike projections. Villous (papillary) and tubulovillous adenomas are three times more likely to become malignant than tubular adenomas. Overall, only a small percentage of colon polyps develop into carcinomas.

Differential Diagnosis

- Not all colorectal polyps have malignant potential, but visual inspection cannot predict polyp histology; accordingly, all visualized polyps should be removed and evaluated by surgical pathology. Hyperplastic polyps consist of hyperplastic mucosal proliferation and are considered to have no malignant potential. Approximately one third of colon polyps are hyperplastic. A subset of large hyperplastic polyps may be premalignant, and are felt to progress to carcinoma through the pathway of serrated adenomas. Juvenile polyps (also known as hamartomas) are tumors of the mucosa, in contrast to epithelial proliferation in hyperplastic and adenomatous polyps. Other polypoid lesions in the colon can include lymphoma, carcinoid, Kaposi's sarcoma, or metastatic disease.
- Symptoms of colorectal cancer are nonspecific and other colonic diseases, including diverticulosis and inflammatory bowel disease, can present with similar symptoms of abdominal pain, hematochezia, and change in bowel habits.

Natural History

It is widely accepted that **adenomatous polyps lead to colon cancer.** This is supported by several studies including the National Polyp study, which found that removal of adenomas resulted in a significantly lower incidence of CRC. In confirmed colon cancers, residual adenomatous tissue can be found within cancerous tissue. Surgically resected colorectal cancer may contain adjacent adenomatous polyps in one-third of cases.

Mechanism

The progression from adenoma to carcinoma occurs as a result of a series of DNA mutations. The exact sequence of mutations necessary for malignant progression is unclear. Among the earliest mutations is inactivation of the adenomatous polyposis coli (APC) gene. Other later changes include mutations of the K-ras proto-oncogene, DNA hypomethylation, 18q inactivation, and p53 (tumor suppressor gene) inactivation. The accumulation of abnormalities results in a stepwise progression over approximately 10 years from normal mucosa to adenoma to carcinoma. Detection of these mutations from sloughed cells in stool samples may eventually prove to be a useful screening test for early CRC.

Presentation

Risk Factors

- For screening purposes, individuals are stratified into average or high risk. High-risk populations include those with prior CRC or adenoma, family history of CRC, family history of adenoma before age 60, and ulcerative colitis. Average risk individuals are those with no family or personal history of CRC or adenoma and no history of ulcerative colitis. Hereditary cancer syndromes will be discussed in the Special Topics section of this chapter.
- The overall colon cancer risk in those with multiple first-degree relatives or a single first-degree relative diagnosed before age 45 years is three to four times that of the general population. In patients with a single first-degree relative with CRC or adenoma diagnosed before age 60 years, risk of developing CRC is increased to two

times that of the general population. Risk for colon cancer in this group begins at an earlier age, so that recommended screening should begin at age 40 years.

- Individuals deemed to be high risk should be screened starting at age 40, or 10 years before the age of the youngest CRC diagnosis in the family. Current recommendations do not take into account race, gender, dietary, or environmental risks modifiers. Tobacco and alcohol use may increase the risk but are not accounted for in current screening recommendations. Medical conditions including diabetes mellitus, obesity, acromegaly, prior cholecystectomy, ureterocolic anastomoses, and pelvic radiation, have also been associated with an increase risk of developing CRC.

- Intense interest surrounds the issue of prevention and risk reduction with lifestyle modification and supplementation. At present, calcium and aspirin have been demonstrated to reduce colorectal neoplasia risk in randomized controlled trials. Hormone replacement therapy and estrogen, statins, nonsteroidal anti-inflammatory drugs (NSAIDs), magnesium, vitamin B_6, folic acid, and physical activity have all been thought to be protective against CRC, but data are inconclusive. Folic acid was recently evaluated in a randomized double-blind, placebo-controlled trial for secondary prevention of adenoma with negative results. The timing of folate administration appears to be important, because folate may be preventative if given before preneoplastic lesions arise, but it may increase tumor development if given after a preneoplastic lesion exists.

Clinical Presentation

Most patients with colonic polyps are asymptomatic but may occasionally present with occult or overt bleeding from the GI tract. Villous adenomas >3 cm can cause a secretory diarrhea, which can lead to volume depletion and electrolyte abnormalities. Many adenocarcinomas are asymptomatic, but may present with symptoms, depending on location. Right-sided cancers may grow large before producing symptoms because of the larger luminal caliber of the cecum and ascending colon. Iron-deficiency anemia is often the only manifestation of right-sided cancer. Tumors in the left side of the colon may present with symptoms of partial or complete obstruction, including abdominal distention, bloating, and constipation. Rectal or sigmoid cancers often cause hematochezia, constipation, or thinning of the stools. Tenesmus, melena, or weight loss may also be symptoms. An infection with *Streptococcus bovis* or *Clostridium septicum* also warrants evaluation of the colon because these individuals often have CRC. Consequently, new onset of hematochezia, anemia, or change in bowel habits, especially in older patients, mandates colonoscopic evaluation.

Management

Diagnosis

- Diagnostic colonoscopy is the test of choice for identifying CRC and adenomas. Barium enema and computed tomography (CT) colonography can suggest CRC or adenoma, but only colonoscopy allows for tissue sampling of tumors and removal of adenomatous polyps.

- Screening for CRC should begin at age 50 years for average risk individuals and earlier for high risk individuals. CRC screening is unique, in that national organizations provide a "menu" of screening options from which to choose, and generally do not endorse one screening test over another. Options for screening include fecal immunochemical testing (FIT), fecal occult blood testing (FOBT), flexible sigmoidoscopy (FS), double contrast barium enema, and colonoscopy. These tests used alone and in combination reduce CRC incidence and mortality. Screening colonoscopy is the most sensitive and specific but involves the greatest cost and carries a small risk of complications. FIT and FOBT are relatively sensitive, but nonspecific, and are associated with minimal initial cost. FS is very low risk and of moderate cost, but only examines approximately one fourth of the colon. Individuals who have an abnormal FIT, FOBT, or FS should have further evaluation with colonoscopy. Multiple studies, however, have shown extremely low population screening rates, generally <50%. Extensive public education of the community has modestly increased screening rates.

Fecal Occult Blood Testing and Fecal Immunochemical Testing. As a screening test, FOBT or FIT should be performed yearly. Two samples from each of three consecutive stools should be evaluated during FOBT. Two samples from two consecutive stools should used for FIT. There is no need to rehydrate the slide because this increases the false-positive rate. For FOBT, a restricted diet and avoidance of red meat for 3 days before testing is recommended. A study in the United States showed that only 30% of individuals with a positive test underwent follow-up colonoscopy.

Sigmoidoscopy. Sigmoidoscopy should be offered every 5 years when used as a screening test. Case-controlled studies have shown a reduced mortality for CRC in individuals who undergo FS; however, there is no reduction in CRC risk in the area beyond the scope. Patients having FS should have a diagnostic colonoscopy if an adenoma is identified because distal adenomas (within reach of FS) are associated with high rates of more proximal adenomas. Up to one half of individuals with a proximal adenoma have no distal adenoma, raising concern about the use of FS as a screening modality.

Colonoscopy. Colonoscopy as a screening method should be offered every 10 years. Studies evaluating the use of screening colonoscopy in average risk individuals are lacking. By extrapolating from the FS studies, however, it is safe to say colonoscopy is at least as good as FS at reducing the incidence or mortality from CRC. Colonoscopy allows examination of the entire colon; however, it does have greater risks and more cost. Detection rates of adenomas appear to be directly related to longer times for scope withdrawal.

Double Contrast Barium Enema. Double contrast barium enema (DCBE) can be offered every 5 years. No randomized trials have shown a reduction in CRC mortality with DCBE screening. DCBE has a lower sensitivity than colonoscopy; it must be combined with FS to offer complete colonoscopic evaluation and is generally not utilized as a CRC screening tool. A positive result requires follow-up with colonoscopy.

CT Colonography. Computed tomography colonography (CTC) is still under investigation as a screening tool. Once this is widely available for screening, it is anticipated that screening will be recommended every 5 years. CTC requires oral contrast as well as colonic catharsis. A small-caliber, flexible rectal catheter is used for colonic distension, generally with CO_2. The colonic preparation does allow for same day colonoscopy if colon polyps are found. Patients with large polyps (>10 mm) or multiple moderate size polyps (>6 mm) are referred for colonoscopy. Polyps <5 mm are not reported. Colonoscopy is recommended for patients with one to two polyps between 6 mm and 9 mm, although some advocate enrolling those patients in a CTC surveillance program every 1 to 2 years. Many factors limit CTC use for screening at this time, including lower sensitivity of detecting small polyps, cost-effectiveness, bowel preparation, risks of cumulative radiation exposure, and questions regarding management of the small polyps seen on CTC. Intense debate rages about the wisdom of CTC surveillance for polyps 6 to 9 mm, because polyps this size carry a small but real risk of advanced neoplasia. Additionally, the issue of extracolonic findings on CTC adds to the complexity and cost of the procedure.

Workup
- Most polyps found at flexible sigmoidoscopy or colonoscopy can be resected completely using electrocautery techniques. Current guidelines for treatment of adenomatous polyps include complete resection by colonoscopy or surgery, when necessary. Positive findings on other screening tests require referral for colonoscopy.

TABLE 15-1	COLONOSCOPIC SURVEILLANCE FOR COLORECTAL POLYPS	
	Risk	Repeat Colonoscopy
One or two adenomas, <1 cm, low-grade dysplasia	Low	5–10 yr
Three or more adenomas, or any adenoma ≥1 cm, or any adenoma with villous architecture, high-grade dysplasia, or both	Moderate	3 yrs
Malignant polyps, large sessile adenomas, multiple adenoma	High	Complete removal is mandatory; then revert to 3-year surveillance. Consider genetic counseling when hereditary syndrome suspected.
Hyperplastic polyps (unless hyperplastic polyposis syndrome, then treat as moderate risk)	None	10 yr

- Evaluation of a newly diagnosed CRC requires a chest x-ray, CT of the abdomen and pelvis, complete blood count, chemistry panel, and carcinoembryonic antigen (CEA) level.

Follow-Up
- The recommended interval for repeat surveillance colonoscopy depends on the findings on the initial examination. Table 15-1 lists the surveillance recommendations for patients with colorectal adenomas. Surveillance intervals after polypectomy should be based on the number, size, and histology of polyps. Screening intervals for individuals at high risk because of family history is generally every 5 years, unless an inherited syndrome is suspected or confirmed. Individuals with hyperplastic polyps are not at increased risk for development of CRC, and colonoscopy every 10 years is sufficient. The exceptions are individuals felt to have hyperplastic polyposis syndrome, wherein many or large hyperplastic polyps are present. These individuals should be screened similarly to individuals with adenomas.
- Surveillance after resection of CRC is generally at 1 year, followed by 3 years, and then every 5 years if no subsequent adenomas or tumors are found. Surveillance intervals should be modified if subsequent adenomas or cancers are found, if a family history of CRC is present, or if a hereditary cancer syndrome is suspected.
- Genetic counseling is recommended for any individual in whom a hereditary cancer syndrome is suspected. Features of hereditary cancer syndromes are outlined in the Special Topics section.

Treatment
- For patients diagnosed with CRC, the treatment of choice is **surgical resection.** The goal of surgery is removal of the affected segment of bowel as well as surrounding lymph nodes, with the extent of resection determined by the distribution of blood vessels and lymphatic drainage. For patients with rectal cancers, surgical treatment depends on the

TABLE 15-2	TUMOR, NODE, METASTASIS (TNM) STAGING SYSTEM FOR COLORECTAL CANCER	
Stage	Criteria	Estimated 5-year Survival (%)
I	T1-2, N0, M0	>90
IIA	T3, N0, M0	60–85
IIB	T4, N0, M0	60–85
IIIA	T1-2, N1, M0	25–65
IIIB	T3-4, N1, M0	25–65
IIIC	T(any), N2, M0	25–65
IV	T(any), N(any), M1	5–7

TX, primary tumor cannot be assessed; Tis, carcinoma in situ; T1, tumor invades submucosa; T2, tumor invades muscularis propria; T3, tumor penetrates muscularis propria and invades subserosa; T4, tumor directly invades other organs or structures or perforates visceral peritoneum.

NX, regional lymph nodes cannot be assessed; N0, no metastases in regional lymph nodes; N1, metastases in one to three regional lymph nodes; N2, metastases in four or more regional lymph nodes.

MX, presence or absence of distant metastases cannot be determined; M0, no distant metastases detected; M1, distant metastases detected.

location, size, and extent of involvement. Therapies include low anterior resection for upper rectal cancers. Low-lying and locally advanced rectal cancers are treated with neoadjuvant chemoradiotherapy followed by low anterior resection. Abdominoperineal resection is rarely performed in the current era.

- In patients with CRC, synchronous polyps can occur in 20% to 40% of cases and synchronous cancers in 3% to 5%. Preoperative colonoscopy is recommended in patients before undergoing resection. If the tumor is obstructing and cannot be traversed by the colonoscope, barium enema may be performed to evaluate the proximal colon. CRC tend to metastasize to regional lymph nodes, liver, and lung. Thus, CT scanning is recommended for patients with an abnormal liver examination or liver enzymes, but whether routine CT should be performed for staging remains controversial. Anatomic staging of cancers occurs at the time of surgery, using the TNM (tumor, node, metastasis) universal system (Table 15-2) Previously CRC was staged with the Dukes system (modified Astler Coller).

- Preoperative and intraoperative staging directs pre- and postoperative treatments. Prospective studies show prolonged survival and enhanced quality of life for patients with metastatic disease who receive chemotherapy. Adjuvant chemotherapy usually uses 5-fluorouracil and leucovorin or capecitabine (Xeloda), which is an oral fluoropyrimidine. Adjuvant therapy has been shown to have a survival benefit and increases the probability of remaining tumor free in patients with stage III disease. Adjuvant therapy in patients with stage II disease is controversial because 5-year survival is 80% with or without treatment. It is thought that a subgroup of these patients with high risk prognostic factors (adherence of tumor to an adjacent organ or bowel perforation) may benefit from chemotherapy. Irinotecan and oxaliplatin are used in combination with fluoropyrimidines for treatment of metastatic disease. Targeted therapies are being developed and applied for CRC. These include cetuximab (Erbitux) and bevacizumab (Avastin). Patients with obstructing metastatic cancers can have palliative resection or endoscopic stenting to prevent complete obstruction.

Prognosis

Colorectal cancer survival is excellent for those with limited stage disease at time of diagnosis. The development in the past decade of new chemotherapeutic agents has led to a significant increase in treatment options for CRC and improved survival. Survival for advanced CRC has increased from a median survival of 10 to 12 months with fluoropyrimidines only to >20 months with combination therapy (fluropyrimidine, irinotecan, and oxaliplatin or cytotoxic chemotherapy with targeted therapy).

SPECIAL TOPICS

Hereditary Nonpolyposis Colorectal Cancer

Also known as **Lynch syndrome,** hereditary nonpolyposis colorectal cancer (HNPCC) is an autosomal-dominant familial CRC syndrome. HNPCC is further divided into Lynch I and II, the latter being associated with cancers of the uterus, ovary, kidney, stomach, small bowel, and biliary tract. HNPCC accounts for 2% to 6% of CRC. The diagnosis is based on the Amsterdam Criteria (Table 15-3). An estimated 68% to 75% of patients with HNPCC develop CRC by the age of 65 years, with the average age at diagnosis being 45 years. In addition, the risk of endometrial carcinoma is 30% to 39% by age 70 years, compared with 3% in the general population. Surveillance colonoscopy for HNPCC should begin at age 20 to 25 years or 10 years earlier than the youngest affected family member, and it should be performed every 1 to 2 years. Screening should involve all members of a family who meet the Amsterdam Criteria. Genetic testing for germline mutations in DNA mismatch repair genes (MLH1 and MSH2) is also available. A different approach is to examine the cancerous colon tissue from a patient for microsatellite instability (MSI). MSI indicates frequent genetic mutations throughout the genome, a feature seen in nearly all cancers from HNPCC, as opposed to approximately 15% of sporadic colon cancers. If MSI is found, genetic testing should be performed. It is now encouraged that both Amsterdam Criteria-positive families and those with strong but Amsterdam Criteria-negative family histories undergo genetic counseling, MSI testing, and mutation testing.

Familial Adenomatous Polyposis

- Familial adenomatous polyposis (FAP) is the most common inherited polyposis syndrome, with a prevalence of 1 of 5000 to 7500. It is an autosomal-dominant disease, but can occur spontaneously and involves a deletion in the long arm of chromosome 5 in the APC gene, leading to the loss of tumor suppressor genes. It is characterized by hundreds to thousands of adenomatous polyps in the colon, with a 100% progression to CRC if not resected. Patients with FAP usually report symptoms after puberty, with the average age for diagnosis at 36 years and death from cancer at 42 years. Despite this, the natural history of onset of polyposis to CRC is estimated to be 10 to 15 years. Screening of known FAP gene carriers with

TABLE 15-3	AMSTERDAM CRITERIA FOR HEREDITARY NONPOLYPOSIS COLORECTAL CANCER

- Three relatives with colon cancer, two of whom must be first-degree relatives of the third
- Colon cancer in two consecutive generations
- One case diagnosed before age 50 years

yearly sigmoidoscopy has allowed clinicians to identify polyps in 50% of patients. Screening of carriers should begin at age 10 to 12 years and colectomy should be performed when polyps are found.

- In addition to colonic polyps, patients with FAP may have upper GI manifestations. Gastric polyps occur in 30% to 50% of cases, but most are non-neoplastic, characterized by hyperplasia of fundic glands without epithelial dysplasia. Duodenal adenomas occur in 60% to 90% of patients with FAP, and the lifetime incidence of duodenal cancer is 4% to 12%, >100 times the risk of the normal population. Most duodenal adenomas involve the periampullary region and may obstruct the biliary system. Patients with a history of duodenal polyps should undergo yearly surveillance upper endoscopy.

Gardner's Syndrome

Gardner's syndrome, a less common variant of FAP, includes the same genetic lesions and GI manifestations as FAP. Gardner's variant is associated with additional extraintestinal features, such as osteomas in the mandible, skull, and long bones. In addition, >90% of patients with Gardner's syndrome have congenital hypertrophy of the retinal pigmented epithelium (CHRPE), consisting of pigmented ocular fundus lesions. CHRPE is seen in only 5% of controls, so presence of such lesions bilaterally, especially in those with a family history, could serve as a reliable marker for gene carriage in adenomatous polyposis. Other abnormalities found in Gardner's syndrome include benign soft tissue tumors and tumors of the thyroid, adrenal gland, and hepatobiliary system. Another complication is the development of diffuse mesenteric fibromatosis, or desmoid tumors, which are found in 8% to 13% of patients with Gardner's syndrome. These tumors can cause GI obstruction or constriction of the mesenteric vasculature or ureters. The mechanism of the development of desmoid tumors is unclear, so there is no single approach proven to prevent or treat this condition, which ranks second behind metastatic disease among the lethal complications of polyposis syndromes. Despite their variable manifestations, FAP and Gardner's syndrome involve the same genetic locus, the APC gene, and no patterns of mutation exist to distinguish between the two syndromes.

Attenuated Familial Adenomatous Polyposis

Attenuated FAP is a rare variant of FAP, consisting of fewer colonic adenomas. These adenomas often have a flat rather than polypoid growth pattern and tend to cluster in the proximal colon. Also known as *hereditary flat adenoma syndrome*, this condition is more aptly termed *attenuated FAP* for the finding of germline mutations in the APC gene. Much like FAP, patients are susceptible to upper GI adenomas and fundic gland polyps, but CRC tend to occur in patients at a later age (approximately 55 years).

Turcot's Syndrome

Turcot's syndrome, also known as *glioma-polyposis*, is a syndrome of familial polyposis along with primary tumors of the CNS. APC mutations are found in these patients, but no association can be found between specific mutations and the development of brain tumors. CNS tumors found in Turcot's syndrome are of different histologic types, depending on the particular genetic mutation. Those with germline mutations of the APC gene tend to have medulloblastomas, whereas those with mutations in DNA base mismatch repair genes typically have glioblastoma multiforme tumors.

Peutz-Jeghers Syndrome

- Peutz-Jeghers syndrome (PJS) is an autosomal-dominant disease consisting of mucocutaneous pigmentation and GI polyposis. Patients manifest mucocutaneous pigmentation in infancy and childhood, with melanin deposits around the nose, lips, hands, feet, and buccal mucosa. Lesions are green-black to brown and fade during puberty, with the exception of buccal lesions. Hamartomatous polyps can be found in the stomach, small intestine, and colon but most commonly appear in the small intestine. Polyps in PJS are unique hamartomas characterized by glandular epithelium supported by an abnormal framework of smooth muscle that is contiguous with the muscularis mucosa.

- Although hamartomas are not true neoplasms, these polyps may grow in size and cause bleeding, small bowel obstruction, or intussusception. Cancer in the small bowel or colon is seen with increased frequency in patients with PJS. Also, benign polyps can be found in the nose, bronchi, bladder, gallbladder, and bile duct. In 5% to 12% of female patients with PJS, ovarian cysts and ovarian sex chord tumors can be seen. Similarly, Sertoli cell testicular rumors can be observed in young boys, causing feminizing features. Management of cases of PJS includes screening of potential family members with colonoscopy, upper GI series films to evaluate for small bowel polyps, and pelvic ultrasound for girls and physical examination of the genitalia in boys.

Juvenile Polyposis

- Juvenile polyposis, an autosomal-dominant disorder, encompasses at least three different forms: familial juvenile polyposis coli, familial juvenile polyposis of the stomach, and generalized juvenile polyposis. Histologically, juvenile polyps are hamartomas, consisting of an excess of lamina propria and dilated cystic glands.
- Normally, these polyps are solitary and located in the rectum of children. An increased risk of colon cancer exists in these patients, arising in mixed juvenile adenomatous polyps or synchronous adenomatous polyps. Other complications include bleeding, obstruction, or intussusception in childhood, seen mostly in childhood as the polyps increase in size.
- Management for potentially affected family members includes colonoscopy and careful histologic examination of polyps with adenomatous foci. Juvenile polyps should generally be removed because of their tendency to bleed or obstruct.

Cowden's Disease

Cowden's disease, or multiple hamartoma syndrome, is a rare autosomal-dominant disorder. It is characterized by multiple hamartomatous polyps and the presence of mucocutaneous lesions, including lichenoid and verrucous facial papules, acral keratoses, and oral papillomas. Other manifestations include breast lesions, ranging from fibrocystic disease to breast cancer in 50% of patients, and thyroid abnormalities, including cancer and multinodular goiter, seen in 10% to 15% of patients. Polyps in the GI tract pose no increased risk for colon cancer, however, so clinical surveillance in patients with Cowden's disease is unnecessary.

Inflammatory Bowel Disease

Surveillance colonoscopy is effective in reducing the mortality from CRC for patients with Crohn's colitis or ulcerative colitis. Risk of dysplasia is associated with duration, extent, and activity of disease; current recommendations are to perform surveillance colonoscopy every 1 to 3 years on patients with pancolitis for >8 years or left-sided colitis for >15 years. Patients should have random biopsies taken every 10 cm throughout the entire colon. Patients with ulcerative colitis may have inflammatory polyps as well as adenomas. Sporadic adenomas that are not associated with active inflammation can be managed similarly to polyps in patients without ulcerative colitis. Adenomas or flat lesions with dysplasia found in the setting of active inflammation should be managed by proctocolectomy. The finding of high-grade dysplasia mandates colectomy, whereas low-grade dysplasia is more controversial, with many experts also recommending colectomy.

KEY POINTS TO REMEMBER

- Annually, approximately 140,000 new cases and 55,000 deaths are attributed to CRC, the second leading cause of overall cancer-related mortality.
- Depending on the type of polyp found, the estimated time from adenoma to malignancy is 5 to 10 years, making screening a vital tool in the treatment and prevention of CRC.
- Risk factors for CRC include a family or personal history of CRC or colorectal adenomas, long-standing inflammatory bowel disease involving the colon, and familial polyposis syndromes.
- Screening should start at age 50 in an average risk individual and at age 40 or earlier for an individual with a family history.
- Surveillance colonoscopy should be performed on patients with IBD who have had pancolitis for 8 years or left-sided colitis for 15 years.
- Patients with FAP have a 100% risk of developing CRC by age 40 years and should undergo colectomy as soon as polyposis is found.
- Adjuvant chemotherapy with 5-fluorouracil and leucovorin is recommended for patients with stage III disease and may be indicated in a subset of stage II disease.

REFERENCE AND SUGGESTED READINGS

Barclay R, Vicari JJ, Doughty AS, et al. Colonoscopic withdrawal times and adenoma detection during screening colonoscopy. *N Engl J Med* 2006;355:2533–2541.

Burt RW, et al. *Preventing Colorectal Cancer: A Clinician's Guide*. Bethesda, Maryland: AGA Press; 2004.

Burt RW. Impact on family history on screening surveillance. *Gastrointest Endosc* 1999;49:S41.

Cole BF, Baron JA, Sandler RS, et al. Folic acid for the prevention of colorectal adenomas. *JAMA* 2007;297:21.

Correa P. Epidemiology of polyps and cancer. In: Morson B, ed. *The Pathogenesis of Colorectal Cancer*. Philadelphia: WB Saunders; 1978:126.

Kim DH, Pickhardt PJ, Hoff G, et al. Computed tomographic colonography for colorectal screening. *Endoscopy* 2007;39:545–549.

Lieberman DA, Weiss DG, Bond JH, et al. Use of colonoscopy to screen asymptomatic adults for colorectal cancer. *N Engl J Med* 2000;343:162.

Lieberman, D. Colorectal cancer screening in primary care. *Gastroenterology* 2007;132:7.

Meyerhardt J, Mayer R. Systemic therapy for colorectal cancer. *N Engl J Med* 2005; 352:476–487.

Muto T, Bussey HJR, Morson BC. The evolution of cancer of the colon and rectum. *Cancer* 1975;36:2251.

Rex, DK. Colonoscopy: the dominant and preferred colorectal cancer screening strategy in the United States. *Mayo Clin Proc* 2007;82:662–664.

Rhodes M, Bradburn DM. Overview of screening and management of familial adenomatous polyposis. *Gut* 1992;33:125.

Vogelstein B, Fearon ER, Hamilton S, et al. Genetic alterations during colorectal-tumor development. *N Engl J Med* 1988;319:525.

Winawer SJ, Fletcher RH, Miller RH, et al. Colorectal cancer screening: clinical guidelines and rationale. *Gastroenterology* 1997;112:594.

Winawer SJ, Fletcher RH, Rex D, et al. Colorectal cancer screening and surveillance: clinical guidelines and rationale. *Gastroenterology* 2003;124:544.

Winawer SJ, Zauber AG, Gerdes H, et al. Prevention of colorectal cancer by colonoscopic polypectomy. *N Engl J Med* 1993;329:1977.

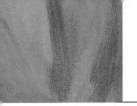

Inflammatory Bowel Disease

T. J. Paradowski and Matthew A. Ciorba

INTRODUCTION

Background

In 1932, Burrill Crohn, Leon Ginzburg, and Gordon Oppenheimer described an idiopathic disorder they designated as *terminal ileitis*, later to be named *regional enteritis*. *Granulomatous colitis* was also described before the eventual eponym of *Crohn's disease* was adopted. These were the beginnings of our ongoing investigation of inflammatory bowel disease.

Definition

- **Inflammatory bowel disease (IBD)** is a spectrum of chronic intestinal inflammation of uncertain etiology. **Crohn's disease (CD)** and **ulcerative colitis (UC)** comprise the two main clinical entities of IBD, often discussed together for ease of comparison and contrast, but most experts believe that these are not two distinct diseases but a continuum of disease represented by several clinical phenotypes. **Microscopic colitis is a less common form of IBD that lacks the characteristic endoscopic findings of CD and UC.**
- IBD is relatively common; it causes substantial morbidity and often initially affects younger people. Advances in understanding IBD continue to shape clinical management, leading to improved quality of life for the individual, and to many additional functional years for society as a whole. New genetic discoveries, enteric flora analysis, and clinical trials as part of translational research have all been important contributors to these advances.

Epidemiology

IBD is more common in well-developed areas, particularly within the northern regions of North America and northern Europe, where incidence rates are about 7 per 100,000 for CD and 11 per 100,000 for UC. The prevalence rates of CD and UC in these areas are about 20 to 100 per 100,000 and 50 to 80 per 100,000, respectively. IBD is rare in Asia and South America. The peak incidence of IBD occurs between ages 15 and 30 years, with a second minor peak between ages of 50 and 80 years. There is no gender specificity. In the United States, an increased frequency is observed in the Jewish population, particularly in Ashkenazi Jews; followed decreasingly by non-Jewish Caucasians, African Americans, Hispanics, and Asians. Urban areas and higher socioeconomic classes are associated with a higher prevalence of IBD as well. Cigarette smoking is associated with an increased risk for CD but a decreased risk for UC. ✗ Smoking ⟹ ↓ UC.

Pathophysiology

Despite being a known clinical entity for 75 years, the precise etiology of IBD has not yet been defined. The current leading hypothesis is that in *genetically predisposed* individuals,

127

TABLE 16-1	COMPARISON BETWEEN CROHN'S DISEASE AND ULCERATIVE COLITIS	
	Crohn's Disease	**Ulcerative Colitis**
Disease location	Anywhere in GI tract; terminal ileum most common	Colon only; begins in rectum
Clinically	Abdominal pain or mass, diarrhea, weight loss, vomiting, perianal disease	Rectal bleeding, diarrhea, passage of mucus, crampy pain
Endoscopy	Rectal sparing, skip lesions, aphthous ulcers, cobblestoning, linear ulceration	Rectal involvement, continuous, friability, loss of vascularity
Radiology	Small bowel and terminal ileal disease, segmental, strictures, fistulae	Colon disease, loss of haustra, continuous ulceration, no fistulae
Histology	Transmural disease, aphthous ulcers, noncaseating granulomas	Abnormal crypt architecture, superficial inflammation
HLA antigen association	HLA-A2, HLA-DR1, HLA-DQw5	HLA-DR2
IBD genes	IBD-1: NOD-2/CARD-15; IL23R	IL23R
Cigarette smoking	Increases risk and recurrence rate	Current smoking decreases risk
Appendectomy	No effect	Decreases risk (if prior to onset)
Antibiotics	Response	No response
p-ANCA/ASCA	ASCA associated	p-ANCA associated
PSC	Not associated	5% develop PSC

ASCA, anti-Saccharomyces cerevisiae antibodies; HLA, human leukocyte antigen; IBD, inflammatory bowel disease; p-ANCA, perinuclear antineutrophil cytoplasmic antibodies; PSC, primary sclerosing cholangitis.

both *exogenous factors* (e.g., normal lumenal flora or infectious agents) and *endogenous host factors* (e.g., intestinal epithelial cell barrier function) may cause a state of *dysregulated mucosal immune function* that is further modified by specific environmental factors.

Many studies and observations support a genetic component to IBD susceptibility. Although most affected patients have no family history of IBD, first-degree relatives of patients with IBD are more likely to develop the disease compared with the general population. Twin studies also support higher concordance rates of IBD, greater in CD than in UC. The clinical features such as location (e.g., ileal versus colonic) and type (e.g., fibrostenotic, fistulizing) are also commonly heritable. IBD is a polygenic disorder. Mutations in the *NOD-2/CARD-15* gene, also called IBD-1, confer increased risk for CD. This gene, expressed in intestinal epithelial cells and mononuclear cells, normally encodes a protein that senses bacterial peptidoglycan and regulates macrophages and nuclear factor-kappa B expression. Recently, mutations in the gene *IL23R*, which normally codes for a component of the immune cell receptor for IL-23 (a proinflammatory cytokine), have been found to be associated with *both* CD and UC.

Genetically modified mouse models of IBD have revealed several important observations. Colitis is a nonspecific phenotype that can be produced from alterations in many different genes involved in the mucosal barrier epithelium or mucosal immune system, backing up the polygenic hypothesis. Also, even a single gene alteration can have variable phenotypes, such as the variable clinical presentations of IBD. Furthermore, genetically susceptible mice raised in sterile conditions do not develop IBD, suggesting that although genes confer susceptibility, the disease development is dependent on the presence of certain environmental factors. Thus far, no specific infectious agent has been clearly linked to IBD.

Crohn's Disease

- CD is characterized by chronic, potentially transmural inflammation with mucosal damage and fissuring that can lead to fibrosis, strictures, fistulae, and obstructive clinical presentations that are not typically seen in UC. Another classic feature of CD is the sharp demarcation (both grossly and microscopically) between diseased and adjacent unaffected bowel. Noncaseating granulomas can be seen on histopathology.

- CD can affect any portion of the gastrointestinal (GI) tract, from mouth to anus, but commonly affects the distal small bowel and colon. Approximately 80% of patients have small bowel involvement, a third with exclusively ileitis (usually distal ileum involvement), and 50% have ileocolitis. Approximately 20% have CD limited to the colon, and about one-half of these patients have sparing of the rectum. Only about 7% have predominant oral or gastroduodenal involvement, and even fewer (5%) have esophageal or proximal small bowel involvement. Oral, esophageal, gastroduodenal, and proximal small bowel involvement is much less common (5% to 7%), and patients are typically younger at disease onset. About a third of patients have perianal disease. Extraintestinal manifestations are common, often related to inflammatory disease activity, and are more frequent with colonic involvement.

- CD appears to be perpetuated by a chronic delayed-type hypersensitivity reaction induced by the interferon-gamma (IFN-γ) -producing T_H1 cells. A role for enteric flora or an unidentified fecal toxin is supported by observations that fecal stream diversion from an involved segment of bowel attenuates the mucosal inflammation, and that antibiotics may be effective in the treatment of CD.

Ulcerative Colitis

- UC is a chronic, relapsing, ulceroinflammatory disease limited to the colon, with continuous lesions affecting predominantly the mucosa and submucosa. Well-formed granulomas are absent in UC, and fistulas are generally not seen. Islands of regenerating mucosa bulge upward to create pseudopolyps. Mucosal damage is continuous from the rectum and extends proximally, a key feature that distinguishes it from CD. *Ulcerative proctitis* refers to disease limited to the rectum. *Distal colitis* or *proctosigmoiditis*, refers to UC extending to the mid-sigmoid colon, usually reachable by the flexible sigmoidoscope. *Left-sided colitis* means disease extending up to the splenic flexure. *Extensive colitis* extends beyond the splenic flexure but to the cecum. *Pancolitis* is the term used when UC extends to the cecum. As with CD, UC is a systemic disorder with common extraintestinal manifestations and the possibility of hepatic involvement and primary sclerosing cholangitis.

- UC is likely a complex interaction between an impaired mucosal immune system, defects in cellular or humoral immunity, dysregulation of cytokines, and microbial flora. Animal models suggest that UC is caused by excessive activation of T_H2 cells; in humans, however, the classic T_H2 cytokine, IL-4, has not been found in UC lesions.

DIFFERENTIAL DIAGNOSIS

The differential diagnosis of IBD is extensive (Table 16-2); it includes infectious as well as noninfectious causes and is based on the chronicity of symptoms. It is important to distinguish CD from UC, because the therapies of these can differ, but when CD involves the colon, this can be difficult. Some findings suggestive of CD in this setting are rectal sparing; small bowel involvement; absence of gross bleeding; presence of perianal disease; and the presence of skip lesions, granulomas, or fistulae. In about 10% to 15% of patients with IBD, the distinction between CD and UC cannot be made, and these are termed *indeterminate colitis.* At initial presentation and during exacerbations it is important to rule out infectious disease. *Salmonella, Shigella, Campylobacter, Aeromonas, Escherichia coli* 0157:H7, *Clostridium difficile,* and sexually transmitted diseases (STD) can all cause bloody diarrhea.

TABLE 16-2	INFLAMMATORY BOWEL DISEASE DIFFERENTIAL DIAGNOSIS	
Infectious Etiologies		
Bacterial	**Mycobacterial**	**Viral**
Salmonella	Tuberculosis	Cytomegalovirus
Shigella	*Mycobacterium avium*	Herpes simplex
Toxigenic *Escherichia coli*	**Parasitic**	HIV
Campylobacter	Amebiasis	**Fungal**
Yersinia	*Isospora*	Histoplasmosis
Clostridium difficile	*Trichuris trichura*	*Candida*
Gonorrhea	Hookworm	*Aspergillus*
Chlamydia trachomatis	*Strongyloides*	
Noninfectious Etiologies		
Inflammatory	**Neoplastic**	**Drugs and Chemicals**
Appendicitis	Lymphoma	NSAID
Diverticulitis	Metastatic carcinoma	Phosphosoda
Diversion colitis	Carcinoma of the ileum	Cathartic colon
Collagenous/lymphocytic colitis	Carcinoid	Gold
Ischemic colitis	Familial polyposis	Oral contraceptives
Radiation colitis/enteritis		Cocaine
Eosinophilic gastroenteritis		Chemotherapy
Neutropenic colitis		
Behçet's syndrome		
Graft-versus-host disease		

HIV, human immunodeficiency virus; NSAIDs, nonsteroidal anti-inflammatory drugs.

NATURAL HISTORY

- Both CD and UC are chronic diseases with intermittent exacerbations of mild to severe symptoms alternating with periods of varying levels of remission.
- About 10% to 20% of patients with CD will experience a very prolonged remission after initial presentation. Conversely, predictors of a severe course include age younger than 40 years, presence of perianal disease, initial requirement of corticosteroids, and recurrent perforations. CD can be associated with a modest decrease in overall life expectancy.
- The course of UC depends on extent of disease. Proctitis and distal colitis usually have a more benign course, resolving spontaneously in about 20% of cases. Increased relapse rates are seen in younger patients (ages 20–30 years), older patients (>70 years), women, those with more than five prior relapses, and those with basal plasmacytosis on rectal biopsy. Approximately 30% undergo colectomy after 15 to 25 years of disease. Overall mortality is only slightly increased compared with the general population.

PRESENTATION

Risk Factors

Understanding the epidemiology of IBD is important in identification stratification of patients with IBD (see above). In addition, several interesting environmental influences have been observed, with cigarette smoking being the strongest. The risk of developing UC in *current* smokers is lower, about 40% that of nonsmokers, and hospitalization rates are lower in nonsmokers at the onset of UC. *Former* smokers, however, have a 1.7 times increased risk for UC than those who have never smoked. Smoking is associated with a twofold increased risk of CD, and increases the chance of recurrence. Some, but not all, studies have also shown an increased risk of IBD with the use of oral contraceptives. Interestingly, appendectomy before age 20 for appendicitis or lymphadenitis may protect against developing UC, but not CD. Concomitant infections (intestinal and extraintestinal) can exacerbate IBD. Nonsteroidal anti-inflammatory drugs (NSAIDs) are often cited as worsening IBD, but the data are conflicting. Short courses of cyclooxygenase 2 (COX-2) inhibitors (e.g., celecoxib) may be safer than nonselective NSAID in patients with IBD whose disease is in remission. Neither stress nor psychopathology have been shown to be clearly related to the onset of IBD, but stress may have a role in the exacerbation of symptoms, possibly via activation of the enteric nervous system and elaboration of proinflammatory cytokines.

History

A careful history should be taken, focusing on the epidemiology and risk factors discussed above, the duration and severity of symptoms, the presence of constitutional symptoms or extraintestinal manifestations, and signs of infection. The patient's quality of life and impairment of daily activities should be addressed. Any prior clinical course should also be elicited.

Physical Examination

A full physical examination should be performed. Vital signs should be reviewed to help determine the general condition of the patient. The abdomen should be auscultated for high-pitched or absent bowel sounds, possibly indicating an obstruction. Peritoneal signs are concerning for an intestinal perforation. The abdomen may be tender in both CD and UC, but the location can be helpful. Right lower quadrant tenderness is classic in CD. A palpable mass is also more common in CD than UC. A rectal examination should be performed to rule out gross or occult blood. Perianal disease, if found, suggests CD over UC. Skin, joint, and eye examinations should also be performed to evaluate for the presence of extraintestinal manifestations.

Clinical Presentation

Crohn's Disease

The clinical manifestations of CD are more variable than those of UC because of the transmural nature and the variability of disease locations in CD. CD may present with GI symptoms, extraintestinal symptoms, or both. The hallmark symptoms of Crohn's ileitis, ileocolitis, or colitis are chronic diarrhea, abdominal pain, weight loss, fatigue, and fever, with or without rectal bleeding. Signs can include cachexia; abdominal tenderness or mass, most commonly in the right lower quadrant; or perianal fissures, fistulas, or abscess. Gastric and duodenal CD may present with nausea and vomiting, epigastric pain, or gastric outlet obstruction. Extraintestinal manifestations can parallel active gut involvement or be independent of intestinal disease activity.

Ulcerative Colitis

Patients with UC can have varying symptoms and signs dictated by anatomic extent and disease severity. Mild proctitis or distal colitis may present with intermittent rectal bleeding and mild diarrhea (less than four loose stools per day) and mucus passage. Tenesmus (the constant feeling of the need to empty the bowel), pain, and cramping are common. Moderate UC is characterized by up to 10 loose bloody stools per day, mild anemia, abdominal pain, and fever. Patients with severe UC typically have more than 10 loose stools per day, severe cramps, higher fevers, bleeding that requires blood transfusion, and weight loss. Extraintestinal manifestations are also common in UC.

MANAGEMENT

Diagnosis

- The diagnosis of IBD is made with a combination of clinical, laboratory, radiographic, endoscopic, and pathologic findings.
- In a patient with a history and physical examination findings compatible with IBD, certain laboratory tests can help support, but not confirm, the diagnosis. Elevated levels of C-reactive protein are nonspecific, but are observed in active IBD and are generally higher in CD than in UC. The two most commonly used antibody tests are antineutrophil cytoplasmic antibodies (p-ANCA) and anti-Saccharomyces cerevisiae antibodies (ASCA). These two tests are somewhat helpful in distinguishing patients with IBD from those who do not, but may be more helpful in differentiating CD from UC. If ASCA-positive and p-ANCA-negative, the patient is more likely to have CD (95% PPV). Conversely, if p-ANCA–positive and ASCA-negative, UC is more likely (88% PPV). The anti-OmpC antibody reacts to the outer membrane porin of *E. coli*, increases the sensitivity of p-ANCA and ASCA in diagnosing IBD, and may correlate to an internal perforating type of CD. Antibodies against CBir1 flagellin have also been associated with CD.
- Endoscopy is used to assess disease location and severity, confirm the IBD diagnosis, and obtain tissue for histologic evaluation. Colonoscopy with ileoscopy and biopsy can usually differentiate CD, UC, and disorders that mimic IBD. Endoscopic features common to both CD and UC include pseudopolyps, loss of haustral folds, fibrotic strictures, and linear superficial scars. Three major endoscopic findings more specific to CD are discrete aphthous ulcers, "cobblestoning" (formed by deep linear

ulcers), and discontinuous "skip" lesions. In an untreated patient, a normal rectum or isolated involvement of the terminal ileum is also highly suggestive of CD over UC. Endoscopic findings in UC consist of contiguous and circumferential involvement, beginning at the anal verge and extending proximally to a gradual transition to normal mucosa. Erythema, loss of the fine vascular pattern, mucosal granularity, friability, and edema are typical endoscopic findings in UC. Colonoscopy should not be performed in patients with severe colitis or toxic megacolon. Flexible sigmoidoscopy can sometimes be performed with less risk than full colonoscopy. Capsule endoscopy can be useful in diagnosing CD of the small bowel if unreachable by endoscopy, but intestinal obstruction can result if the capsule is caught in a tight stricture.

- Radiologic studies are adjunctive diagnostic tools in IBD. Small bowel follow-through can be useful to evaluate the small bowel in CD. Typical small bowel CD features are lumenal narrowing with "string" sign, nodularity and ulceration, a "cobblestone" appearance, and fistulae or abscess formation. Air contrast barium enema may be used to confirm the anatomic pattern and extent of disease in UC and Crohn's colitis. Barium studies may be normal despite endoscopically evident mild disease, and are also susceptible to false-positive results, especially in infectious conditions. Barium enema must be avoided in severely ill patients because of the risk of precipitating ileus with toxic megacolon. Computed tomography (CT) and magnetic resonance imaging (MRI) (and more recently, CT and MR enterography) have been particularly useful in evaluating specific complications (e.g., abscesses and fistulas).
- Pathologic specimens can help establish the diagnosis and differentiate between CD and UC. Aphthoid ulcers, focal crypt abscesses, and chronic transmural inflammatory infiltrates can be seen in CD. Noncaseating granulomas are pathognomonic for CD, but are seen in <50% of biopsies. Continuous, diffuse inflammatory infiltrate confined to the mucosa and submucosa, cryptitis, and crypt abscesses are common in UC.

Treatment

With advances in newer biologic therapies as well as improved understanding of existing medications, treatment of moderate or severe IBD is best orchestrated in specialized centers focusing on IBD.

Crohn's Disease

- Management of CD depends on disease location, severity, and existing complications. Treatment can be divided into induction therapy and maintenance therapy.
  - **5–Aminosalicylic Acid Compounds.** Aminosalicylates are used for induction of remission in mild to moderate active CD, maintenance of remission, and reduction of postoperative recurrence.

    Sulfasalazine (2–6 g daily in divided doses) is a diazo-compound consisting of the sulfonamide sulfapyridine and 5-aminosalicylic acid (5-ASA). Colonic bacteria are required to cleave the azo bond, releasing sulfapyridine and 5-ASA into the colon. Therefore, sulfasalazine is effective in colonic CD, but much less effective in small bowel CD. The therapeutic effects are derived primarily from the 5-ASA moiety (mesalamine), whereas side effects are mostly caused by its sulfa moiety. Nausea, vomiting, malaise, anorexia, and headache are dose related, whereas hypersensitivity reactions (rash, fever, hemolytic anemia, agranulocytosis, hepatitis, pancreatitis, and worsening of colitis) are idiosyncratic. In some patients with arthritis or spondyloarthropathy, sulfasalazine has the additional benefit of being a disease-modifying antirheumatic drug.

    Nonsulfa 5-ASA derivatives are better tolerated than sulfasalazine. Mesalamine (up to 4.8 g daily in divided doses) is effective in active CD and has been shown to facilitate steroid withdrawal after induction of remission. Optimal use of available

5-ASA preparations involves consideration of the site of disease involvement. Sustained-release preparations of 5-ASA (e.g., Pentasa) may be used for small bowel involvement, whereas delayed-release preparations (e.g., Asacol) should be used for inflammation in the terminal ileum and colon. A new once-daily formulation of colonically released mesalamine (i.e., Lialda) using multi matrix (MMX) technology is now available, and may improve patient adherence. Balsalazide (i.e., Colazol) is a 5-ASA moiety linked to an inert unabsorbed carrier molecule and requires colonic bacteria for bond cleavage. The mesalamine compounds are modestly effective for maintenance of remission (2–4 g daily) and for reducing postoperative relapse rates.

- **Antibiotics.** For patients who do not respond to (or do not tolerate) 5-ASA drugs, one of several antibiotics can be used as primary therapy before using corticosteroids. Metronidazole (10 or 20 mg/kg/day) with or without ciprofloxacin (500 mg PO BID) may be useful in the treatment of active lumenal CD. Metronidazole, ciprofloxacin, tetracycline, or combinations thereof are often used for extended periods in patients who have fistulas, abscesses, or perianal disease. Antibiotics are indicated for bacterial overgrowth, seen with small bowel strictures or after ileo-colic resection. Patients taking long-term metronidazole need to be monitored closely for peripheral neuropathy, which can be irreversible. The onset of new neurologic symptoms mandates immediate discontinuation of metronidazole.

- **Corticosteroids.** Corticosteroids have been a mainstay of treatment for mild to moderate IBD unresponsive to the above measures, or for severe presentations. Although useful for *inducing* remission, steroids are ineffective in *maintaining* remission or *preventing* relapse. Superimposed infections, such as cytomegalovirus (CMV) or *C. difficile*, and complications, including toxic megacolon or perforation, must be considered before starting steroids. Both oral prednisone (40–60 mg daily) and intravenous (IV) methylprednisolone (40–60 mg daily) induce remission in patients with active disease compared with placebo. Doses are typically tapered (about 5 mg/wk) when a clinical response has been achieved. Budesonide (up to 9 mg daily) is a controlled-release corticosteroid with poor absorption and a high first-pass hepatic metabolism. It is an alternative to prednisone in patients with distal small bowel disease to reduce systemic side effects. Because many patients treated acutely with steroids become steroid dependent or refractory, the treating physician always needs to consider a maintenance strategy at the time of initiating steroids.

- **Immunomodulator Therapy.** Oral azathioprine (2.5 mg/kg/day) and its metabolite 6-mercaptopurine (6-MP; 1.0–1.5 mg/kg/day) have been demonstrated to be effective in both induction and maintenance of remission in CD. These agents are effective for use as steroid-sparing agents and in fistulous disease, and also have a role in preventing postoperative relapses.

  The use of azathioprine or 6-MP also has disadvantages. Onset of action is generally delayed for as long as 6 to 10 weeks. Agranulocytosis, pancreatitis, allergic reactions, hepatitis, and life-threatening infections have been reported, but are usually reversible on discontinuation of therapy. Allergic symptoms, such as joint aches, fevers, nausea, and malaise, typically occur within the first 1 to 2 weeks of use; pancreatitis occurs around week 3 and leukopenia by week 4. Susceptibility to early, severe leukopenia can be predicted before initiation by measuring thiopurine s-methyltransferase (TPMT) enzyme activity, which is responsible for drug metabolism. Weekly blood counts should be followed the first 4 weeks and after any dose increases. Once the goal dose has been reached, a complete blood count (CBC) should be checked every 2 to 3 months. If the leukocyte count falls below 3000 cells/µL, the dose should be lowered or held. There appears to be an increased risk of lymphoma with azathioprine or 6-MP, but overall the absolute risk still remains quite low. Although controversial, experts feel the risk of harm to a developing fetus is low. The ultimate recommended length of therapy is unclear, because some experts consider drug withdrawal after 3 to 4 years whereas others suggest a longer-term continuation.

Subcutaneous or intramuscular methotrexate is more effective than placebo in inducing remission in patients with severe CD, although the data are less compelling than with azathioprine or 6-MP. Studies evaluating methotrexate for maintenance of remission have produced mixed results. Cyclosporine probably has little role in most cases of CD. The roles of tacrolimus and mycophenolate mofetil require further study.

- **Tumor Necrosis Factor Antagonists.** Infliximab (Remicade) is a chimeric monoclonal antibody to tumor necrosis factor (TNF), effective in fistulizing CD and in moderate to severe CD refractory to 5-ASA, antibiotics, corticosteroids, and immunomodulatory agents in adequate doses. The induction dose sequence is 5 mg/kg IV infusion over 2 hours at weeks 0, 2, and 6. Maintenance of remission can be achieved by retreatment every 8 weeks. Acute infusion reactions and delayed-type hypersensitivity reactions are more common with repeat infusions given after a prolonged interval since the last dose (over 12 weeks). Development of antichimeric antibodies, now termed antibodies to infliximab (ATI), occur in 10% to 15% of cases. Reactivation of latent tuberulosis (TB) can occur; therefore, a purified protein-derivative (PPD) skin test must be placed and confirmed negative before therapy. Congestive heart failure has also been reported. Other mild and self-limited side effects include headache, upper respiratory infection, and nausea.

  Adalimumab (Humira) is a recombinant human monoclonal antibody to TNF, used for rheumatoid arthritis, which has now been approved for treatment of active CD. Efficacy has been shown in those who have lost responsiveness or developed intolerance to infliximab. Subcutaneous administration offers dosing advantages over infliximab. Therapeutic induction consists of a loading dose of 160 mg followed by 80 mg at week 2, then 40 mg every other week. Side effects are similar to infliximab, with injection site reactions or pain seen instead of infusion reactions. Clinical experience with infliximab and adalimumab demonstrates that increases in dosing or dose frequency are sometimes required to maintain therapeutic effect.

- **Antidiarrheal Agents.** Antidiarrheal agents, such as loperamide (Imodium) or codeine, may decrease the frequency and volume of diarrhea. These agents should be withheld if intestinal infection or severely active disease is suspected.

- **Nutritional Therapy.** Maintenance of adequate nutrition is essential in the therapy of CD. Vitamin and nutrient supplementation are needed after bowel resection or with extensive small bowel involvement. For example, patients with ileitis may need vitamin B_{12} supplementation.

  Enteral nutrition is favored over total parenteral nutrition (TPN). TPN with bowel rest, however, may be an effective therapy alone or in combination with corticosteroids in refractory CD, with remission rates up to 80%. Discontinuation of TPN, however, leads to high relapse rates of 60% within 2 years.

- **Surgical Management.** Surgical management is often necessary for complications of intractable hemorrhage, perforation, persistent obstruction, abscess, or disease activity intractable to medical therapy. Abscesses often require drainage under radiographic guidance or with surgical management. Surgical resection is not curative in CD, with clinical recurrence rates of 10% to 15% per year. Postoperative prophylaxis with azathioprine or 6-MP, metronidazole, or mesalamine may lower recurrence rates.

  Suppurative perianal disease is often treated surgically with the placement of a noncutting seton (silastic band). Therapeutic options for strictures include strictureplasty, endoscopic balloon dilation, and local injection of steroids or biologic glues. All strictures should be biopsied to exclude malignancy.

Ulcerative Colitis

- Management of UC depends on extent and location of disease involvement and severity. Therapy may again be divided into induction therapy and maintenance therapy.
  - **5-Aminosalicylic Acid Compounds.** Salicylates are used for induction of remission in mildly to moderately active UC and for maintenance of remission. Considerations specific to UC include the option of rectally administered drugs and improved therapeutic effects seen with adjunctive mucosal drug delivery. Induction therapy in ulcerative proctitis can include topical 5-ASA (mesalamine) suppositories (e.g., Canasa) or enemas (e.g., Rowasa), which can also be used for maintenance. Topical therapies can be used together with orally administered 5-ASA preparations such as mesalamine (e.g., Asacol, lialda), balsalazide (e.g., Colazal), or sulfasalazine (up to 6 g daily in divided doses) in the treatment of more extensive colitis. Once remission is achieved, lower doses of sulfasalazine (2 g daily) or mesalamine (2.4 g daily) may maintain remission. Maintenance 5-ASA treatment has been shown to reduce risk of colorectal cancer.
  - **Antibiotics.** Except in fulminant colitis and pouchitis, antibiotics have little role in the management of UC.
  - **Corticosteroids.** Corticosteroids are sometimes necessary for mild to moderate UC. Steroid enemas (e.g., Cortenema) or foams (e.g., Cortifoam) can be used to treat distal disease in the short term. Oral corticosteroids are useful in more extensive moderate disease, especially if response to salicylates is slow or absent. Oral or IV corticosteroids can be considered for severe disease. If tapering leads to a return of symptoms despite 5-ASA treatment, an immunomodulator should be considered. Steroids, topical or systemic, have not been shown to be effective in maintaining remission in UC.
  - **Immunomodulator Therapy.** Oral azathioprine (2.5 mg/kg/day) and its metabolite 6-mercaptopurine (6-MP; 1.0–1.5 mg/kg/day) are effective in the induction and maintenance of remission and as steroid-sparing agents in chronic active UC. Their slow onset of action, often over 2 months, makes them relatively unhelpful in treating an acute UC flare. Current evidence is insufficient to support the use of methotrexate for UC. Intravenous cyclosporine (2–4 mg/kg/day) has been shown effective in fulminant UC, but side effects include grand mal seizures, opportunistic infection, and bowel perforation.
  - **Tumor Necrosis Factor Antagonists.** Infliximab (Remicade) is now approved for the treatment of UC that does not respond to conventional therapy. The dosing is the same as for CD. Maintenance dosing can be considered for those who respond to induction therapy.
  - **Antidiarrheal Agents.** Drugs, such as loperamide, tincture of opium, and codeine, are helpful in decreasing diarrhea but are contraindicated in severe UC exacerbations because of the risk of toxic megacolon.
  - **Surgical Management.** Medically refractory disease activity is the most common reason for surgery in UC. Less commonly, surgical consultation and total colectomy are required for acutely ill patients with megacolon or systemic toxicity not responding to medical therapy within 48 hours. Proctocolectomy or colectomy with rectal preservation is curative in UC, and the mortality of colectomy even in severe cases is low. Advances in surgical technique allow for the creation of an ileal pouch-anal anastomosis, and a permanent ileostomy is typically not required. *Pouchitis,* or inflammation of the surgically created ileal reservoir, is the most common complication of this surgery and occurs in 7% to 44% of the population. Symptoms include increased stool frequency, urgency, hematochezia, abdominal pain, and fever, but the diagnosis is made endoscopically and with histology. First-line therapy is typically with antibiotics (metronidazole); probiotics may be useful for prevention.

SPECIAL TOPICS

Microscopic Colitis

- Microscopic colitis (MC) is a group of diseases characterized by chronic, watery, nonbloody diarrhea, with largely normal endoscopic findings. The two main types of MC are collagenous colitis and lymphocytic colitis, although mixed forms and variants have also been described. On histology, a thickened subepithelial collagenous band is seen in collagenous colitis. Lymphocytic colitis is marked by a subepithelial lymphocytic infiltrate. Etiology is unknown, and it is doubtful that a single pathogenetic mechanism exists. MC is less common than CD and UC. Collagenous colitis has a female-to-male predominance of 9 to 15:1, whereas lymphocytic colitis has equal incidence in both genders. Collagenous colitis may be caused by abnormal collagen metabolism, particularly reduced matrix degradation rather than enhanced synthesis. Vascular endothelial growth factor (VEGF) may play a role in this collagen balance. Bacterial toxins, NSAID, selective serotonin reuptake inhibitors (SSRI), and other drugs have been linked to the development of MC.
- The clinical presentation of collagenous and lymphocytic colitis is similar. Progressively increasing watery diarrhea refractory to over-the-counter antidiarrheal agents is a common presentation. Associated symptoms can include nausea, abdominal pain, and fecal urgency. Many patients are diagnosed with irritable bowel syndrome with diarrhea until colonic pathology is examined, stressing the importance of colonoscopy and random biopsies of normal-appearing mucosa.
- Although the disease course is generally benign, relapsing and remitting symptoms can be debilitating. Patients should be reassured that MC is not associated with severe disease, increased mortality, or an increased risk of colorectal cancer. NSAIDs or other drugs associated with MC should be discontinued. Patients should be tested for celiac disease. Antidiarrheal agents, such as loperamide, can be tried; bismuth subsalicylate has also been demonstrated effective in MC. If response is inadequate, budesonide at a dose of 9 mg daily or 5-ASA compounds can be initiated. Other options include cholestyramine, systemic corticosteroids, and immunomodulators.

Extraintestinal Manifestations

Extraintestinal complications are frequent in IBD, involving almost any organ system, and contributing considerably to patient morbidity (Table 16-3). Usually seen with UC or with colonic CD, extraintestinal manifestations are associated with a family history of IBD, and certain major histocompatibility complex (MHC) or HLA antigen loci have been linked. Having one manifestation increases the chance of having another, with four common sites of involvement: skin, joints, eyes, and biliary tract. A proposed pathogenesis is an autoimmune-related process with antibodies forming against antigens shared among the colon and these four common sites, associated with imbalanced cytokine production. A variety of hepatobiliary manifestations can be seen in IBD. Primary sclerosing cholangitis (PSC) is seen in about 5% of patients with UC. Extraintestinal manifestations may parallel or be independent of intestinal disease activity. Generally, manifestations that parallel disease activity are addressed first by intensification of intestinal IBD therapy, whereas the other conditions are treated independently.

Osteoporosis

Osteoporosis is a source of significant morbidity, impaired quality of life, and costs in IBD. Risk factors include corticosteroid use (the greatest risk factor), malnutrition, low body weight, and low intake or absorption of dietary calcium and vitamin D. Bone densitometry (DEXA) is the current gold standard for measuring bone mass and is the best predictor of

TABLE 16-3	EXTRAINTESTINAL MANIFESTATIONS OF INFLAMMATORY BOWEL DISEASE	
Manifestation		**Parallels Intestinal Disease**
Erythema nodosum		Yes
Pyoderma gangrenosum		Yes
Peripheral arthropathy		Yes
Episcleritis or scleritis		Yes
Anterior uveitis		No
Spondyloarthropathy (ankylosing spondylitis, sacroiliitis)		No
Osteoporosis (often steroid-induced)		No
Primary sclerosing cholangitis (usually ulcerative colitis)		No
Nephrolithiasis (usually Crohn's disease)		No
Cholelithiasis (after ileal resection)		No

in vitro skeletal strength. Other useful tests include a CBC, alkaline phosphatase, calcium level corrected for serum albumin, creatinine, testosterone level (males), and 25-OH-vitamin D level. IBD itself only modestly lowers bone mineral density, but increases the risk of fractures by 40% over the general population. All patients should be educated about the importance of regular weight-bearing exercise and avoiding smoking and excessive alcohol intake. Adequate intake of vitamin D (at least 400–800 IU daily) and calcium (1000–1500 mg daily) are recommended. Bisphosphonates are used in patients at highest risk for fractures.

Malignancy

Patients with IBD are thought to be at increased risk for colorectal cancer (CRC) compared with the general population. The level of risk is related to the duration, severity, and colonic extent of inflammation. Because CRC is generally preceded by dysplasia, surveillance is recommended to detect and intervene when dysplasia is found.

In patients with UC with pancolitis, CRC risk seems to increase after 8 to 10 years of symptoms. The cumulative incidence of CRC in UC is 5% to 10% after 20 years and 12% to 20% after 30 years of disease, although recent studies report lower incidences. For left-sided colitis, CRC risk may increase after 15 to 20 years. Distal colitis and proctosigmoiditis probably do not increase the risk of CRC. Patients with UC with PSC have an even higher increased risk for CRC. Surveillance colonoscopy with random biopsies is recommended beginning after 8 years of pancolitis and after 15 years of left-sided colitis, and then repeated every 1 to 3 years thereafter. No screening is recommended for ulcerative proctitis. Colectomy is generally recommended for carcinoma, high-grade dysplasia, and multifocal low-grade dysplasia.

Patients with Crohn's colitis also have an increased risk of colonic adenocarcinoma compared with the general population. Patients with long-standing colitis or age above 30 years at diagnosis are at greatest risk. Recommended surveillance strategies are similar to those for UC.

KEY POINTS TO REMEMBER

- In genetically susceptible individuals, IBD may develop from dysregulation of the normal immune system directed against luminal bacteria or from an appropriate immune response, not normally expressed, elicited by alterations in gut flora or mucosal barrier function.
- Crohn's disease consists of transmural skip lesions involving any part of the GI tract, most commonly ileum and colon, and can present with abdominal pain, diarrhea, and weight loss.
- Ulcerative colitis, which is characterized by continuous superficial ulceration of the rectum and varying proximal amounts of colon, commonly presents with diarrhea and rectal bleeding.
- Smoking has been associated with reduced risk of UC, but complicates the course of CD.
- 5-ASA compounds, corticosteroids, and immunomodulators are useful for inducing remission in mild to moderately active CD and UC.
- Steroids are ineffective in maintaining remission in IBD and the side effects of long-term use are unacceptable; initiation of steroids should be accompanied by a plan for taper and discontinuation, as well as a suitable alternate maintenance regimen.
- Azathioprine or 6-MP as well as infliximab may be used as steroid-sparing agents.
- Surgical resection is curative in UC, but must be considered carefully in the context of symptom severity, response to full medical therapy, and patient preferences.
- Surgical resection is not curative in CD, but is often necessary for refractory disease or complications of intractable hemorrhage, perforation, persistent obstruction, or abscess.
- Surveillance colonoscopy with mucosal biopsies should be performed after 8 years of pancolitis or Crohn's colitis, after 15 years of left-sided colitis, and repeated every 1 to 3 years thereafter.

REFERENCES AND SUGGESTED READINGS

American Gastroenterological Association Consensus Development Conference on the Use of Biologics in the Treatment of Inflammatory Bowel Disease, *Gastroenterology* 2007;133(1):312–339.

American Gastroenterological Association Institute medical position statement on corticosteroids, immunomodulators, and infliximab in inflammatory bowel disease. *Gastroenterology* 2006;130(3):935–939.

Baumgart DC, Sandborn WJ. Inflammatory bowel disease: clinical aspects and established and evolving therapies. *Lancet* 2007;369(9573):1641–1657.

Rothfuss KS, Stange EF, Herrlinger KR. Extraintestinal manifestations and complications in inflammatory bowel diseases *World J Gastroenterol* 2006;12(30):4819–4831.

Lichtenstein GR, Sands BE, Pazianas M. Prevention and treatment of osteoporosis in inflammatory bowel disease. *Inflamm Bowel Dis* 2006;12(8):797–813.

Strober W, Fuss I, Mannon P. The fundamental basis of inflammatory bowel disease. *J Clin Invest* 2007;117:514–521.

Targan SR, Shanahan F, Karp LC. *Inflammatory Bowel Disease: From Bench to Bedside*. 2nd ed. New York: Springer-Verlag; 2003.

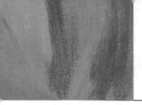

Irritable Bowel Syndrome

Vilaas Shetty and Gregory S. Sayuk

INTRODUCTION

Background and Definition

Collectively, the functional gastrointestinal disorders (FGID) comprise chronic or recurrent conditions wherein alterations in bowel sensitivity, motility, or both are predominant manifestations. Despite a lack of identifiable structural abnormalities on diagnostic evaluations, these common conditions impose substantial burdens on patient well-being and, in turn, account for large portion of visits to both primary care physicians and gastroenterologists. The FGID represent a complex interface between abnormal GI motility, visceral hypersensitivity, altered central nervous system (CNS) processing of peripheral stimuli, and psychosocial factors. FGID symptoms can arise from any portion of the GI tract, and frequently multiple FGID may be identified in the same individual. These functional syndromes are listed in Table 17-1. The prototypical and most common functional GI disorder is irritable bowel syndrome (IBS), which is defined as abdominal pain or discomfort associated with defecation or a change in bowel habit with features of disordered defecation.

Epidemiology

Worldwide, it is estimated that 10% to 20% of adolescents and adults report symptoms consistent with IBS at any given time. As few as one in three individuals affected with IBS, however, actually seek medical attention in the United States. IBS is frequently seen in both primary care and speciality care settings, comprising 12% of the diagnoses made in primary care practices and >25% of those made by gastroenterologists. Population surveys of adults have shown IBS to be more prevalent in women than in men with a ratio of 3 to 4:1, typically with a first presentation between the ages of 20 and 50 years. The cost to society is considerable, accounting for approximately 3 million physician visits and $1.6 billion in direct medical costs each year in the United States alone. Indirect costs in the form of work absenteeism may reach as high as $19 billion per annum.

CAUSES

Pathophysiology

- No single pathophysiologic abnormality has been found that adequately explains the manifestations of IBS. Given the symptomatic basis on which the diagnosis is made, it is conceivable that more than one pathophysiologic mechanism may be operative. Multiple factors, including abnormalities of intestinal motility, visceral hypersensitivity, GI tract inflammatory processes, disturbances along the brain–gut axis, and psychological factors, have been examined as potential pathophysiologic bases for IBS.

TABLE 17-1	THE FUNCTIONAL GASTROINTESTINAL DISORDERS (FROM ROME III)

Functional Esophageal Disorders
  Heartburn
  Chest pain of presumed esophageal origin
  Dysphagia
  Globus

Functional Gastroduodenal Disorders
  Functional dyspepsia
  Belching disorders
  Nausea and vomiting disorders
  Rumination syndrome

Functional Bowel Disorders
  Irritable bowel syndrome
  Functional bloating
  Functional constipation
  Functional diarrhea
  Unspecified functional bowel disorder

Functional Abdominal Pain Syndrome
Functional Gallbladder and Sphincter of Oddi (SO) Disorders
  Functional gallbladder disorder
  Functional biliary SO disorder
  Functional pancreatic SO disorder

Functional Anorectal Disorders
  Functional fecal incontinence
  Functional anorectal pain
  Functional defecation disorders

- In a proportion of patients with IBS, exaggerated motility and sensory responses to stressors, meals, and balloon inflation in the GI tract can be identified. These motility responses, however, are neither uniformly identifiable in patients with IBS nor consistently present in affected individuals and, thus, cannot be used as diagnostic markers. Nevertheless, accelerated transit times may be seen in diarrhea-predominant IBS and slowed transit times in constipation-predominant IBS. IBS may result from sensitization of afferent neural pathways from the gut in such a fashion that normal intestinal stimuli induce pain. It has been demonstrated that patients with IBS have a lower pain threshold to balloon distention of the colon as compared with healthy volunteers, while retaining normal sensitivity to somatic stimuli.
- Intestinal inflammation has also been hypothesized as playing a role in the development of IBS, particularly as it relates to persistent neuroimmune interactions after infectious gastroenteritis. Approximately one-third of patients with IBS report that symptoms began after an episode of acute gastroenteritis, and 7% to 30% of patients presenting with an acute enteric infection go on to develop IBS-like symptoms. Psychological distress (particularly somatization) seems to be an important cofactor in determining who retains symptoms after an enteric infection. Although additional studies are needed, recent publications have raised a possible mechanistic role of small intestinal bacterial overgrowth in the development of IBS.
- The CNS (and its interpretation of peripheral enteric nerve signals) is receiving increasing attention because of the potential mechanistic significance in IBS. Differential

—not needed for diagnosis

TABLE 17-2	THE ROME III IRRITABLE BOWEL SYNDROME CRITERIA

Recurrent abdominal pain or discomfort at least 3 days per month in the last 3 months associated with two or more of the following:
1. Improvement with defecation
2. Onset associated with a change in frequency of stools
3. Onset associated with a change in form (appearance) of stool

responses of brain activation to both noxious rectal stimulation and anticipated rectal discomfort can be appreciated in patients with IBS compared with a control population. As such, these connections are both the focus of intense research and the target of novel therapies. Psychological factors (anxiety, depression, somatization) are important in their potential to further modulate this afferent pain network, but by themselves are not sufficient explanations of IBS pathogenesis. In addition to amplifying both visceral and somatic pain experiences, the patient's psychological framework may also influence illness behaviors, such as seeking health care.

Classification

Several historical diagnostic criteria for IBS exist, but the most commonly cited is the Rome criteria. The Rome III criteria (Table 17-2) are the most recent and encompassing criteria, asserted primarily as a tool for devising clinical studies in the area. In clinical practice, these criteria have a 98% positive predictive value. Although they are not necessary for IBS diagnosis, several supporting symptoms (Table 17-3) help to solidify the diagnosis and further characterize the disorder into IBS with constipation (IBS-C), IBS with diarrhea (IBS-D), mixed IBS (IBS-M), or unsubtyped IBS.

PRESENTATION

History and Physical Examination

Irritable bowel syndrome is a symptom-based diagnosis founded on a chronic reporting of abdominal discomfort and a temporal association with alterations in stool pattern, improvement with bowel movement, or both. The diagnosis of IBS should be made after organic causes have been considered, so a careful search for alarm symptoms should be conducted. Important alarm symptoms include weight loss of 10 lb, recurrent fever, persistent diarrhea, hematochezia, age older than 50 years, and family history of GI malignancy, inflammatory bowel disease, or celiac sprue. In addition, a short history of rapidly progressive symptoms suggests organic disease. The presence of any such features warrants a more entailed investigation before establishing a diagnosis of IBS.

TABLE 17-3	SUPPORTIVE SYMPTOMS OF IRRITABLE BOWEL SYNDROME

Abnormal stool frequency (*abnormal* defined more than three bowel movements per day or fewer than bowel movements per week)

Abnormal stool form (lumpy/hard or loose/watery stool)

Abnormal stool passage (straining, urgency, or feeling of incomplete evacuation)

Passage of mucus

Bloating or feeling of abdominal distention

Likewise, the physical examination should be focused to exclude organic disease. Diffuse abdominal tenderness is commonly present because of the heightened visceral sensitivity noted in this population. Physical examination alarm signs include the presence of ascites, jaundice, organomegaly, abdominal mass, adenopathy, or heme-positive stool.

MANAGEMENT

Diagnostic Evaluation

- Laboratory and invasive testing should be kept to a minimum, because extensive or repetitive investigations may be costly and serve only to reinforce illness behavior. Initial laboratory testing should include a complete blood count (CBC), and fecal occult blood test when appropriate. If clinically indicated, a complete metabolic profile, thyroid-stimulating hormone, sedimentation rate, and stool for *Clostridium difficile*, culture, and ova or parasites examination may be ordered. Testing for celiac sprue should be considered in diarrhea-predominant patients with risk factors such as family history, ethnicity, or presence of other autoimmune disease processes.
- Endoscopy may be unnecessary in young patients presenting with classic features of IBS. Colonoscopy can be performed with the following advantages: (a) to rule out inflammation or tumors (especially in patients older than 50 year), (b) to identify melanosis coli indicative of laxative abuse, and (c) to allow detection of visceral hypersensitivity to visceral pain via endoscopic insufflation of the colon.

Treatment

The approach to therapy in IBS is multifaceted and should be tailored to the individual patient given the constellation and severity of symptoms. Two key factors that determine therapy are (a) dominant symptom (diarrhea, constipation, pain, other) and (b) symptom severity. Current management approaches include peripherally acting agents, centrally acting agents, and psychological-behavorial therapy. Cases with mild or intermittent symptoms can be managed with symptomatic treatment using simple peripheral agents administered as needed. Patients with moderate symptoms (as designated by intermittent interference with daily activities) benefit from regular use of peripheral agents as an initial approach, with the option of introducing centrally acting agents if this approach fails. Patients with severe symptoms (regular interference with daily activities, and concurrent affective, personality, and psychosomatic disorders) benefit from combinations of peripheral and central agents, but may also need contemporary pharmaceutical agents and cognitive-behavioral therapy to manage their overlapping affective, personality, and psychosomatic disorders.

General Points

Although medical therapy is available and new drugs are currently in development, IBS is a lifelong condition with exacerbations and remittances, and medications should be minimized to the extent possible. Clearly, narcotics have no role in the management of IBS. Given the lack of identifiable biomarkers, trials of medications are frequently part of the IBS diagnostic process. These trials should be pursued for ≥4 weeks before moving on to different therapy. If failure to respond to a single agent in a drug class is experienced, response to a different drug in the same class may still be observed. Finally, in managing IBS it is important to recognize the substantial (up to 50%) placebo response rates present in this patient population. Consequently, patient education and reassurance while establishing a therapeutic relationship are cornerstones in the management of this condition. The strength of the physician's relationship with the patient correlates to higher rates of patient satisfaction and fewer return visits. Table 17-4 summarizes general management principles for patients with IBS or other functional bowel disorders.

...ve testing, targeted to exclude other disorders as appropriate
- Avoid repetitive testing unless necessary
- Determine patient expectations and goals
- Education and reassurance with emphasis on benign nature of condition
- Dietary modifications and fiber supplementation are first-line therapy
- Medications for more persistent or difficult cases
- Behavioral or psychological interventions for refractory and motivated patients with IBS

Peripherally Acting Agents
- Increasing the amount of dietary fiber can be considered in mild constipation-predominant IBS, but randomized controlled studies have failed to demonstrate benefit in global symptom relief with this approach. Nevertheless, fiber supplementation is an inexpensive approach, and can be instituted as an early option. Natural fiber sources (e.g., psyllium) or synthetic fiber (e.g., methylcellulose) are available. In patients who complain of bloating or gas, fiber supplementation can be associated with an increase in those symptoms and exclusion of flatulogenic foods should be encouraged.
- Osmotic laxatives such as milk of magnesia, sorbitol, lactulose, or polyethylene glycol may be considered in patients with IBS-C. These agents are generally safe for long-term use and are preferable to stimulant laxatives. Lactulose and sorbitol can induce bloating symptoms. Lubiprostone (Amitiza) is a chloride channel activator indicated in the treatment of chronic constipation at a dosage of 24 μg BID. Women of child-bearing age should have a negative pregnancy test before starting therapy, and should be capable of complying with effective contraception while on this medication. Tegaserod (Zelnorm) is a partial 5-hydroxytryptamine-4 receptor agonist that exerts GI stimulatory effects and had been indicated for short-term treatment of women with constipation-predominant symptoms. In 2007, however, it was withdrawn from the market because of a small but statistically significant increase in cardiovascular events in patients taking it. Its role is currently being re-evaluated in a restricted access program.
- In diarrhea-predominant IBS, loperamide (2–4 mg up to QID) or diphenoxylate 2.5 mg with atropine 0.025 mg (Lomtil, upto QID) may be used. Suspension forms of these medications are available for patients who need dose titrations. Cholestyramine (Questran) and colesevelam (WelChol) should be considered for patients with diarrheal symptoms exacerbated by cholecystectomy. Alosetron (Lotronex), a selective 5-hydroxytryptamine-3 receptor antagonist, was approved for treatment of women with IBS-D. It was withdrawn from the market in 2000 because of an unclear relationship with acute ischemic colitis in 0.1% to 1% of patients, but was reapproved by the U.S. Food and Drug Administration (FDA) in 2002 under restrictive guidelines for its use. Frequently prescribed drugs in the treatment of IBS are the anticholinergics or antispasmodic agents. Hyoscyamine (Levsin), 0.125 to 0.25 mg PO or sublingual, dicyclomine (Bentyl) 10 to 20 mg PO, up to TID, glycopyrrolate (Robinul) 1 to 2 mg BID to TID, and methscopolamine (Pamine) 2.5 to 5 mg BID are available. The latter two agents have decreased CNS side effect potential. These agents are most useful in patients with postprandial symptoms of abdominal pain, bloating, diarrhea, or fecal urgency. They should be prescribed to circumvent symptoms, such as before meals. These agents often become less effective with chronic use.

- The use of antibiotic regimens, such as the gut-selective antibiotic rifaximin or neomycin, have been proposed in patients with IBS for whom bacterial overgrowth is suspected, particularly in those with significant gas-bloat symptoms. Similarly, randomized-controlled data have emerged in support of the use of probiotics such as *bifidobacterium infantis* (Allign) in the management of IBS symptoms. These studies involved small sample sizes and lack long-term follow-up, however, and corroborative studies are needed.

Centrally Acting Agents

Antidepressant medications are most useful in patients with chronic, refractory symptoms. They are particularly helpful with those who have concomitant psychiatric and somatic complaints, although their efficacy is independent of any direct influence on these comorbid conditions. It is thought that antidepressants serve to interrupt or modulate the CNS interpretation of peripheral gut signaling. Tricyclic antidepressants (TCA), such as nortriptyline, amitriptyline, imipramine, and desipramine are the best studied agents, and they are used in doses much lower than those traditionally used in depression management (starting dose, 10–25 mg at bedtime). The anticholinergic properties of TCA may be beneficial in IBS-D, but should not dissuade use in patients with IBS-C. Side effects can include sedation, dry mouth, and dizziness. Individuals experiencing such side effects may tolerate use of agents with fewer anticholinergic effects, such as desipramine. Selective serotonin reuptake inhibitors (SSRI) are also being used increasingly, although experience in IBS is more limited. Citalopram may be selected because of its low side-effect profile and its effect on colonic tone and sensitivity. Paroxetine may be useful in patients with IBS-D because of its anticholinergic effect. Patient perceptions and expectations should be adequately addressed in using antidepressants in the management of IBS in order to optimize compliance.

Cognitive and Behavioral Therapy

Psychological and behavioral therapies, such as cognitive behavioral therapy (CBT), may be useful in IBS management, particularly in patients who correlate an increase in severity of symptoms with life stressors. CBT has been demonstrated to be beneficial in IBS in randomized, controlled trials, particularly in its positive influence on global well-being. Although response is sporadic, factors favoring a good response include high patient motivation, diarrhea or pain as the predominant symptom, overt psychiatric symptoms, and intermittent pain exacerbated by stress.

KEY POINTS TO REMEMBER

- IBS comprises a group of functional bowel disorders in which abdominal discomfort or pain is associated with defecation or a change in bowel habits.
- The Rome III criteria help to separate functional from organic disease, and the history, physical examination, and limited laboratory and invasive testing increase the specificity of the diagnosis.
- A very high placebo response rate is seen in treatment of IBS; the most important components of therapy are patient education and reassurance and establishment of a therapeutic physician–patient relationship.
- Dietary and supplemental fiber and osmotic laxatives are recommended in constipation-predominant IBS, although these can increase symptoms of bloating and gas in some patients. Newer agents, such as lubiprostone, and antibiotic-probiotic regimens remain therapeutic options.
- Low-dose TCA and SSRI may be helpful in modifying aberrant brain–gut interactions important to the functional GI disorders.

REFERENCES AND SUGGESTED READINGS

Drossman DA, Camilleri M, Mayer E, et al. AGA Technical Review on Irritable Bowel Syndrome. *Gastroenterology* 2002;123:2108–2131.

Drossman DA, Corazziari E, Tally NJ, et al., eds. *Rome III: The Functional Gastrointestinal Disorders. Diagnosis, Pathophysiology and Treatment: A Multinational Consensus.* 3rd ed. McLean, VA: Degnon Associates; 2006.

Drossman DA, Toner BB, Whitehead WE, et al. Cognitive-behavioral therapy versus education and desipramine versus placebo for moderate to severe functional bowel disorders. *Gastroenterology* 2003;125:19–31.

Posserud I, Stotzer PO, Bjornsson ES, et al. Small intestinal bacterial overgrowth in patients with irritable bowel syndrome. *Gut* 2007;56:802–808.

Spanier JA, Howden CW, Jones MP. A systematic review of alternative therapies in the irritable bowel syndrome. *Arch Intern Med* 2003;163:265–724.

Whitehead WE, Palsson O, Jones KR. Systematic review of the comorbidity of irritable bowel syndrome with other disorders: what are the causes and implications? *Gastroenterology* 2002;122:1140–1156.

Acute Liver Disease

Anil B. Seetharam and Kevin M. Korenblat

INTRODUCTION

Acute liver disease encompasses a wide range of disorders from asymptomatic aminotransferase elevations to acute liver failure (ALF). Most commonly, it is the result of viral hepatitis or drug-induced liver injury. Histologic changes to the liver are typically those of acute inflammation with varying degrees of necrosis and collapse of the liver's architectural framework. These features are in contrast to the changes of cirrhosis and complications of portal hypertension that dominate chronic liver disease.

CAUSES

Viral Hepatitis

Hepatitis A

- **Hepatitis A** virus (HAV), an enterically transmitted RNA virus, is the most common cause of acute hepatitis worldwide. Infection is associated with unsanitary living conditions or improper food handling techniques. Both the morbidity and mortality (case-fatality rate) of infection are determined by the age of onset. In developing countries, infection in childhood is universal and typically asymptomatic for those younger than 6 years of age. Adults are more likely to be symptomatic and infection is characterized by a 1-week prodrome of malaise, abdominal pain, and fever followed by jaundice. Aminotransferase elevations range from 10 to 100 times the upper limits of the reference range (ULR). The disease is diagnosed by the detection of IgM anti-HAV. Resolution of the illness is associated with replacement of IgM with IgG anti-HAV, and this change provides the basis for distinguishing acute from convalescent infection. Treatment is supportive; however, careful attention should be paid to identifying those at risk for ALF. Most symptoms of infection, including jaundice, resolve by 3 to 4 months. Although there is no chronic phase of HAV infection, a polyphasic form of the disease can occur associated with relapse of symptoms. Postexposure prophylaxis with hyperimmune globulin is available and effective if administered within 2 weeks of exposure. Vaccination against HAV should be encouraged in child care providers, food handlers, individuals with chronic liver disease, and nonimmune subjects traveling to endemic areas.

Hepatitis B

- **Hepatitis B** virus (HBV) is a blood-borne DNA virus that is estimated to occur in more than 300 million individuals worldwide. In comparison to HAV, hepatitis B is associated with both acute and chronic infection. Perinatal transmission from mother to child (most common in Asia) is associated with asymptomatic infection and high rates of chronic infection. Infection acquired in adulthood is associated with injection drug use and sexual intercourse, particularly in men who have sex with men.

- The period from exposure to symptoms ranges from 60 to 180 days and the disease can vary from asymptomatic infection to an icteric hepatitis rarely culminating in ALF. Serologic markers of acute infection include hepatitis B surface antigen (HBs antigen), hepatitis B e-antigen (HBe antigen), and HBV DNA. These markers are detectable 6 weeks after exposure and precede the onset of symptoms. Aminotransferase elevations are also detectable during the prodromal phase and are usually >10 times ULR. With the onset of symptoms, antibodies to the hepatitis B core protein (anti-HBc) become detectable. Serologic assays for anti-HBc detect either IgM or total (IgM and IgG) subtypes. Anti-HBc IgM typically becomes detectable with the onset of symptoms and can persist for 6 to 12 months. Concomitantly, IgG antibodies are produced and these antibodies (anti-HBc total) are the most durable antibody marker of exposure to HBV. The typical symptoms of acute infection include fatigue and jaundice. Extrahepatic signs of rash, arthralgias, and vasculitis can also occur.
- The most devastating consequence of acute infection is acute liver failure, which occurs in <1% of cases. Most cases of symptomatic, acute HBV infection in adults resolve with the development of antibodies to the surface protein (anti-HBs), the central neutralizing antibody to HBV. Thus, generally no role exists for antiviral therapy with acute infection; however, case reports have suggested a potential role for oral antiviral therapy in subjects who develop signs that they may progress to ALF. Effective postexposure prophylaxis consists of the simultaneous administration of the HBV vaccine and hyperimmune globulin. These treatments can also be given to newborns of infected mothers to prevent vertical transmission.
- The development of chronic infection represents the second major consequence of HBV infection. Chronic infection is defined as the presence of HBs antigen beyond 6 months from infection and the risk of chronic infection is determined by the age and immune status of the host. Both young age—particularly perinatal transmission—and immunocompromised hosts are at substantial risk of chronic infection. Vaccination continues to represent the best approach for disease prevention and should be offered to all newborns, health care works, household contacts of infected subjects and carriers, injection drug users, hemodialysis recipients, and men who have sex with men.

Hepatitis C

- **Hepatitis C** virus (HCV) is a blood-borne RNA virus. In the United States, the prevalence of infection is estimated at 1% of the population and chronic infection with HCV is the most frequent indication for liver transplantation. The most common modes of transmission are injection drug use or transfusion of infected blood products. The latter route was made uncommon by screening procedures introduced in the early 1990s. Other groups associated with infection include those receiving hemodialysis and users of intranasal cocaine. Neither sexual intercourse nor vertical infection is a robust route of transmission. Symptomatic, acute infection is unusual and <15% of infected subjects develop an icteric hepatitis. When symptoms do occur—typically 6 to 12 weeks from exposure—they can be mild and nonspecific with symptomatic hepatitis uncommon and ALF distinctly rare. The two most relevant serologic markers of hepatitis C infection are antibody testing (anti-HCV) and polymerase chain reaction (PCR)-based assays of HCV RNA. Anti-HCV is nearly uniformly present in all infected subjects; however, it may require 3 to 6 months from exposure to develop. Thus, testing for HCV RNA should be performed even if antibody testing is negative in situations in which a suspicion exists for acute infection. HCV RNA should also be assayed to confirm chronic infection when a reactive anti-HCV is discovered.
- The development of chronic HCV infection occurs in as many as 85% of subjects following acute infection. What makes the detection of acute infection important is

that the introduction of antiviral therapy within 6 month of exposure appears to result in dramatically higher rates of viral clearance than treatment during the chronic phase and, thus, treatment should be strongly considered in all acutely infected patients. In contrast to HAV and HBV, neither vaccination nor an established postexposure prophylaxis (PEP) regimen exists in the case of HCV.

Hepatitis D

The **hepatitis D** virus (HDV) or delta agent requires coinfection with hepatitis B for replication and expression. HDV may be acquired with HBV (coinfection) or after an established HBV infection (superinfection). In both situations, the clinical picture can be that of an acute hepatitis. Antibodies to HDV (anti-HDV) can be assayed for diagnosis.

Hepatitis E

Hepatitis E virus (HEV) is an enterically transmitted RNA virus. Infection with HEV is typically a self-limited icteric hepatitis, although it can be associated with acute liver failure in pregnant women. Available tests to detect HEV infection include assays for antibodies to HEV antigens and the reverse transcriptase-polymerase chain reaction (RT-PCR) to detect HEV RNA. Outbreaks and sporadic cases of HEV have been documented in the Indian subcontinent, Asia, Africa, and Mexico. In the United States, nearly all reported cases of HEV have been in travelers returning from endemic areas. The first case of sporadic hepatitis E in the United States was reported in 1997. Isolation of HEV in domestic sheep, cattle, and hogs has raised the possibility of hepatitis E being a zoonotic infection. Other viruses implicated in acute liver disease, particularly in immunocompromised populations, include cytomegalovirus, Epstein-Barr virus, human herpes virus, and varicella zoster virus.

Alcohol   *AST >ALT (2:1)*

- Excessive consumption of alcohol can result in a spectrum of liver diseases that include fatty liver, alcoholic hepatitis, and cirrhosis. Typical features of alcoholic hepatitis include jaundice, hepatomegaly, and fever. Leukocytosis is common, as are elevated hepatic aminotransferases (although they are typically under five times the limit of the reference range). The ratio of aspartate aminotransferase (AST) to alanine aminotransferase (ALT) is typically 2:1 or greater. Alcoholic hepatitis can be clinically indistinguishable from cirrhosis because in both cases complications of portal hypertension (ascites, portal hypertensive-related bleeding, and encephalopathy) can occur. In some cases, features of cirrhosis and alcoholic hepatitis can occur simultaneously, particularly in patients with more than one cause of liver disease, for example chronic hepatitis C infection and alcohol use. Although clinical assessment is frequently sufficient to make the diagnosis of alcoholic hepatitis, in cases of uncertainty, liver biopsy is appropriate.
- The severity of alcoholic hepatitis and the mortality risk can be estimated from a discriminant function formula (Maddrey score):

Discriminant function (DF) = 4.6 × [measured prothrombin time − control prothrombin time] + total bilirubin (mg/dL).

A DF score >32 is considered severe alcoholic hepatitis and associated with a high 30-day mortality rate, mostly from sepsis, multiorgan failure, or gastrointestinal hemorrhage. For DF scores <32, alcohol abstinence and supportive care are sufficient. In those with severe disease (DF ≥32), treatment options include corticosteroids or pentoxifylline. Individual studies and meta-analysis of trials of corticosteroids for alcoholic hepatitis have resulted in conflicting results. Currently, corticosteroids (prednisolone 40 mg daily for 30 days) should be considered in patients with alcoholic hepatitis and a DF >32 or encephalopathy. Even with treatment, mortality rates of at least 40% exist and at least seven patients need to be treated to prevent one death. The efficacy and safety of corticosteroids has not been studied in patients with gastrointestinal bleeding, active infection, or pancreatitis. Treatment with pentoxifylline 400 mg PO TID, the subject of one study, resulted in a reduction in the 30-day mortality rate. The improvement was attributed to a reduction in renal dysfunction in treated patients.

Acetaminophen

- Acetaminophen (APAP) toxicity is the most common cause of toxic medication-related ingestion in the United States. It is most frequently a consequence of intentional ingestion; however, unintentional overdoses do occur and can result in severe liver injury. APAP is a safe and generally well-tolerated analgesic medication. Significant hepatic injury generally requires ingestions above a threshold value of 150 mg/kg body weight. Chronic, excessive alcohol use may predispose to liver injury, although only with overdoses of acetaminophen.
- The antidote to treatment, N-acetylcysteine (NAC) administered within 8 hours of ingestion, is indicated in those with acetaminophen levels above the "possible" toxicity line on the Rumack-Matthew nomogram (line connecting 150 μg/mL at 4 hours with 50 μg/mL at 12 hours) (Fig. 18-1). NAC can be given orally (loading

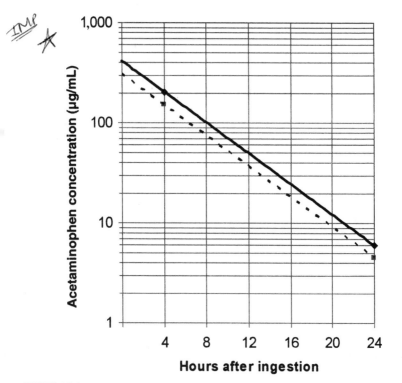

FIGURE 18-1. Acetaminophen toxicity nomogram. The area below the *dashed line* represents nontoxic ingestion. The area between the two lines is potentially toxic, and the area above the *solid line* is likely to be toxic. Treatment should be initiated for any level above the *dashed line*. (Adapted from Rumack BH, Matthews H. Acetaminophen poisoning. *Pediatrics* 1975;55:871–866, with permission.)

dose of 140 mg/kg followed by 70 mg/kg every 4 hours for a total of 17 doses) or intravenously (loading dose 150 mg/kg in 5% dextrose over 15 minutes; maintenance dose 50 mg/kg over 4 hours followed by 100 mg/kg over 16 hours). For ingestions that present late (>10 hours) a longer duration of intravenous (IV) treatment is recommended (loading dose, 140 mg/kg IV over 1 hour; maintenance, 70 mg/kg IV every 4 hours for 12 doses). Hypophosphatemia is a frequent finding in APAP-related liver injury and should be treated. In addition to APAP's effects on the liver, acute renal failure can occur independently of hepatic injury.

Drug-Induced Liver Injury

Drug-induced liver injury (DILI) encompasses a wide range of medication-related injuries. In some cases, the injuries reflect dose-dependent phenomena. More commonly, the effect may be idiosyncratic and occur independent of the dose or duration of exposure. Many of the specifics, particularly those regarding prognosis and treatment, of DILI are unique to the responsible medication. It is important to be particularly attuned to the development of jaundice because this sign is associated with case fatality rates of 10% to 50%. This prognostic indicator is known as "Hy's law" named after the hepatopathologist Hyman Zimmerman.

Autoimmune, Vascular, and Metabolic Disease

- **Autoimmune hepatitis** can present as an acute hepatitis with elevated transaminases, jaundice, and synthetic dysfunction. Typical serologic studies include the presence of antinuclear antibodies and elevated gamma globulins. The diagnosis can be substantiated by liver biopsy findings. Prompt treatment with oral prednisone 40 to 60 mg daily may prevent the development of ALF.
- Vascular events associated with the development of acute liver disease include **ischemic hepatopathy**; also known as "shock liver." This syndrome occurs after periods of profound systemic hypotension, particularly in those with preexisting hepatic venous congestion. The diagnosis is often apparent from the clinical context and is characterized by hypertransaminasemia that resolves rapidly with improvements in hemodynamics.
- The **Budd-Chiari syndrome** (hepatic venous thrombosis) should be suspected in patients with hepatomegaly, ascites, jaundice, and elevated aminotransferases. Hypercoagulable states, including those resulting from malignancy or myeloproliferative disorders, are frequently implicated as the cause. The diagnosis can be confirmed by radiographic imaging of the hepatic veins by Doppler ultrasonography or venography. Prompt venous decompression, either by placement of a transjugular portosystemic shunt (TIPS) or surgical shunting is the treatment; in the presence of liver failure, however, shunting should be avoided in favor of liver transplantation.
- **Wilson's disease** is a metabolic disorder of tissue copper overload that, although rare, is an important cause of ALF. The fulminant presentation of the disorder is very dramatic, often occurring in young women unaware that they have the disease. Clinical findings of the fulminant presentation include jaundice, coagulopathy, rapidly progressive renal failure, and a Coombs-negative hemolytic anemia. Aminotransferase elevations are typically modest and the alkaline phosphatase is either normal or below the lower limit of the reference range (alkaline phosphatase to bilirubin ratio <2). Serum ceruloplasmin is usually decreased and serum copper (including ceruloplasmin free serum copper) and 24-hour urinary copper excretion are increased. Prompt diagnosis is critical; although the fulminant presentation is often the first indication of disease, advanced liver disease is invariably present and liver transplantation is the only treatment option.

TABLE 18-1	GRADES OF ENCEPHALOPATHY

I Behavioral changes
II Disorientation, drowsiness, inappropriate behavior
III Confusion, somnolence but retained response to painful stimuli, incoherent speech
IV Comatose, unresponsive to noxious stimuli

ACUTE LIVER FAILURE

Acute liver failure is a syndrome characterized by jaundice, coagulopathy, and encephalopathy occurring within 26 weeks of first symptoms in individuals without preexisting liver disease. The acute presentation of Wilson's disease is also considered in this definition even though cirrhosis is commonly present. ALF is a dramatic illness with a high mortality rate. In comparison to decompensated cirrhosis, ALF is associated with hepatic collapse rather than fibrosis and complications of portal hypertension (varices, ascites) are uncommon. The treatment of ALF is mostly supportive, although in cases in which a cause is known, therapies should be directed at that proximate cause. These treatments include NAC for acetaminophen overdosage, silymarin or penicillin G for Amanita poisoning, antiviral therapy for acute hepatitis B, and corticosteroids for autoimmune hepatitis.

Treatment

- In the absence of an identifiable diagnosis and therapy, the treatment of ALF is directed at the syndrome's major complications. Evidence-based guidelines for the management of ALF have been published and are available at https://www.aasld.org/eweb/docs/practiceguidelines/Acuteliverfailure.pdf. Complications of ALF include **hepatic encephalopathy**, which is graded on a scale of I to IV (Table 18-1) for both acute and chronic liver disease. Grades I and II encephalopathy may be manifested by either agitation or somnolence. The initial evaluation should search for potential causes, such as structural lesions of the brain, infection, and hypoglycemia. Sedation should be avoided unless required to prevent self-harm. The patient should be observed in an intensive care unit and stimulation avoided.

- Progression to grade III and IV encephalopathy carries the risk of cerebral edema. With these higher grades of encephalopathy, tracheal intubation is appropriate for airway protection. The patient should rest with the head at 30 degrees and endotracheal suction should be minimized. The necessity of intracranial pressure monitoring is controversial, although general agreement is that it be utilized for liver transplant candidates. Frequent assessment of neurologic function is needed, particularly looking for signs of impending uncal herniation.

- If cerebral edema develops, prompt treatment is required. Intravenous mannitol (0.5 to 1 g/kg), hyperventilation to $PaCO_2$ 25 to 30 mm Hg, moderate hypothermia (32°C–34°C), and maintenance of a hypertonic state (either by permissive hypernatremia or by hypertonic sodium chloride infusions to maintain serum sodium of 145–155 mEq/L) are all potential treatment strategies. Although lactulose is the mainstay of treatment of hepatic encephalopathy in cirrhosis, its role in ALF is not established and the resulting gaseous abdominal distention from its use may complicate liver transplantation. Seizure activity should be controlled with phenytoin. (anti-convulsant).

- **Renal failure** is common and usually multifactorial in origin, with poor perfusion from septic shock or volume depletion. Maintenance of renal perfusion and avoidance of nephrotoxic agents are imperative. If all reversible causes of renal failure have been addressed and renal failure persists, then the patient likely has an acute form of the hepatorenal syndrome. If the patient survives to transplantation, renal function usually returns to normal.

- **Hypoglycemia** is frequently seen because of poor hepatic glucose production and consumption of glycogen stores and may be refractory to IV dextrose. Regular blood glucose monitoring should be performed.
- **Acid-base disturbances** may be seen, especially metabolic acidosis in acetaminophen overdose, lactic acidosis, or renal failure, or alkalosis secondary to hyperventilation. Hypophosphatemia and hypomagnesemia are also frequently seen.
- **Coagulopathy** is secondary to poor synthesis of clotting factors, particularly factor VII, leading to an elevated prothrombin time (PT). Patients with severe liver failure often do not respond to vitamin K, although supplementation can be attempted with 10 mg subcutaneously daily for 3 days. Fresh frozen plasma (FFP) should be used for bleeding or before invasive procedures. Recombinant activated factor VII (rFVIIa) 90 μg/kg body weight can also be used in treating the coagulopathy of ALF, particularly in the setting of renal failure in which the excessive administration of FFP may result in volume overload.
- **Infection** is commonly seen in ALF because of the impaired reticuloendothelial system, decreased opsonization, and the frequent need for indwelling catheters and tracheal intubation. A high index of suspicion for infection is critical, with appropriate use of tissue culture and empiric antibiotic therapy as necessary.

Liver Transplantation

Liver transplantation is the ultimate therapy for those with acute liver failure. Several criteria have been proposed to identify those unlikely to recover spontaneously and in whom liver transplantation would be lifesaving. The King's College Criteria are most commonly used (Table 18-2). In the United States, patients with ALF listed for transplantation are given United Network for Organ Sharing status 1, which permits them to receive organ donation ahead of those with chronic liver failure.

TABLE 18-2 KINGS COLLEGE CRITERIA (for transplant in ALF).

Acetaminophen induced
Arterial pH <7.3
    OR
All three of the following
    Prothrombin time >100 seconds (INR >6.5)
    Serum creatinine >3.4 mg/dL
    Grade III or IV encephalopathy

Nonacetaminophen induced
INR >6.5 irrespective of coma grade
        OR
Three of the following five criteria
    Patient age <10 years or >40 years
    Serum bilirubin >17.5 mg/dL
    Prothrombin time >50 seconds (INR ≥3.5)
    Unfavorable cause (seronegative hepatitis or DILI)
    Jaundice >7 days before encephalopathy

DILI, drug-induced liver injury; INR, international normalized ratio.

KEY POINTS TO REMEMBER

- There are many causes of acute hepatitis. The most common causes are from viruses and toxic (alcohol or medication) exposures.
- Among the viral causes, HAV and HBV are the two viruses most commonly associated with symptomatic acute infection. The management of most cases is supportive; however, a small percentage of acutely infected patients are at risk for ALF. Vaccination and postexposure prophylaxis are available for both viruses.
- Alcohol can cause a wide spectrum of liver disease, including acute alcoholic hepatitis. The severity of the acute alcoholic hepatitis is determined by the Maddrey Discriminant Function, and scores >32 are associated with high rates of mortality. Treatments for alcoholic hepatitis include supportive care, corticosteroids, and pentoxifylline.
- Significant hepatic injury from acetaminophen generally requires ingestions above a threshold value of 150 mg/kg body weight. Chronic, excessive alcohol use may predispose to liver injury.
- Acetaminophen levels should be drawn >4 hours after ingestion plotted on the Rumack-Matthews nomogram. For patients falling into the potentially toxic range, treatment with NAC should be initiated.
- Drug-induced liver injury is a common cause of acute liver disease. The development of jaundice from a medication-related injury is associated with increased mortality rate.
- ALF is a syndrome characterized by jaundice, coagulopathy, and encephalopathy occurring within 26 weeks of first symptoms in individuals without preexisting liver disease.
- The King's College Criteria can be used a guide to help identify those unlikely to recover spontaneously and in whom liver transplantation would be lifesaving.

REFERENCES AND SUGGESTED READINGS

Jaeckel E, Cornberg M, Wedemeyer H, et al. Treatment of acute hepatitis C with interferon alfa-2b. *N Engl J Med* 2001;345:1452–1457.

Korenblat KM, Dienstag JL. Viral hepatitis. In: Richman DD, Whitley RJ, Hayden FG, eds. *Clinical Virology*. Washington, DC: ASM Press; 2002:59–77.

Lee WM. Acute liver failure in the United States. *Semin Liver Dis* 2003;23:217–226.

Lee WM. Drug-induced hepatotoxicity. *N Engl J Med* 2003;349:474–485.

McCullough AJ, O'Connor JF. Alcoholic liver disease: proposed recommendations for the American College of Gastroenterology. *Am J Gastroenterol* 1998;93:2022–2036.

Murphy N, Auzinger G, Bernel W, et al. The effect of hypertonic sodium chloride on intracranial pressure in patients with acute liver failure. *Hepatology* 2004;39:464–470.

O'Grady J, Alexander G, Hayllar K, et al. Early indicators of prognosis in fulminant hepatic failure. *Gastroenterology* 1989;97(2):439–445.

Polson J, Lee WM. AASLD position paper: the management of acute liver failure. *Hepatology* 2005;41:1179–1197.

Rumack BH. Acetaminophen misconceptions. *Hepatology* 2004;40:10–15.

Chronic Liver Disease

Pari M. Shah and Mauricio Lisker-Melman

CHRONIC VIRAL HEPATITIS

Chronic viral hepatitis is defined by the persistence of viral infection for longer than 6 months resulting in liver necroinflammatory and fibrotic changes, which can lead to cirrhosis. Histopathologic classification of chronic liver disease is based on etiology, grade, and stage, with grade representing the severity of necroinflammatory changes and stage representing the severity of fibrosis. The two most frequent viruses that result in chronic hepatitis are the hepatitis B virus (HBV) and the hepatitis C virus (HCV).

CHRONIC HEPATITIS B

Introduction

- While 2 billion people worldwide have been in contact with the HBV, 350 million people are chronic carriers. Chronic carriers are positive for hepatitis B surface antigen (HBsAg) for longer than 6 months. Infection with HBV can result in acute disease, chronic hepatitis, inactive carrier state, or resolved hepatitis. Patients with hepatitis B can have a fluctuating disease course and may progress from one stage to another. Approximately 30% of all patients with chronic hepatitis B infection will have progressive liver fibrosis and develop cirrhosis with complications of end-stage liver disease (ESLD). Chronic HBV infection is associated with approximately 15% of all hepatocellular carcinomas (HCC) in the United States. HBV infection can be prevented with vaccination.
- The HBV has a DNA genome and belongs to the *Hepadnavirus* family. In endemic world regions, such as Asia and sub-Saharan Africa, hepatitis B infection is acquired from mother to child (vertical transmission), whereas in Western countries, where chronic hepatitis B is relatively rare, infection is acquired in adulthood from adult to adult (horizontal transmission). Infection is transmitted through **parenteral routes** (e.g., needle stick, injection drug use, and blood transfusions), **sexual contact**, or **perinatal transmission**. High-risk groups include individuals with a history of multiple blood transfusions, hemodialysis patients, health care workers, men having sex with men, patients with a history of sexual promiscuity, intravenous (IV) drug users, residents and employees of residential care facilities, travelers to endemic areas (>6 months), and natives of Alaska, Asia, or the Pacific Islands.

Clinical Presentation

- Chronic hepatitis B infection is generally defined with the following characteristics: HBsAg positive for more than 6 months, serum HBV DNA >20,000 IU/mL (although lower levels can be seen in patients with HBeAg-negative chronic hepatitis B), persistent or intermittent elevation in alanine aminotransferase (ALT) or aspartate aminotransferase (AST) levels, and liver biopsy showing chronic hepatitis with moderate or severe necroinflammation and fibrosis.

- Chronic hepatitis B usually courses with few nonspecific symptoms until complications develop from cirrhosis or HCC. Approximately 30% of all patients with chronic HBV will develop cirrhosis and 5% to 10% of all patients with chronic HBV will develop HCC with or without cirrhosis. Risk factors for HCC development include high viral replication, male gender, older age, presence of HBeAg, presence of cirrhosis, HBV genotype C, core promoter mutation, and coinfection with HCV.

- Patients with chronic hepatitis B may also have immune-mediated **extrahepatic manifestations,** including polyarteritis nodosa, glomerulonephritis, cryoglobulinemia vasculitis, serum sickness-like illness, papular acrodermatitis (predominantly in children), and aplastic anemia. Approximately 1% patients with chronic hepatitis B will spontaneously clear HBsAg annually.

Diagnosis

- Diagnosis of chronic hepatitis B is based on the detection of antigens of the hepatitis B virus or their corresponding antibodies and HBV DNA. Additional testing includes genotype and liver biopsy.
- Patients with chronic HBV infection are evaluated for the presence or absence of markers of infection. These markers include the following:
  - **Hepatitis B surface antigen (HBsAg)** is detectable in serum or hepatocyte cytoplasm (immunoperoxidase staining) in acute or chronic HBV infection and disappears if the virus is cleared. The persistence of HBsAg is the diagnostic hallmark of chronic HBV infection.
  - **Antibody against HBsAg (anti-HBs)** appears after the disappearance of HBsAg and after vaccination. The presence of anti-HBs demonstrates clearance or immunity to the disease. In rare cases of chronic hepatitis B, low titers of heterotypic anti-HBs can be present.
  - **Hepatitis B core antigen (HBcAg)** is not detectable in serum but can be found in the hepatocyte nuclei by immunoperoxidase staining during active viral replication.
  - **IgM Antibody against HBcAg (IgM anti-HBc)** is usually present in acute infection and during periods of high viral replication in chronic disease (flares).
  - **IgG Antibody against HBcAg (IgG anti-HBc)** is usually present in patients with chronic disease and in conjunction with anti-HBs in patients who have had acute hepatitis B and cleared the disease. In rare cases, patients with isolated IgG anti-HBc can activate the HBV after immunosuppression.
  - **Hepatitis B e antigen (HBeAg)** appears in the serum shortly after HBsAg and its persistence is indicative of active viral replication and high infectivity. Patients harboring HBV infection with precore or basal core promoter mutations are HBeAg negative despite high viral replication.
  - **Antibody against HBeAg (anti-HBe)** usually indicates low level of replication and a lower degree of infectivity. The best known exception is the patient infected with precore or basal core promoter mutations (HBeAg negative but anti-HBe positive).
  - **HBV DNA is the most accurate and sensitive marker of viral replication.** It is detected by polymerase chain reaction (PCR) and reported as international units per milliliter (IU/mL).
- Based on these markers, patients with chronic HBV infection can be subdivided into one of the following clinical profiles:
  - **Immune tolerant** is generally seen in patients with perinatally acquired infection. Patients generally have subclinical or mild disease and normal ALT levels.

Within this clinical profile, HBV is actively replicating. HBV DNA and HBeAg are present, usually in high titer. Liver biopsy will generally be normal or with mild inflammatory changes. Some of these patients may clinically and histologically develop active liver disease later in life.

- **HBeAg positive chronic hepatitis B** is characterized by active liver disease with elevated ALT levels, high viral load ($>10^5$ IU/mL), and progressive necroinflammation and fibrosis on liver biopsy.
- **HBeAg negative chronic hepatitis B** is characterized by precore or basal core promoter mutations with defective production of HBeAg (HBeAg negative). These patients have increased HBV DNA levels, although generally lower levels than HBeAg-positive patients, and persistently elevated ALT levels with active and progressive liver histology. Generally, HBeAg-negative patients are older and have more advanced liver disease.
- **Inactive HBsAg carrier** is characterized by the loss of HBeAg and seroconversion to anti-HBe. In this clinical group, HBV DNA levels typically fall to $<10^3$ IU/mL. HBsAg persists, but ALT levels and liver histology return to normal.
- Patients with previously known hepatitis B in the presence of positive anti-HBc and anti-HBs, with normal levels of ALT, undetectable serum HBV DNA, and negative HBsAg are diagnosed with **resolved hepatitis B**.

- **Genotype determination** of HBV is slowly becoming a standard marker in clinical practice and its clinical significance is growing. **Liver biopsy** is useful in determining the degree of inflammation (grade) and fibrosis (stage) in patients with chronic hepatitis B.

Treatment

- Treatment of chronic HBV infection is targeted at the following goals: clearance of HBV DNA, HBeAg and HBsAg seroconversion, normalization of serum ALT, and normalization of liver histology.
- Treatment should be considered in **HBeAg-positive** patients if ALT levels are elevated (ideally >2 times the upper limit of normal) and HBV DNA is $>20,000$ IU/mL. Treatment should be considered in **HBeAg-negative** patients if ALT levels are elevated (ideally >2 times the upper limit of normal) and HBV DNA is >2000 IU/mL. Patients with less elevated ALT levels or persistently elevated DNA levels should be evaluated for possible treatment on a case-by-case basis. Liver biopsy may be useful in this clinical setting to evaluate extent of necroinflammatory changes and fibrosis. Patients with moderate or severe inflammation or significant fibrosis may benefit from treatment. HBV carriers who are at high risk for HCC should be screened every 6 to 12 months with ultrasound and α-fetoprotein.
- Current treatment options include **interferon (IFN) therapy** or **nucleoside or nucleotide analogs**. The IFN are glycoproteins with antiviral, immunomodulatory, and antiproliferative actions. The addition of polyethylene glycol (PEG) to the standard IFN (α2a or α2b) molecules results in prolonged half-life with improved bioavailability. IFN-α2a or IFN-α2b is administered subcutaneously three times per week for 4 to 6 months or peginterferon-alfa (PEG IFN-α) is administered once a week for 48 weeks. HBeAg seroconversion occurs in 30% of treated patients. HBsAg seroconversion occurs in 5% to 10% of patients. No antiviral-resistance mutations are induced with these medications. Interferon is contraindicated in patients with decompensated liver disease. Side effects include a flu-like syndrome (headache, fatigue, myalgias, arthralgias, fever, and chills), neuropsychiatric disorders (depression, irritability, and concentration impairment), reversible bone marrow suppression, and other effects (alopecia, thyroiditis, injection site reactions).

- Nucleoside or nucleotide analogs are better tolerated than IFN-based therapy; however, the major concern for long-term use of these agents is the selection of antiviral-resistant mutations.
  - **Lamivudine** is a nucleoside analog with antiviral activity. It is administered orally at 100 mg daily. Treatment success is proportional to treatment duration. This medication is safe to use in patients with advanced or decompensated liver disease. The high rate (15%–20%/year of treatment) of induction of antiviral-resistant mutations has led to diminished use of this medication as monotherapy.
  - **Adefovir** is a nucleotide analog with antiviral activity. It is administered orally at 10 mg daily. Treatment success is proportional to treatment duration. Clinical studies have shown that adefovir can be used successfully to treat naïve and lamivudine-resistant HBV. Dose adjustment is needed in patients with renal disease. Approximately 15% to 29% of patients who are nucleotide naïve will develop resistance after 4 to 5 years of treatment. The use of adefovir and lamivudine in combination leads to a significant reduction of adefovir-induced, antiviral-resistant mutations.
  - **Entecavir** is a nucleoside analog with potent antiviral activity. It is administered orally at 0.5 mg daily in treatment naïve patients and 1 mg daily in patients with known lamivudine resistance. Dose adjustment is needed in patients with renal disease. Resistance mutations are very rare in entecavir-naïve patients after 3 years of treatment. In patients with lamivudine resistance, resistant mutations to entecavir will develop in about 40% of patients after 4 years of therapy.
  - **Telbivudine** is a nucleoside analog. It was recently U.S. Food and Drug Administration (FDA)-approved for treatment of HBV in the United States. Preliminary data report good antiviral activity with a moderate rate of resistant mutations at 2 years of therapy (HBeAg positive 21%, HBeAg negative 9%).
  - Other newer therapies are investigated in clinical trials. Emtricitabine is a potent inhibitor of human immunodeficiency virus (HIV) and HBV replication and has been approved for treatment of HIV. Initial studies suggest promising HBV response to this treatment; however, because of its structural similarity to lamivudine, emtricitabine selects for the same resistant mutations. Tenofovir is a nucleotide analog used for the treatment of HIV. Tenofovir is structurally similar to adefovir and clinical studies suggest promising activity against HBV with possible increased efficacy and lower induction of antiviral-resistant mutations when directly compared with adefovir. Clevudine is a pyrimidine nucleoside analog that is effective in inhibiting HBV replication in animal models. Clinical studies have shown promising results with significant decline in HBV DNA levels and longer durability of viral suppression.
- **Liver transplantation** is indicated in patients with decompensated cirrhosis caused by HBV. Given that there can be recurrence after transplant, immunoprophylaxis with hepatitis B immunoglobulin (HBIg) combined with a nucleoside or nucleotide analog is used to diminish this possibility.

Prophylaxis

- **Pre-exposure prophylaxis** with HBV vaccine should be considered for everyone, but particularly for individuals with a history of multiple blood transfusions, patients on hemodialysis, health care workers, injection drug users, household and heterosexual contacts of hepatitis B carriers, men having sex with men, residents and employees of residential care facilities, travelers to hyperendemic areas, and natives of Alaska, Asia, and the Pacific Islands. The Centers for Disease Control recommends universal vaccination programs for infants and sexually active adolescents in the United States. Vaccination is administered as a three-shot series at time 0, 1, and 6 months. For patients who require rapid immunity, vaccination can be administered at 0, 1, and 2 months with a follow-up booster shot at 6 months for long-lasting immunity.

Additional doses, higher doses, or revaccination can be considered in nonresponders and hyporesponders (anti-HBs <10 IU/mL) to elicit protective anti-HBs levels and long-lasting immunity. Booster doses may be needed in immunocompromised individuals in whom anti-HBs levels fall below 10 IU/mL on annual testing.

- **Postexposure prophylaxis** should be considered in infants born to HBsAg-positive mothers. Newborns should receive HBV vaccine and HBIg within 12 hours of birth. Immunized infants should be tested at 12 months of age for HBsAg, anti-HBs, and anti-HBc. Susceptible sexual partners and needle-stick injuries with HBV contamination should receive HBIg (0.04–0.07 mL/kg) and the first dose of HBV vaccine at different body sites as soon as possible. A second dose of HBIg should be administered at 30 days postexposure and the vaccine series should be completed.

CHRONIC HEPATITIS C

Introduction

- Approximately 200 million carriers of hepatitis C virus (HCV) are found worldwide. In the United States, about 3 million people have chronic hepatitis C and 8000 to 10,000 people die annually of HCV-related cirrhosis and hepatocellular carcinoma. Chronic liver disease secondary to HCV is the leading indication for liver transplantation in the United States.
- Hepatitis C virus is an RNA virus that belongs to the *Flaviviridae* family. HCV is transmitted **parenterally** via transfusion, injection drug use, or needle-stick injury, and less frequently through **sexual** or **vertical transmission** (from mother to child). Risk factors for HCV infection include a history of multiple blood transfusions, hemodialysis, injection drug use, use of intranasal cocaine, tattooing, body piercing, multiple sexual partners, and occupational exposure. In the United States, injection drug use is the leading mode of transmission.

Clinical Presentation

- The incubation period after exposure to HCV is 15 to 150 days. Children and young adults are more likely to have silent presentation. Symptoms can include malaise, fatigue, pruritus, headaches, abdominal pain, myalgias, arthralgias, nausea, vomiting, anorexia, and fever. Of patients infected with HCV, 15% will experience spontaneous resolution, whereas chronic hepatitis infection will occur in approximately 85% of infected individuals. **Chronic hepatitis** has an indolent clinical course with fatigue as the most common symptom. Approximately 25% of patients with chronic HCV will develop cirrhosis over two to three decades of life, and 30% of persons with HCV-related cirrhosis will develop ESLD over a 10-year period. Risk factors for the development of cirrhosis include male gender, older age, drinking more than 50 g of alcohol per day, obesity or hepatic steatosis, and HIV coinfection. HCC develops in 1% to 2% of patients per year and rarely occurs in the absence of cirrhosis.
- **Extrahepatic manifestations** of hepatitis C include mixed cryoglobulinemia vasculitis (10%–25% of patients with HCV), glomerulonephritis, porphyria cutanea tarda, cutaneous necrotizing vasculitis, lichen planus, lymphoma, and other autoimmune diseases. The result of induction of abnormal circulating proteins, mixed cryoglobulinemia vasculitis presents with skin manifestations and internal organ damage, predominantly involving the kidneys.

Diagnosis

Diagnosis of HCV infection is based on the presence of antibodies against HCV (anti-HCV) and confirmed with the detection of HCV RNA. Anti-HCV antibodies may be undetectable for the first 8 weeks after infection and diagnosis of **acute HCV** must be made with HCV RNA in this time frame. A **false–positive anti-HCV** result can be seen in the setting of hypergammaglobulinemia or autoimmune hepatitis. A **false–negative** test finding may be seen in patients who are immunocompromised or on hemodialysis. HCV RNA can be detected with PCR amplification of serum as early as 1 to 2 weeks after infection. Different HCV RNA assays are available and vary in sensitivity and specificity. This test is useful both for diagnosis and for assessment of sustained virologic response after treatment. **HCV genotype** determination influences the duration, dosage, and predicted response to treatment. Genotype 1 accounts for 75% of infections in the United States and generally has a poorer susceptibility to treatment. Genotypes 2 and 3 account for 20% of HCV infection in the United States and generally are more treatment sensitive. **Liver biopsy** is most useful in determining the grade (degree of inflammation) and stage (degree of fibrosis) of liver disease. In some patients, this information may be helpful in determining when to start therapy and as a prognosis adjuvant. In most studies, extent of liver fibrosis is an independent predictor of treatment response. Most clinicians routinely obtain liver biopsy in patients with genotype 1 to guide treatment, whereas they may not obtain liver biopsy in all patients with genotypes 2 and 3.

Treatment

- The goal of treatment is to clear the hepatitis C virus and prevent complications of chronic HCV infection, including cirrhosis, HCC, and ESLD. Treatment response is assessed by following virologic response. **Sustained virologic response (SVR)** is defined as undetectable HCV RNA levels 6 months after treatment discontinuation. Infection is considered eradicated when an SVR is obtained. SVR is generally achieved in 55% of all patients who are treated. **Early virologic response (EVR)** is defined as a 2-log drop or an undetectable HCV RNA level 12 weeks into therapy. EVR can be used to predict whether an SVR will be obtained. In clinical studies, 97% to 100% of patients who failed to obtain an EVR did not obtain an SVR. Approximately 65% to 75% of patients who demonstrated an EVR subsequently achieved an SVR. In addition to EVR, patients are also evaluated for response at 4 weeks after the initiation of treatment; **rapid virologic response (RVR)** is defined as undetectable HCV RNA levels at 4 weeks of therapy. RVR is increasingly being used to predict treatment outcomes and may replace the use of EVR. **End of treatment response (ETR)** is defined as undetectable HCV RNA levels at the termination of treatment.

- **Nonresponders** are patients whose HCV RNA levels remain unchanged despite antiviral therapy. **Partial responders** are patients whose HCV RNA levels decline on therapy by >2 logs, but never become undetectable. When a patient develops detectable HCV RNA levels after an initial positive response to treatment, **relapse** is diagnosed. Many of these individuals will generally achieve re-response after a second course of treatment.

- Chronic HCV infection is optimally treated with a combination of **subcutaneous pegylated-interferon (PEG-IFN) and oral ribavirin** (800–1200 mg/day) for a period of 6 to 12 months. Peginterferon α-2a at 180 μg/week and peginterferon α-2b at 1.5 μg/kg/week are both efficacious. Side effects to IFN include flu-like syndrome (headache, fatigue, myalgias, arthralgias, fever, and chills), neuropsychiatric disorders (depression, irritability, and concentration impairment), reversible bone marrow suppression, and other effects (alopecia, thyroiditis, injection site reactions). Interferon is contraindicated in patients with decompensated liver disease. Side effects to ribavirin include teratogenicity, hemolytic anemia, and pulmonary symptoms. Contraindications include pregnancy, chronic renal insufficiency, and inability to tolerate anemia.

- **Specifically targeted antiviral therapies** for hepatitis C are in different phases of clinical development and include proteases, nucleoside, and non-nucleoside agents. Most likely, these new agents will be used in combination with standard of care treatments, including PEG-IFN and ribavirin.
- Treatment outcomes are based on clinical status (acute versus chronic), HCV genotype, viral load at initiation of therapy, and degree of fibrosis. Genotype 1 HCV infection is less susceptible to treatment and requires 12 months of therapy and an estimated 35% to 45% of patients achieve an SVR. Genotypes 2 and 3 are more susceptible to treatment and usually require 6 months of therapy with an estimated 80% to 85% of patients achieving an SVR.
- **Liver transplantation** may be indicated in patients with advanced viral disease and manifestations of cirrhosis refractory to treatment. HCV is the most common indication for liver transplantation in the United States at present. Disease recurrence after transplantation is frequent.

★ hep C = most common reason for liver transplant.

ALCOHOLIC LIVER DISEASE

Introduction

- Liver toxicity induced by alcohol generates a spectrum of different liver disease entities. A single patient can be affected by more than one of the following conditions: **alcoholic fatty liver, alcoholic hepatitis, or alcoholic cirrhosis.** Only 10% to 20% of chronic alcohol users (over a decade of alcohol consumption) will develop significant liver damage. Fatty liver disease, the most common manifestation of alcoholic liver disease, is present in 90% of chronic alcohol users. Cirrhosis and HCC are common causes of ESLD attributable to chronic alcohol intake.
- Average alcohol consumption can be measured in units per week. One unit is equal to 7 g of alcohol, one glass of wine, or one 240-mL can of 3.5% to 4% beer. Approximately 30 to 40 units per week can result in cirrhosis in 3% to 8% of patients with >12 years of alcohol use. Alcoholic liver disease can develop at much lower doses in women and in patients with chronic hepatitis C infection. It has been estimated that 90% to 100% of heavy drinkers will show evidence of fatty liver disease; however, only 10% to 35% will develop alcoholic hepatitis and 8% to 20% will develop cirrhosis.

Clinical Presentation

- Clinical presentation varies by diagnosis at the time of presentation. In **fatty liver disease,** patients are usually asymptomatic. Clinical findings include hepatosplenomegaly and mildly elevated alkaline phosphatase and liver enzymes. Fatty liver disease may be reversible with abstinence.
- **Alcoholic hepatitis,** which is defined as the presence of hepatic inflammation, presents with a spectrum of clinical consequences. Patients may have clinically silent disease or severe disease with rapid development of hepatic failure and death. Clinical findings include fever, right upper quadrant abdominal pain, anorexia, nausea, vomiting, weight loss, and jaundice. In severe cases, patients may develop hepatic encephalopathy, ascites, and gastrointestinal (GI) bleeding. Patients frequently give a history of drinking up until the onset of symptoms. Short- and long-term prognosis depends on the severity of presentation and the degree of alcohol abstinence, respectively. In-hospital mortality is as high as 50% for severe cases.
- Patients with **alcoholic cirrhosis** may present with clinically silent disease or with decompensated cirrhosis and complications of portal hypertension, including ascites, hepatic encephalopathy, or GI bleeding. Patients have a history of current or past long-term drinking. Prognosis is variable and depends on the degree of decompensation, alcohol abstinence, and availability of treatment options.

Diagnosis

- All patients should be screened for alcoholic liver disease with a thorough history of drinking and sometimes with random alcohol levels. The CAGE questionnaire can be helpful to screen patients for alcohol dependency. The CAGE questionnaire consists of the following four questions: (1) Have you ever felt you needed to Cut down on your drinking? (2) Have people Annoyed you by criticizing your drinking? (3) Have you ever felt Guilty about drinking? (4) Have you ever felt you needed a drink first thing in the morning (Eye-opener) to steady your nerves or to get rid of a hangover? Two "yes" responses indicates a need to evaluate the patient further.
- Diagnosis is based on clinical findings, liver enzymes, and sometimes liver biopsy. Patients with alcoholic hepatitis generally present with a hepatocellular pattern of liver damage with enzyme elevation including AST greater than ALT. Patients may additionally have a cholestatic picture characterized by elevated alkaline phosphatase (AP) and total bilirubin (predominantly conjugated) or abnormal coagulation parameters. Patients have poorer prognosis with renal failure, leukocytosis, marked cholestasis, and coagulopathy that does not improve with vitamin K administration. In alcoholic cirrhosis, liver abnormalities vary with disease severity.

- A **discriminant function** (DF) can be determined to assess in-hospital mortality. DF = 4.6 × (PTpatient − PTcontrol) + serum total bilirubin. DF >32 is associated with poor prognosis. Liver biopsy is rarely indicated during the acute phase of alcoholic hepatitis. In later stages, it may be used to assess the extent of liver damage. In alcoholic liver disease, typical histology includes Mallory hyaline bodies, neutrophilic infiltrate, necrosis of hepatocytes, collagen deposition, and fatty change.

Treatment

- **Abstinence from alcohol is the hallmark of treatment.** Treatment in alcoholic liver disease also includes nutritional support. In the absence of hepatic encephalopathy or a nonfunctioning GI tract, enteral feeding should be administered. In patients with hepatic encephalopathy or gastric ileus, total parenteral nutrition (TPN) should be given and has been shown to confer a mortality benefit. Treatment of alcoholic hepatitis with corticosteroids is controversial. Evidence suggests, however, that patients with a DF >32 and hepatic encephalopathy may benefit from steroid therapy. Oral prednisone can be started at 40 to 60 mg/day and subsequently tapered as clinically indicated. Treatment with pentoxifylline 400 mg PO TID, a nonselective phosphodiesterase inhibitor with anti-inflammatory properties, has been shown to improve survival in severe (DF >32) alcoholic hepatitis. Treatment with S-adenosylmethionine, antioxidants, tumor necrosis factor (TNF) inhibitors, and glutathione prodrugs are under investigation.
- Liver transplant is indicated for patients with advanced liver disease from alcohol. Patients, however, are required to be abstinent from alcohol for a minimum of 6 months and under rehabilitation before candidacy is considered.

AUTOIMMUNE LIVER DISEASE

Autoimmune liver disease encompasses a spectrum of illnesses, including autoimmune hepatitis, primary sclerosing cholangitis, primary biliary cirrhosis, and overlap syndromes. These diseases have varying presentations and the diagnosis is often challenging to the physician. Patients with autoimmune liver disease may also have other nonhepatic autoimmune illnesses at the same time.

Autoimmune Hepatitis

Introduction

- Autoimmune hepatitis (AIH) is a chronic inflammatory disease of the liver with no known cause. Ongoing inflammation results in progressive fibrosis and cirrhosis. AIH is associated with circulating auto-antibodies and hypergammaglobulinemia.
- Autoimmune hepatitis occurs worldwide. It occurs most commonly in women aged 10 to 30 years and after the age of 60 years. In the United States, cirrhosis is the initial clinical presentation more commonly in black than in white patients. Approximately 20% of patients will present with a clinical picture of AIH after the age of 60 years. These patients generally have greater degree of fibrosis, cirrhosis, and a higher frequency of ascites at the time of presentation. Additionally, these patients are generally more responsive to treatment. Genetic studies have demonstrated different HLA antigen alleles in the older population versus the younger population, indicating that genetic factors may influence the varying presentation of AIH in different age groups.

Clinical Presentation

- Clinical presentation may vary at initial diagnosis. In approximately 30% of cases, the clinical presentation is acute with symptoms similar to viral hepatitis. Patients may present with asymptomatic elevation of serum ALT or may present in fulminant hepatic failure. In 25% of patients, AIH will present as cirrhosis. The most common symptoms at presentation include fatigue, jaundice, myalgias, anorexia, diarrhea, acne, menstrual abnormalities, and right upper quadrant abdominal pain.
- Extrahepatic manifestations may be found in 30% to 50% of patients and they include celiac sprue, Coombs' positive hemolytic anemia, autoimmune thyroiditis, Graves' disease, rheumatoid arthritis, ulcerative colitis, and others. Patients with AIH may also have findings consistent with other liver diseases (e.g., primary biliary cirrhosis [PBC], primary sclerosing cholangitis [PSC], autoimmune cholangitis).

Diagnosis

- Diagnosis is made by detection of elevated serum aminotransferases, circulating autoantibodies, elevated immunoglobulin levels, and liver biopsy. The most commonly elevated antibodies include: **antinuclear antibody (ANA), smooth muscle antibody (SMA), and liver-kidney microsomal antibody (LKMA)**. Hypergammaglobulinemia can also be detected.
- Liver biopsy is essential for the diagnosis of AIH. "Piecemeal necrosis" or interface hepatitis with lobular or panacinar inflammation along with lymphocytic and plasmacytic infiltration are the histologic hallmarks. Liver biopsy may also demonstrate bridging necrosis or fibrosis or well-developed cirrhosis.

Treatment

- Treatment is directed at achieving remission of disease. Therapy is initiated with **prednisone** (40–60 mg/day) alone or prednisone with **azathioprine** (1–2 mg/kg/day). Prednisone is tapered when biochemical and clinical improvement is noted. Some patients require lifelong low-dose prednisone and azathioprine therapy. Remission (normalization of serum bilirubin, immunoglobulin levels, AST, ALT; disappearance of symptoms; resolution of histologic changes) occurs in 65% of patients within 1 year and 80% within 3 years. Relapses occur in 20% to 50% of patients after cessation of therapy. Refractory disease may require "salvage" therapy with cyclosporine, tacrolimus, or mycophenolate mofetil.
- Liver transplantation is considered for patients with decompensated cirrhosis. After transplantation, recurrent AIH is seen in 17% of patients. De novo AIH (AIH in patients receiving transplant for non-autoimmune diseases) is seen in 3% to 5% of transplant recipients.

Primary Sclerosing Cholangitis

Introduction

- Primary sclerosing cholangitis (PSC) is a cholestatic liver disorder characterized by chronic inflammation and fibrosis resulting in progressive destruction of the extrahepatic and intrahepatic biliary duct system and ultimately in cirrhosis. PSC is frequently associated with inflammatory bowel disease (IBD).
- Primary sclerosing cholangitis occurs mainly in the fourth or fifth decade of life in adults and is more frequent in men than in women. PSC is frequently associated with IBD, although the clinical course of one has no correlation with the clinical course of the other. In the United States, 70% of patients with PSC have ulcerative colitis and approximately 2% to 4% of patients with IBD have PSC. Genetic associations have been described in PSC and complex family inheritance patterns have been demonstrated. A 100-fold increased risk of PSC exists among siblings.

Clinical Presentation

Classic clinical manifestations include intermittent episodes of jaundice, hepatomegaly, pruritis, weight loss, and fatigue in a patient with ulcerative colitis. As many as 30% of patients will develop cholangitis; this complication presents in patients with severe biliary duct strictures caused by inflammation and fibrosis. Cirrhosis can occur with disease progression. Cholangiocarcinoma can occur in 6% to 20% of patients with PSC and may occur before the onset of cirrhosis. Patients with PSC can be subdivided into those with small duct disease versus patients with large duct disease. Approximately 75% of patients have involvement with both; 15% have small duct disease affecting bile ducts that are too small to see with endoscopic retrograde cholangiopancreatography (ERCP) and 10% have large duct disease. Patients with small duct disease have a more favorable prognosis. Patients with PSC may also have concomitant features of autoimmune hepatitis.

Diagnosis

Diagnosis is supported by liver chemistry, imaging to visualize the biliary tree, and sometimes with liver biopsy. **Alkaline phosphatase** is the most commonly elevated liver test. ALT and AST are often elevated to lesser degrees. Patients with IBD and increased AP should be evaluated for PSC even in the absence of symptoms. ANA is positive in up to 50% of cases and **perinuclear antineutrophil cytoplasmic antibody (p-ANCA)** is positive in 80% of cases. PSC is confirmed by demonstration of multiple strictures or irregularities of the intrahepatic or extrahepatic bile ducts by **ERCP or magnetic resonance cholangiopancreatography (MRCP)**. Liver biopsy can be helpful in the diagnosis of small duct PSC and in excluding other diagnoses. Characteristic findings include concentric periductal fibrosis ("onion-skinning") that progresses to narrowing and obliteration of small bile ducts.

Treatment

- High-dose **ursodeoxycholic acid** (20–25 mg/kg) may be beneficial in reducing ductal damage and liver fibrosis. Episodes of cholangitis require antibiotics and may require endoscopic therapy to dilate or stent dominant biliary duct strictures. Other therapies under research include TNF inhibitors, antifibrotic agents, and inhibitors of formation of toxic bile.
- Liver transplantation is a treatment alternative in patients with advanced disease or recurrent cholangitis. In the United States, 5% of all liver transplants are for patients with PSC. With a few exceptions, cholangiocarcinoma is considered a contraindication for liver transplantation. Recurrent PSC after liver transplantation has been documented.

Primary Biliary Cirrhosis

Introduction
- Primary biliary cirrhosis (PBC) is a cholestatic liver disorder of unknown etiology with autoimmune features. In patients with PBC, granulomatous destruction of interlobular bile ducts results in progressive ductopenia, cholestasis, fibrosis, and cirrhosis.
- Primary biliary cirrhosis most commonly affects women in the fourth and fifth decades of life. PBC is seen worldwide, but is more commonly described in North America and northern Europe. PBC has a worldwide prevalence of approximately 5 per 100,000 and an annual incidence of approximately 6 per 1,000,000.

Clinical Presentation
- The clinical course of PBC is highly variable from patient to patient. Many patients will be asymptomatic at the time of diagnosis. As disease progresses, the most common clinical features of PBC include fatigue and pruritus. Patients with PBC may develop noncirrhotic portal hypertension and have complications, including ascites, GI bleeding, and hepatic encephalopathy. Additionally, patients with PBC and chronic cholestasis have a significantly higher risk of osteoporosis, which may present with bone pain in the axial bones or increased number of fractured bones. Extrahepatic manifestations associated with PBC include keratoconjunctivitis sicca, renal tubular acidosis, gallstones, thyroid disease, scleroderma, Raynaud's phenomenon, and CREST syndrome (**C**alcinosis, **R**aynaud's phenomenon, **E**sophageal hypomotility, **S**clerodactyly, and **T**elangiectasia).
- Patients with PBC also develop clinical complications secondary to bile duct obstruction and chronic cholestasis. Jaundice, the most common clinical manifestation associated with chronic cholestasis, will often be the first noted symptom in PBC. Jaundice will worsen as disease progresses. Decreased secretion of bile acids and bile salts into the small bowel results in malabsorption of fat and fat-soluble vitamins, including vitamins A, D, E, and K. The most notable clinical consequences include the development of osteoporosis and, less frequently, osteomalacia from vitamin D deficiency and increased risk of bleeding from elevated prothrombin time secondary to vitamin K deficiency. Additionally, chronic cholestasis results in hypercholesterolemia and associated development of xanthomas. Xanthomas are more common in PBC than in other diseases with chronic cholestasis. Cholestasis can also increase the production of melanin in the skin resulting in hyperpigmentation.
- Patients with PBC typically develop cirrhosis and complications of progressive liver failure 10 to 15 years after diagnosis.

Diagnosis
- Diagnosis of PBC is based on laboratory studies and liver biopsy. Elevated AP is the most common abnormality seen in PBC; elevated conjugated bilirubin, cholesterol, hyperglobulinemia (specifically IgM), and bile acids are also noted. As disease continues to worsen, patients may also develop elevated ALT and AST. **Antimitochondrial antibody** is present in >90% of patients and is a major serologic hallmark for the diagnosis of PBC.
- Liver biopsy may be helpful for both diagnosis and staging. Stage 1 disease is characterized by portal hepatitis with granulomatous destruction of bile ducts. Stage 2 disease is characterized by periportal hepatitis and bile duct proliferation. Stage 3 disease is characterized by fibrosis or bridging necrosis. Stage 4 disease is characterized by cirrhosis.

Treatment
- **Ursodeoxycholic acid** (13–15 mg/kg/day) may improve liver function test abnormalities and appears to delay progression of disease and time to liver transplantation

when given long term (>4 years). Symptom-specific therapy for pruritus, steatorrhea, and malabsorption can be given. Immunosuppressive therapies (azathioprine, cyclosporine, prednisolone, methotrexate) continue to undergo research, but none have yet been shown to have long-term clinical benefit.

- Liver transplant is indicated with advanced cirrhosis. Recurrent PBC after transplantation has been documented.

NONALCOHOLIC FATTY LIVER DISEASE

Introduction

- Nonalcoholic fatty liver disease is a clinicopathologic syndrome that encompasses several clinical entities, including simple steatosis, steatohepatitis, fibrosis, and ESLD in the absence of significant alcohol consumption. Nonalcoholic steatohepatitis (NASH), which is part of the spectrum of NAFLD, is defined by the combination of steatosis, hepatocellular ballooning, lobular inflammation, and pericellular or perisinusoidal fibrosis.
- The exact mechanisms that lead to excessive hepatic fatty infiltration and hepatic cellular damage are incompletely understood. NAFLD is usually associated with insulin resistance and features of the metabolic syndrome (central obesity, insulin resistance, high blood pressure, high triglycerides, and low high-density lipoprotein [HDL] cholesterol). Secondary causes include hepatotoxic drugs (amiodarone, nifedipine, estrogens) surgical procedures (jejunoileal bypass, extensive small bowel resection, pancreatic and biliary diversions), and miscellaneous conditions (total parenteral nutrition, hypobetalipoproteinemia, environmental toxins).
- A worldwide phenomenon, NAFLD is a common liver disease in the United States affecting 20% to 35% of the adult population. NAFLD affects both children and adults and its incidence increases with age.

Clinical Presentation

The disease presentation can vary from asymptomatic to advanced ESLD and HCC. Up to 70% of patients with cryptogenic cirrhosis have NASH as the underlying etiology. Approximately 25% of patients with NASH develop cirrhosis over a 10- to 15-year period. Cirrhosis resulting from NASH may also be complicated by HCC. Approximately 13% of all patients with HCC have associated NASH.

Diagnosis

Diagnosis is suspected clinically and confirmed by imaging and liver biopsy. Liver enzymes elevations can occur and are generally mild. Up to 80% of patients will have normal liver enzymes. Imaging studies, such as ultrasonography, computer tomography (CT) scan, and magnetic resonance imaging (MRI) may detect moderate to severe steatosis. Magnetic resonance spectroscopy offers a quantitative measurement of liver fat content, but is not commonly available. Liver biopsy remains the gold standard of diagnosis.

Treatment

- **No specific established therapy** for NAFLD exists. Treatment to correct or control associated conditions are warranted (weight loss through diet and exercise, tight control of diabetes and insulin resistance, appropriate treatment of hyperlipidemia, and discontinuation of possible offending agents).
- Liver transplantation should be considered in patients with ESLD. Recurrence of NAFLD can occur after transplantation.

METABOLIC LIVER DISEASE

The most frequently encountered metabolic liver diseases include hereditary hemochromatosis, α-1-antitrypsin deficiency, and Wilson's disease. These diseases are primarily caused by mutations resulting in progressive liver disease through different mechanisms. These entities can progress to cirrhosis.

Hereditary Hemochromatosis

Introduction
- Hereditary hemochromatosis (HH) is an autosomal recessive disorder of iron overload. This systemic disorder is related to abnormal iron absorption in the duodenum that leads to excessive and damaging iron deposition in the liver, heart, pancreas, skin, and endocrine system.
- Hereditary hemochromatosis is primarily caused by a missense mutation (C282Y) in the *HFE* gene located on chromosome 6. HH is transmitted in an autosomal recessive gene pattern. Approximately 90% of patients with HH are homozygote for the C282Y mutation. In one study, however, only 58% of homozygotes for the HH mutation had the full phenotype with tissue iron overload. Less frequent mutations include H63D and S65C and the compound heterozygous C282Y/H63D mutation. HH is the most common inherited form of iron overload affecting white populations; 1 of 200 to 400 white individuals is homozygous for the *HFE* gene mutation.

Clinical Presentation
Clinical presentation varies from asymptomatic disease to cirrhosis. In stage 1 disease (age 0–20 years), patients have clinically insignificant iron accumulation. In stage 2 disease (age 20–40 years), there is iron overload with clinical disease. After the age of 40 years, stage 3, patients present with clinical signs of iron overload with organ damage. Clinical manifestation includes liver dysfunction, slate-colored skin, diabetes, cardiomyopathy, arthritis, and hypogonadism. Patients with significant liver iron overload will develop fibrosis and cirrhosis. Patients with cirrhosis caused by HH are at increased risk of HCC, despite adequate iron depletion therapy.

Diagnosis
- The degree of iron overload has a direct impact on life expectancy in individuals with HH; thus, diagnosis is targeted at identifying individuals before they become symptomatic. Early treatment of HH is highly effective at preventing morbidity and mortality. Diagnosis is based on laboratory testing, imaging, and liver biopsy. **High fasting transferrin saturation** (>45%) is highly predictive of the diagnosis. Other nonspecific laboratory tests include **serum iron** and **ferritin** levels. The diagnosis is confirmed by the presence of specific mutations in the *HFE* gene. Iron overload in the presence of genotypes not associated with HH requires further assessment with ancillary tests. **MRI** is the imaging of choice for noninvasive quantification of iron storage in the liver. In confirmed HH, ferritin >1000 ng/mL is an accurate predictor of the presence of cirrhosis.
- Liver biopsy is not required to establish the diagnosis of HH; however, it is helpful in staging the disease, especially in individuals who are at increased risk of having advanced fibrosis or cirrhosis and in patients with iron overload without typical *HFE* gene mutations.

Treatment
- Therapy consists of **phlebotomy** (500 mL blood/week) until iron depletion is confirmed by a ferritin level of <50 ng/mL and a transferrin saturation of <40%.

Maintenance phlebotomy of 1 to 2 units of blood three to four times a year is continued for life. Treatment with phlebotomy before the onset of cirrhosis or diabetes has been shown to significantly reduce the morbidity and mortality of HH. Asymptomatic individuals homozygous for the *HFE* gene mutation with iron overload should be treated. Symptomatic individuals should also be treated to minimize extent of end-organ damage. **Deferoxamine** is an iron-chelating agent used in the setting of HH if the patient's hemodynamics cannot tolerate phlebotomy. It binds free iron and facilitates urinary excretion.

- Patients with appropriately treated HH without cirrhosis have a survival rate that is identical to that of the general population. Liver transplantation may be considered in cases of HH with cirrhosis. Patients who undergo liver transplantation for HH tend to have poorer 1- and 5-year survival rates when compared with other liver transplant recipients.

Screening
Family members of patients with HH should be screened for the diagnosis of HH with fasting transferritin saturation and ferritin levels. Genetic testing may be performed.

α-1-Antitrypsin Deficiency
Introduction
- α-1-Antitrypsin (α1AT) deficiency is an autosomal recessive disease that presents as neonatal cholestasis or, later in life, as chronic hepatitis, cirrhosis, or hepatocellular carcinoma.
- Deficiency of α1AT is the result of accumulation of misfolded α1AT in the endoplasmic reticulum of hepatocytes. The gene associated with this disorder is located on chromosome 14. The most common allele is protease inhibitor M (PiM-normal variant) followed by PiS and PiZ (deficient variants). α1AT deficiency occurs in 1 of 1600 individuals. Blacks have lower frequency of mutant alleles.

Clinical Presentation
Patients may present with cholestasis, mild abnormalities in aminotransferases, or cirrhosis. α1AT deficiency can also present as emphysema in early adulthood, as well as with other extrahepatic manifestations, including panniculitis, pancreatic fibrosis, and membranoproliferative glomerulonephritis. The presence of significant pulmonary and hepatic disease in the same patient is very rare (1%–2%). Chronic hepatitis, cirrhosis, or HCC may develop in 10% to 15% of patients with the PiZZ phenotype during the first 20 years of life. Controversy exists whether liver disease develops in heterozygotes (e.g., PiMZ, PiSZ, PiFZ).

Diagnosis
- Diagnosis is based on laboratory data and liver biopsy. **Low serum α-1-antitrypsin level** (10%–15% of normal) is suggestive of the disease. Other suggestive tests include decreased α-1-globulin level. Patients should be tested for α1AT phenotype.
- Liver biopsy is essential for diagnosis and shows characteristic periodic acid-Schiff positive, diastase-resistant globules in the periportal hepatocytes.

Treatment
- Currently, **no specific medical treatment** exists. Gene therapy for α1AT is a potential future alternative.

- Liver transplantation is curative, with survival rates of 90% at 1 year and 80% at 5 years.

Wilson's Disease

Introduction
- Wilson's disease (WD) is an autosomal recessive disorder that results in progressive copper overload in the liver, kidney, brain, and cornea.
- WD is caused by a mutation in the *ATP7B* gene located on chromosome 13. Absence or reduced function of the *ATP7B* gene results in decreased hepatocyte excretion of copper. This results in copper accumulation within the liver. Progressive copper build-up results in hepatocyte injury, fibrosis, and cirrhosis. Copper is subsequently released into the bloodstream and deposited into other organs, including the brain, kidneys, and cornea. The incidence of WD is 1 in 30,000.

Clinical Presentation
- Wilson's disease can present as chronic hepatitis, cirrhosis, or rarely as fulminant hepatic failure. The diagnosis should be considered in patients with unexplained liver disease with or without neuropsychiatric symptoms, first-degree relatives with WD, or individuals with fulminant hepatic failure. The average age of presentation of liver dysfunction is 6 to 20 years, but it can manifest later in life. Cirrhosis is frequently identified in patients with WD between the age of 10 and 20 years.
- Neuropsychiatric disorders usually occur later in life and generally are associated with cirrhosis. The manifestations include asymmetric tremor, dysarthria, ataxia, and psychiatric features. Other extrahepatic manifestations include Kayser-Fleischer rings on slit lamp examination (gold to brown rings caused by copper deposition in Descemet's membrane in the periphery of the cornea), hemolytic anemia, renal tubular acidosis, arthritis, and osteopenia.

Diagnosis
- Diagnosis is based on laboratory studies, imaging, and liver biopsy. Laboratory findings include **low ceruloplasmin level** (<20 mg/dL), although normal values do not rule out the diagnosis. **Elevated serum copper level** (>25 μg/dL), and **elevated 24-hour urinary copper level** (>100 mg/24 hours) may also be seen, but are dependent on the method of testing. Thus, these laboratory examinations are better used for monitoring treatment in patients with WD than for diagnosis. Brain imaging can demonstrate basal ganglia changes.
- Liver biopsy findings are nonspecific and depend on the presentation and stage of the disease. Liver histology can include massive necrosis, steatosis, glycogenated nuclei, chronic hepatitis, fibrosis, and cirrhosis. Elevated hepatic copper levels >250 μg/g dry weight (normal <40 μg/g dry weight) on biopsy are highly suggestive of WD.

Screening
DNA testing for family members of an affected individual is now becoming commercially available. The analysis requires identification of the patient's *ATP7B* gene mutation or haplotype. This same haplotype is then screened in first-degree relatives. This type of testing does, however, have limitations. Many patients are compound heterozygotes, making identification of mutations more difficult. To date, over 200 mutations of the *ATP7B* gene have been identified.

Treatment

Treatment is with copper chelating agents or zinc salts. Patients require life-long therapy. Zinc salts are used to block copper uptake from the GI tract. **Zinc salts** 50 mg PO TID is indicated in patients with chronic hepatitis and cirrhosis in the absence of hepatic failure. Zinc can be used in association with penicillamine and trientine. Other than gastric irritation, zinc has a very good safety profile. **Penicillamine**, a chelating agent, 1 to 2 g/day PO in divided doses BID or QID plus pyridoxine 2.5 mg/day to avoid deficiency during treatment can be used in patients with hepatic failure. Use may be limited by side effects, including hypersensitivity, bone marrow suppression, proteinuria, systemic lupus erythematosus, or Goodpasture's syndrome. Penicillamine should never be given as initial treatment to patients with neurologic symptoms. **Trientine**, a chelating agent, 1 to 2 g/day PO in divided doses BID or QID can also be given as treatment. The side effects are similar to those of penicillamine, but are seen in lower frequency. The risk of neurologic worsening with trientine is less than with penicillamine. **Tetrathiomolybdate** (TM) 120 mg/day divided as 20 mg TID with meals and 60 mg at bedtime away from food can be given with zinc therapy. TM functions as a general chelator that also blocks copper absorption. This is the treatment of choice for patients presenting with neurologic symptoms. TM has a good safety profile; possible side effects include anemia, leukopenia, and mild elevations of aminotransferases. Dietary limitation of copper-containing food should be used in conjunction with drug treatment.

Liver transplantation is the only therapy for fuminant hepatic failure or in progressive dysfunction, despite chelation therapy. In the absence of neurologic symptoms, liver transplantation has a good prognosis and requires no further medical treatment.

KEY POINTS TO REMEMBER

- Infection with hepatitis B can resolve, progress to chronic hepatitis B or inactive HBsAg carrier state.
- Diagnosis of HBV is based on serum antigen or antibody testing, HBV DNA quantification, and liver biopsy.
- Treatment of HBV with IFN-based therapies and nucleoside or nucleotide analogs are effective in delaying or preventing the progression of liver disease.
- Exposure to HCV results in chronic infection in 85% of individuals of which approximately 25% will develop cirrhosis.
- Diagnosis of HCV is based on antibody testing and is confirmed by HCV RNA and liver biopsy. Patients with HCV genotypes 2 and 3 are more susceptible to antiviral therapy than patients with genotype 1.
- Treatment of HCV is targeted at obtaining an SVR with the use of PEG-IFN in combination with ribavirin.
- The diagnosis of alcoholic liver disease is based on careful history and laboratory studies demonstrating elevated liver enzymes, usually with AST greater than ALT. Liver biopsy is useful for determining diagnosis as well as disease grade and stage.
- The hallmark of treatment for alcoholic liver disease is abstinence. Steroids and pentoxifylline may be indicated in a subgroup of patients with alcoholic hepatitis.

(*continued*)

- Autoimmune hepatitis must be considered in all patients with acute or chronic hepatitis of unknown origin. Diagnosis is based on the presence of autoantibodies (ANA, SMA, and LKMA), hyperglobulinemia, and liver biopsy with characteristic histology.
- Treatment for autoimmune hepatitis is generally with prednisone and azathioprine.
- PSC is frequently associated with inflammatory bowel disease, characterized by inflammation and fibrosis of the extrahepatic and intrahepatic biliary ducts resulting in cirrhosis.
- Diagnosis of PSC is based on demonstration of stricturing or focal dilation of bile ducts with ERCP or MRCP.
- Treatment options for PSC include ursodeoxycholic acid, antibiotics, therapeutic ERCP, and liver transplantation.
- Primary biliary cirrhosis is a cholestatic liver disease with autoimmune features classically affecting middle-aged women. Ursodeoxycholic acid may delay disease progression.
- Nonalcoholic liver disease encompasses several different entities, including simple steatosis, steatohepatitis, fibrosis, and cirrhosis and it is associated with an increasing prevalence of type II diabetes mellitus, metabolic syndrome, and obesity in the United States.
- No established treatment for NAFLD exists. Treatment to correct associated conditions may improve NAFLD.
- Hereditary hemochromatosis is an autosomal recessive genetic disorder that results in abnormal iron absorption and iron deposition in the liver, heart, pancreas, skin, and endocrine system.
- Patients are screened for HH with fasting transferrin saturation levels and ferritin. Diagnosis is confirmed with genetic testing.
- Treatment of HH is with life-long phlebotomy.
- $\alpha 1AT$ deficiency is the result of accumulation of misfolded α-1-antitrypsin in the endoplasmic reticulum of hepatocytes resulting in chronic hepatitis, cirrhosis, or hepatocellular carcinoma.
- Wilson's disease is an autosomal recessive disorder that results in progressive copper overload in the liver, kidney, brain, and cornea.
- Diagnosis of WD is suggested by low ceruloplasmin levels, high serum copper levels, or high 24-hour urinary copper levels. Measurement of hepatic copper levels may be of additional diagnostic value.
- Treatment of WD is with lifelong chelation therapy or zinc.

REFERENCES AND SUGGESTED READINGS

Czaja AJ. Autoimmune liver disease. *Curr Opin Gastroenterol* 2007;23(3):255–262.

Dienstag J, McHutchison JG. American Gastroenterology Association Medical Position Statement on the Management of Hepatitis C. *Gastroenterology* 2006;130(1): 225–230.

Ewing JA. Detecting Alcoholism: The CAGE Questionnaire. *JAMA* 1984;252: 1905–1907.

Heathcote EJ. Management of primary biliary cirrhosis. *Hepatology* 2000;31(4): 1005–1013.

Heathcote, J. Treatment strategies for autoimmune hepatitis. *Am J Gastroenterol* 2006; 101(12 Suppl):S630–S632.

Larusso NF, Shneider BL, Black D, et al. Primary sclerosing cholangitis: summary of a workshop. *Hepatology* 2006;44(3):746–764.

Lazaridis KN, Talwalkar JA. Clinical epidemiology of primary biliary cirrhosis: incidence, prevalence, and impact of therapy. *J Clin Gastroenterol* 2007;41(5):494–500.

Lok A, McMahon M. Chronic Hepatitis B, AASLD Practice Guidelines. *Hepatology* 2007;45(2):507–539.

McCullough AJ, O'Connor B. Alcoholic liver disease: Proposed recommendation for the American College of Gastroenterology. *Am J Gastroenterol* 1998;93(11):2022–2036.

Roberts EA, Schilsky ML. A practice guideline on Wilson disease. *Hepatology* 2003; 37(6):1475–1492.

Strader D, Wright T, Thomas D, et al. Diagnosis, management, and treatment of hepatitis C. *Hepatology* 2004;39(4):1147–1171.

Tavill AS. Diagnosis and management of hemochromatosis. *Hepatology* 2001;33(5): 1321–1328.

Zhang F, Zhang J, Jia J. Treatment of patients with alcoholic liver disease. *Hepatobiliary Pancreatic Disease International* 2005;4(1):12–17.

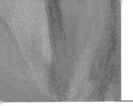

Cirrhosis

Sumeet Asrani and Jeffrey S. Crippin

INTRODUCTION

Background and Epidemiology

Cirrhosis is the common endpoint of a multitude of insults to the liver, with a myriad of complications caused by progressive liver dysfunction and portal hypertension. Chronic liver disease and cirrhosis affects nearly 5.5 million Americans. Males are more commonly affected than females, and Hispanic and Native American populations have a higher prevalence than other ethnic groups. Cirrhosis is the tenth leading cause of death in the United States. In 1998, approximately 31,000 deaths (1.3%) were related to chronic liver disease, with 39% secondary to alcoholic liver disease, 15% to hepatitis C, 4% to hepatitis B, and 44% without a recorded cause.

Definition

Cirrhosis is a pathologic diagnosis. The World Health Organization defines cirrhosis as a "diffuse process characterized by fibrosis and conversion of normal liver architecture into structurally abnormal nodules which lack normal lobular organization." Fibrosis is the common endpoint of a cycle of degeneration, necrosis, apoptosis, inflammation, and attempted regeneration. Histologic characteristics include a diffuse pattern of fibrosis and parenchymal injury, with the presence of fibrous septae between portal tracts and hepatic veins and parenchymal nodules with proliferating hepatocytes.

Etiology

The most common causes are alcohol-related liver disease and chronic viral hepatitis C. Other causes are listed in Table 20-1.

Classification

Liver fibrosis is staged by increasing amounts of collagenous tissue. Cirrhosis represents the most advanced stage of liver fibrosis. Cirrhosis may also be classified based on etiology.

CAUSES

Physiology and Pathophysiology

- The hepatocyte or liver cell has a variety of functions. The fenestrated sinusoids with absent intercellular junctions and basement membranes ensure close interactions between the sinusoidal blood and hepatocytes. Hepatic stellate cells, present in the space of Disse, are in close communication with the hepatocytes and the sinusoidal endothelial cells. Injury to hepatocytes leads to the initiation of an inflammatory cascade with the release of cytokines. This amplifies and sustains the overall response,

TABLE 20-1 EVALUATION OF CIRRHOSIS

Historical Factors	Laboratory Evaluation	Suspected Cause
Excessive alcohol use	Increased AST-to-ALT ratio	Alcoholic liver disease
Intravenous drug abuse, tattoos, multiple sexual partners, sharing of needles, transfusions before 1992	Positive hepatitis B or C serologies	Chronic viral hepatitis
Fatigue, jaundice, pruritus	Antimitochondrial antibody, elevated alkaline phosphatase	Primary biliary cirrhosis
Ulcerative colitis, bacterial cholangitis or cholangiocarcinoma	Elevated alkaline phosphatase	Primary sclerosing cholangitis
Neuropsychiatric symptoms	Kaiser-Fleisher rings, low serum ceruloplasmin, high urinary copper	Wilson's disease
Skin changes, arthritis, diabetes mellitus, hypogonadism	Ferritin, iron studies, hemochromatosis gene (*HFE*) mutations	Hemochromatosis
Autoimmune disease	ANA, increased serum quantitative immunoglobulins, smooth muscle antibody	Autoimmune hepatitis
Diabetes mellitus, obesity, dyslipidemia	Dyslipidemia, elevated sugars	Nonalcoholic fatty liver disease
Emphysema without smoking history, positive family history	Emphysema, phenotype testing (PiZZ phenotype), α-1-antitrypsin level	α-1-antitrypsin deficiency
Methotrexate or amiodarone use		Drug hepatotoxicity
History of anasarca, venous thromboembolism, or malignancy	Hypercoagulable state, nephrotic syndrome, paroxysmal nocturnal hemoglobinuria	Budd-Chiari syndrome
Stem-cell transplant		Veno-occlusive disease
Unknown factors		Cryptogenic cirrhosis

ALT, alanine aminotransferase, ANA, antinuclear antibody; AST, aspartate aminotransferase.

with subsequent activation of effector cells, especially hepatic stellate cells. An autocrine loop of activation is set in motion. Hepatic stellate cells have multiple roles, but are primarily transformed into cells with fibrinogenic, contractile, and proliferative properties. Cytokines, small peptides, and the extracellular matrix serve as crucial mediators of the fibrinogenic response. Bridging fibrosis ensues, leading to "capillarization" of the hepatic sinusoids (a shift from a fenestrated sinusoid to a "nonfenestrated" capillary) and a shift in balance toward vasoconstrictors, such as endothelin, and away from vasodilators, such as nitric oxide. Furthermore, there is an overproduction of endothelin by the damaged liver and decreased nitric oxide production by the sinusoids. Because of increased stellate cell contractility, there is an increased intrahepatic resistance and decreased sinusoidal blood flow. Thrombosis of the microvasculature occurs with formation of intrahepatic arterial shunts. An erratic proliferation of hepatocytes takes place in hypoperfused areas, leading to a nodular pattern of regeneration within areas of fibrosis. Globally, there is an increase in the portal pressure and complications of portal hypertension caused by the formation of portosystemic collaterals, including the formation of gastroesophageal varices and splenomegaly. Arterial flow varies inversely with portal venous flow and shunting of blood leads to an increased dependence on arterial flow for hepatic perfusion. Ongoing destruction leads to a decrease in hepatic synthetic function, with coagulopathy, jaundice, and hypoglycemia. Common endpoints of progressive liver dysfunction and portal hypertension include ascites and hepatic encephalopathy.

- Portal hypertension leads to splanchnic arterial vasodilation caused by an imbalance favoring release of nitric oxide. Homeostatic sensing of this presumed arterial underfilling leads to the activation of the neurohormonal system causing vasoconstriction in nonsplanchnic vascular beds and an increase in arterial blood pressure. The detrimental effect of this compensatory activation of the sympathetic nervous system (SNS), renin-angiotensin-aldosterone system (RAAS) and the arginine vasopressin system leads to a pattern of sodium retention, water retention, and renal vasoconstriction, leading to dilutional hyponatremia, peripheral edema, ascites, and, in severe cases, the hepatorenal syndrome.

Differential Diagnosis

Life-threatening complications of cirrhosis derive from portal hypertension. Normal portal venous pressure ranges from 5 to 10 mm Hg, producing a portosystemic gradient of 2 to 6 mm Hg. An increase in the gradient >12 mm Hg increases the risk of variceal bleeding. Cirrhosis is the most common cause of portal hypertension in the United States, although other causes must be excluded. The etiology of portal hypertension is divided into pre-, intra-, and posthepatic causes. Prehepatic causes include portal and splenic vein thromboses. Intrahepatic causes are viral hepatitis, primary biliary cirrhosis, alcoholic hepatitis, veno-occlusive disease, and schistosomiasis. Common posthepatic causes are hepatic venous thrombosis (Budd-Chiari syndrome), congestive heart failure, and constrictive pericarditis.

Natural History

Compensated cirrhosis has a 10-year survival of 47%, with a higher mortality rate seen in decompensated cirrhosis. Decompensated cirrhosis is characterized by jaundice, variceal hemorrhage, or uncontrolled ascites. Patients usually die from complications of hepatic dysfunction or portal hypertension. Patients develop decompensated disease at the rate of 7% to 10% per year. Ascites develops in approximately 35% to 50% of patients within 5 years. Varices develop in 5% to 10% of patients annually.

PRESENTATION

Risk Factors

Cirrhosis is a common endpoint of chronic diseases that cause hepatic injury. Risk factors for cirrhosis include chronic viral hepatitis, alcohol dependence, iron overload, and chronic inflammatory conditions, such as nonalcoholic steatohepatitis.

TABLE 20-2	MANIFESTATIONS AND PRESENTATION OF CIRRHOSIS
Constitutional	Fatigue, weight loss, anorexia, malaise, muscle wasting
Gastrointestinal	Hematemesis, melena, esophageal or gastric varices, portal hypertensive gastropathy, gastritis, ascites
Pulmonary	Shortness of breath, dyspnea on exertion, hypoxia, hepatopulmonary syndrome, respiratory alkalosis, hepatic hydrothorax, portopulmonary syndrome
Cardiovascular	Hypotension, hyperdynamic circulation
Renal	Hepatorenal syndrome, hyponatremia
Endocrine	Decreased libido, impotence, testicular atrophy, dysmenorrhea, gynecomastia
Neurologic	Confusion, short-term memory loss, hyperirritability, insomnia encephalopathy
Dermatologic	Jaundice, spider angioma, palmar erythema, Dupuytren's contracture, caput medusa
Hematologic	Splenomegaly, thrombocytopenia, anemia, leukopenia, coagulopathy
Infectious	Spontaneous bacterial peritonitis, sepsis

Symptoms

Patients can present with a myriad of symptoms (Table 20-2), including the following:

- Malaise and fatigue
- Hematemesis or melena
- Jaundice
- Pruritus
- Anorexia, nausea, and vomiting
- Confusion
- Hyperirritability
- Abdominal bloating, increase in abdominal girth, lower extremity swelling
- Shortness of breath or dyspnea on exertion
- Change in sleep pattern
- Decreased libido or impotence

History

The history should focus on common causes of liver disease and cirrhosis. Specifically, patients should be asked about duration and quantity of alcohol intake, risk factors for viral hepatitis (parenteral risks, such as intravenous drug use and multiple sexual partners), a family history of liver disease, and prescription and over-the-counter drug use. Also, identify diseases associated with less common causes of cirrhosis. Patients with primary sclerosing cholangitis (PSC) have a high incidence of ulcerative colitis. Obesity, dyslipidemia, hyperglycemia, and the metabolic syndrome can suggest nonalcoholic fatty liver disease (NAFLD). Patients with α-1-antitrypsin deficiency often have a history of premature emphysema, not related to excessive smoking. Women with a history of autoimmune disease raise a high suspicion of autoimmune liver diseases, such as autoimmune hepatitis or primary biliary cirrhosis. A history of a hypercoagulable state or prior malignancy may lead to hepatic vein thrombosis or the Budd-Chiari syndrome. A stem cell or bone marrow transplant increases the risk of veno-occlusive disease. A constellation of skin changes, arthritis, diabetes mellitus, and hypogonadism is seen in individuals with hereditary hemochromatosis.

Physical Examination

The physical examination can reveal complications of cirrhosis. Muscle wasting, jaundice, spider angiomata, gynecomastia, caput medusa, prominent venous collaterals, palmar erythema, Dupuytren's contracture, testicular atrophy, and ecchymoses may be present. The cardiac examination may reveal a bounding pulse. The neurologic examination can reveal encephalopathy and asterixis. Splenomegaly, a coarse liver edge, and evidence of ascites (fluid wave, dullness in flanks, and shifting dullness) may be present on the examination of the abdomen. The rectal examination can show evidence of hemorrhoids, guaiac positive stools, and melena.

Evaluation

- Table 20-1 lists causes of cirrhosis and a suggested laboratory workup to elucidate the cause. Initial laboratory work should assess hepatic synthetic function and complications of portal hypertension. Serum albumin, total bilirubin, and international normalized ratio (INR) reflect synthetic function. A complete blood count may identify leukopenia and thrombocytopenia related to hypersplenism. Electrolytes, blood urea nitrogen (BUN), and serum creatinine are helpful in screening for renal dysfunction and hyponatremia. Disease-specific serologies and levels are used to identify the cause of cirrhosis, in some cases. Cirrhosis of any cause increases the risk of hepatocellular carcinoma. Although relatively insensitive, an elevated α-fetoprotein can be associated with this tumor.
- Imaging studies of the liver are useful in assessing the size and echotexture of the liver, the presence of ascites, biliary ductal dilation, and splenomegaly. Imaging studies also screen for liver masses and hepatocellular carcinoma. Ultrasonography, computed tomography (CT), and magnetic resonance imaging (MRI) are useful, with the specific study tailored to the patient. Additional studies, such as an endoscopic retrograde pancreatography (ERCP), are required for assessment of the biliary tree. A liver biopsy is often helpful for rare cases, such as Wilson's disease, autoimmune hepatitis, and hemochromatosis.

Clinical Presentation

Some patients are incidentally found to have physical findings or laboratory abnormalities suggestive of cirrhosis. In the inpatient setting, however, most patients present with one or more of the following complications of cirrhosis, namely portal hypertension and progressive liver failure. Complications of portal hypertension include ascites, spontaneous bacterial peritonitis (SBP), gastrointestinal bleeding, portopulmonary syndrome (portal hypertension associated with pulmonary hypertension), and hepatorenal syndrome (renal failure associated with cirrhosis). Complications of progressive liver dysfunction can include a myriad of infections, coagulopathy, acute on chronic liver failure, hepatic encephalopathy (Table 20-2), hepatopulmonary syndrome, and hepatocellular carcinoma.

MANAGEMENT

Gastrointestinal Hemorrhage

Diagnosis

Patients present with hematemesis, melena, or both. Variceal bleeding is a consequence of portal hypertension. A hepatic venous portal gradient >12 mm Hg increases the risk of a variceal rupture. Variceal bleeding is often intermittent and endoscopic evaluation is essential for diagnostic and therapeutic purposes.

Workup

Upper gastrointestinal (GI) bleeding in cirrhotic patients is usually caused by variceal rupture, gastritis, portal hypertensive gastropathy, or peptic ulcer disease. Nasogastric (NG) lavage with 500 mL to 1 L of normal saline or water should be considered, if there is any question of bleeding. The risk of variceal rupture with placement of the NG tube is minimal. If the hematemesis was witnessed or the patient has melena, endoscopic evaluation is indicated.

Follow-up

Periodic endoscopic evaluation is essential to identify varices and prevent progression to variceal bleeding. Varices are present in 30% to 40% of patients with compensated cirrhosis and 60% of patients with ascites. The annual incidence of new varices is 5% to 10%. The overall incidence of first variceal bleeding is 25% at 2 years. A high risk exists of rebleeding within the first 5 days of a bleed and the incidence of early rebleeding in the first 6 weeks is 30% to 40%. The incidence of first bleeding with large varices is 15% yearly and is 5% yearly with small varices.

Prevention relies on early identification of varices and decreasing portal pressure by the use of **nonselective beta-blockers**, such as nadolol, propranolol, or timolol. Nonselective beta-blockers decrease cardiac output and produce splanchnic vasoconstriction. The role of beta-blockers for primary prophylaxis in cirrhotic patients without evidence of varices has not been convincingly established. A recent trial with 200 patients followed for 55 months without evidence of prior varices showed an insignificant rate of development of varices (39% vs. 40%) in patients on beta-blockers versus placebo. The role of primary prophylaxis in cirrhotic patients with evidence of varices has been well established. Two separate meta-analyses comparing beta-blockers with placebo showed a 40% to 50% reduction in the risk of bleeding. The second analysis demonstrated lower rates of fatal bleeding in treated patients, but no improvement in overall survival (free from rebleed 78% vs. 65% with survival rate 71% vs. 68%). For secondary prophylaxis after a sentinel bleeding event, a combination of beta-blockers and endoscopic variceal ligation (EVL) versus endoscopic therapy alone was associated with a significantly lower rate of recurrent variceal bleeding with combination therapy (14% vs. 38% at 16 months), but with similar mortality. Side effects of beta-blocker therapy and high rates of discontinuation impede aggressive protection from rebleeding. A proton pump inhibitor should be considered in patients with evidence of gastritis, although acid inhibition does not decrease bleeding from portal hypertensive gastropathy.

Treatment

Hemodynamic stability is essential in the management of variceal bleeding. Intravenous (IV) access must be established and volume repletion should be pursued with crystalloid or colloid solutions. Because of the presence of liver disease, coagulopathy is common and should be corrected with vitamin K, fresh frozen plasma or platelets, as clinically indicated. Variceal bleeding, however, is related to portal hypertension and less so to coagulopathy. Care must be used not to overtransfuse, because increased blood volume has the theoretic risk of increasing bleeding. Octreotide (50–100 μg IV bolus, 25–50 μg/hour) is a somatostatin analog that decreases splanchnic pressure and should be started if variceal bleeding is suspected. It is effective at decreasing bleeding and is much safer than vasopressin and nitroglycerin. Once patients have been adequately resuscitated, upper endoscopy should be performed. This allows both diagnostic and therapeutic interventions. Patients with active hematemesis may require intubation for airway protection. EVL has largely replaced sclerotherapy in the management of acute variceal bleeding. If endoscopy is not

TABLE 20-3	GRADES OF ENCEPHALOPATHY

Grade	Characteristics
I	Sleep reversal pattern, mild confusion, irritability, tremor
II	Lethargy, disorientation, inappropriate behavior, asterixis
III	Somnolence, severe confusion, aggressive behavior, asterixis
IV	Coma

immediately available or if the bleeding cannot be stopped with medical and endoscopic management, balloon tamponade may provide temporary control. This procedure, however, has a high risk of complications, including aspiration and asphyxiation, and must be used cautiously. For patients refractory to these measures, emergent transjugular intrahepatic portosystemic shunts (TIPS) can be placed to decompress the varices.

Patients with upper GI hemorrhage are predisposed to infection. A meta-analysis showed that antibiotic prophylaxis covering enteric organisms was associated with a reduction in infection rate (14% vs. 45%) and a significant decrease in mortality (15% vs. 24%). Patients should be placed on a third generation cephalosporin to prevent spontaneous bacterial peritonitis.

Encephalopathy

Diagnosis and Workup

Hepatic encephalopathy (HE) is a neuropsychiatric disorder associated with severe liver disease. HE is graded by the West Haven criteria, with a range of neurologic manifestations from subtle changes in handwriting to obtundation (Table 20-3). Early recognition is imperative. Based on current understanding, ammonia is central to the pathogenesis of this process because it accelerates astrocyte swelling and cerebral edema, thought to be central to the neurologic manifestations. The diagnosis can usually be made on clinical grounds with altered mental status, asterixis, and hypo- or hyper-reflexia. Other causes of encephalopathy should be excluded. Ammonia levels have very poor specificity and should not be used to diagnose portosystemic encephalopathy (PSE) or monitor treatment response. Management should be directed at identifying and treating possible precipitating factors (Table 20-4).

TABLE 20-4	COMMON PRECIPITANTS OF HEPATIC ENCEPHALOPATHY

Gastrointestinal bleeding

Post-transjugular intrahepatic portosystemic shunt (TIPS)

Constipation

Spontaneous bacterial peritonitis and other infections

Narcotics or benzodiazepine use

Hepatocellular carcinoma

Worsening liver function

Diuretic use

Alkalosis

Hypokalemia

Treatment

Initial treatment is targeted at identifying and treating the precipitating factor (Table 20-4). Treatment is also geared at lowering the ammonia. Disaccharides, such as **lactulose**, are the mainstay of treatment because of their ability to reduce intraluminal pH, converting ammonia to ammonium and allowing it to be purged from the colon. Lactulose can be administered orally, rectally, or through an NG tube, with a typical dose of 60 to 90 g/day, titrated to three to five loose bowel movements daily. Its utility has been questioned, however, as a recent Cochrane database review noted that when compared with placebo or no intervention, nonabsorbable disaccharides did not have a statistically significant effect on mortality (RR 0.41, 95% CI 0.02–8.68), but did appear to reduce the risk of no improvement of hepatic encephalopathy (RR 0.62, 95% CI 0.46–0.84). Nonabsorbable antibiotics, such as **rifaximin** (1200 mg divided TID), have uncertain efficacy in comatose patients, but appear to be effective in patients treated chronically. Probiotics may play an increasing role in the management of HE. Patients with grade III to IV encephalopathy may require endotracheal intubation for airway protection. Frequent neurologic examinations are imperative.

Diagnostic Test and Laboratory Analysis

No correlation is found between the degree of HE and ammonia level, thus, levels should not be checked routinely. Neurologic imaging can be used to identify other causes, such as a subdural hematoma. Laboratory evaluation should focus on ruling out electrolyte abnormalities, peritonitis, bleeding, volume depletion, and other infections as possible precipitants.

Complications

The risk of cerebral edema increases with progression of encephalopathy, with a >75% risk in patients with grade IV encephalopathy. Advanced cerebral edema can lead to uncal herniation and death. This is more common in patients with acute liver failure, although it can be seen in patients with chronic liver disease.

Ascites

Ascites, the most common complication seen in cirrhotic patients, is associated with a high rate of morbidity and mortality. It is intimately associated with the hepatorenal syndrome (HRS) and SBP. Splanchnic vasodilation and arterial underfilling lead to the activation of the renin-angiotensin-aldosterone system and sympathetic nervous system, leading to sodium retention and ascites.

Diagnosis and Workup

Patients may complain of an increased abdominal girth, shortness of breath, and lower extremity edema. Common physical findings include dullness to percussion in the flanks, shifting dullness, pleural effusion, a fluid wave, and an umbilical hernia. A diagnostic and therapeutic **paracentesis** is often necessary. Ascitic fluid should be sent for cell count with differential, aerobic and anaerobic cultures, and albumin. The presence of >250 polymorphonuclear (PMN) cells/mm^3 strongly suggests SBP and should be aggressively treated. A positive culture, regardless of the number of PMN, should also be treated. A difference in albumin concentration (serum albumin to ascitic albumin gradient) of >1.1 supports the diagnosis of portal hypertension. For a ratio <1.1, other causes, such as malignancy, tuberculosis, or pancreatitis, must be considered.

Treatment

Patients should be maintained on a restricted sodium diet to prevent excessive sodium retention. Free water restriction to <1.5 L/day is advisable only in patients with evidence of hyponatremia. Aldosterone antagonists, such as **spironolactone**, 50 to 400 mg daily in a single dose, inhibit sodium reabsorption and are used in combination with **loop diuretics** (furosemide, 20–160 mg daily) that further impair sodium reabsorption. A typical starting dose is spironolactone 100 mg and furosemide 40 mg daily. Doses are increased proportionally. Hyponatremia, hypokalemia, volume depletion, and hepatic encephalopathy can complicate therapy. Therapeutic paracentesis can be used to manage ascites and has an important role in refractory ascites. Removal of 5 to 7 L is well tolerated by patients, but should be accompanied by a plasma volume expander to prevent circulatory dysfunction. One study showed albumin administration at a dose of 6 to 8 g/L of ascitic fluid removed was associated with lower rates of renal impairment.

The goal of therapy is the loss of 0.5 kg/day and 1 kg/day if peripheral edema is present. Refractory ascites can be treated with bimonthly outpatient large volume paracenteses or TIPS. In a meta-analysis, TIPS was more effective at removing ascites without a significant difference in mortality, GI bleeding, infection, and acute renal failure, but with a significantly higher rate of hepatic encephalopathy.

Spontaneous bacterial peritonitis and the hepatorenal syndrome are common complications of ascites and its treatment, such as overdiuresis, and a high index of suspicion should be maintained for aggressive management. Patients should also be considered for liver transplantation. Daily weights should be checked to follow and assess the diuresis.

Spontaneous Bacterial Peritonitis

Diagnosis

Spontaneous bacterial peritonitis is associated with a high rate of morbidity and mortality. Bacterial translocation of enteric organisms is facilitated by decreased gut motility, bacterial stasis, and overgrowth. Mucosal integrity is compromised because of submucosal edema and bacterial endotoxins with bacterial translocation. Presentation may be subtle, with abdominal pain, fever, chills, jaundice, or worsening encephalopathy. Up to half of patients with SBP are asymptomatic and a diagnostic paracentesis with a 22- to 25-gauge needle is imperative, regardless of an elevated prothrombin time and the presence of thrombocytopenia.

Workup

A diagnostic paracentesis is the gold standard diagnostic test. Ascitic fluid should be sent for cell count with differential, gram stain and aerobic and anaerobic blood cultures. The presence of >250 PMN/mm^3 strongly suggests SBP and should be aggressively treated. A positive culture, regardless of the number of PMN, should also be treated. Blood cultures should be pursued to find a causative organism. Although most cases are caused by SBP, secondary causes (e.g., bowel perforation or systemic infections) should also be considered.

Treatment

Because of the predilection of infection by enteric organisms, a **third generation cephalosporin** administered for at least 5 days serves as the standard of care. Traditionally, cefotaxime 1 to 2 g IV every 8 to 12 hours has been used. Ceftriaxone at 1 to 2 g every 24 hours is also effective. A repeat diagnostic paracentesis should be considered at day 3, if there is no clinical improvement. If clinical deterioration is confirmed, coverage should be broadened to cover enterococcus, methicillin-resistant *Staphylococcus aureus*, and anaerobic organisms. Because hepatorenal syndrome is a feared complication, efforts to maintain adequate volume expansion should be pursued. Diuretics and large volume paracentesis should be avoided. Albumin administration should be given to reduce the risk of HRS. In patients treated for SBP with a third generation cephalosporin, with and without albumin, a study has shown albumin administration at 1.5 g/kg on day 1 and 1 g/kg on day 3 was associated with a lower rate of renal failure (10% vs. 33%) and lower in hospital mortality (10% vs. 29%).

Patients can be switched to an oral fluoroquinolone on discharge to complete a 10-day course. Prophylaxis with an oral fluoroquinolone should be considered in patients following the first episode of SBP, because of the decreased risk of additional episodes.

The 2-year survival in patients who develop SBP is 25% to 30% and the median survival is 9 months.

Hepatorenal Syndrome

Introduction

The hepatorenal syndrome is seen in patients with cirrhosis and an identifiable precipitant may be difficult to find. HRS affects 5% of patients hospitalized for GI bleeding, 30% of patients with SBP, and 10% of patients with ascites treated by paracentesis.

Diagnosis

The International Ascites Club developed criteria for the diagnosis of hepatorenal syndrome. In summary, the criteria define a state of oliguria, characterized by decreased glomerular filtration rate (GFR), no obvious cause of renal failure, a lack of response to volume repletion, and progressive renal failure. Laboratory evaluation often reveals a urine sodium <10, hyponatremia, and the absence of granular casts on urine sediment.

Workup

An expedited workup is necessary to rule out reversible causes of renal failure. Common causes include hypovolemia (owing to aggressive diuresis, GI bleeding, or poor nutrition), sepsis, nephrotoxins, obstruction, and acute tubular necrosis. Renal function should be followed closely. Precipitants of the hepatorenal syndrome, such as GI bleeding, SBP, and alcoholic hepatitis must be sought and corrected.

Treatment

Treatment is often disappointing, but is geared toward modifying the underlying triad of arterial underfilling, splanchnic vasodilation, and renal vasoconstriction. A diagnostic paracentesis must be performed to rule out SBP. If identified, albumin as described above should be used. For patients with alcoholic hepatitis, 400 mg of pentoxifilline TID reduces the incidence of HRS. Although its role is controversial, albumin has been used as a plasma expander to blunt the overactive sympathetic nervous system, suppress the RAAS system, and promote renal perfusion. Vasoconstrictors (e.g., octreotide and terlipressin) and alpha agonists (e.g., midodrine [in combination with octreotide]), and albumin have been effective in small cohorts. One analysis showed that in pooled studies of 154 patients with these varied approaches, a reversal of HRS was seen in 61% versus 3% of the untreated population and the 3-month survival was 30% versus 0% in the control group. TIPS and a molecular adsorbent recirculating system are two other options requiring further study. Liver transplantation is another therapy for refractory HRS, with excellent survival rates and improvement in renal function.

Prognosis

Type I hepatorenal syndrome is progressive over a period <2 weeks; it often has a precipitating factor, such as SBP, and is associated with a median survival of 12 days and a >90% mortality at 10 weeks.

Special Considerations

Electrolyte and Metabolic Abnormalities

Cirrhotic patients often have varying degrees of coagulopathy, thrombocytopenia, and leukopenia. Blood products and correction of coagulopathy are not needed unless evidence of bleeding exists. Hyponatremia is also present because of active water retention. Free water restriction of 1 to 1.5 L/day can be implemented. Hypertonic saline should not be administered because this can lead to further ascites and water retention. Vasopressin antagonists are currently being investigated in clinical trials. Hypoglycemia should be aggressively corrected.

Hepatocellular Cancer

Hepatocellular cancer is associated with a 23% annual survival rate. Yearly or semiannual surveillance with ultrasonography is useful in patients who have evidence of cirrhosis. Once a tumor is found, classification is based on the Barcelona Clinic Liver Cancer staging system that stratifies therapy based on tumor size, the patient's functional status, and Child-Turcotte-Pugh

TABLE 20-5   CHILD-TURCOTTE-PUGH SCORING SYSTEM

Criteria	1	2	3
Ascites	None	Slight	Moderate-severe
Encephalopathy	None	Mild	Moderate-severe
Bilirubin (mg/dL)	<2	2–3	>3
Albumin (g/dL)	>3.5	2.8–3.5	<2.8
Prothrombin time (seconds above normal prothrombin time)	1–3	4–6	>6

Note: Child's class determined by adding scores from each of the five criteria together: class A, 5–6 points; class B, 7–9 points; class C, 10–15 points.

stage of cirrhosis (Table 20-5). Treatment options include resection, chemoembolization, and liver transplant. Resection is often contraindicated, because of the lack of adequate hepatic reserve. The Milan criteria (solitary tumor <5 cm or up to three nodules <3 cm) are used to determine whether liver transplantation is an effective option.

Hepatopulmonary Syndrome
Hepatopulmonary syndrome is classically defined by a triad of hypoxia, liver disease, and intrapulmonary shunting. Evaluation reveals hypoxemia, platypnea, and orthodeoxia. Shunts can be revealed by bubble contrast echocardiography and radionuclide scintigraphic scanning with technetium labeled albumin. Orthotopic liver transplantation is a therapeutic option and medical management is not well established.

Indications for Transplantation
Liver transplantation is generally considered after the first episode of decompensation or with an increase in MELD score. The Model for End-Stage Liver Disease (MELD) score applies objective variables to patients listed for transplantation, combining serum creatinine, total bilirubin, and INR in a complicated mathematical formula that provides an objective "score," enabling the allocation of donor livers to "sicker" patients.

KEY POINTS TO REMEMBER

- Treatment of variceal hemorrhage includes volume and red blood cell resuscitation, correction of coagulopathy (as indicated), administration of octreotide, and endoscopic variceal ligation. Patients should be placed on a nonselective beta-blocker for secondary prophylaxis and treated with a third generation cephalosporin to prevent SBP.
- Treatment of hepatic encephalopathy includes administration of nonabsorbable disaccharides, antibiotics, or both. Common precipitants, such as a GI bleed and SBP, must be urgently recognized and treated.
- Ascites can be managed with aldosterone antagonists and loop diuretics or therapeutic paracentesis. Albumin administration should be considered.
- Spontaneous bacterial peritonitis must be suspected in any patient with ascites. A diagnostic paracentesis is required regardless of coagulopathy and thrombocytopenia. Recommended treatment includes a third generation cephalosporin and albumin to prevent renal dysfunction.
- Hepatorenal syndrome is associated with high morbidity and mortality rates and must be recognized and treated urgently.

REFERENCES AND SUGGESTED READINGS

Abraldes JG, Bosch J. Clinical features and natural history of variceal hemorrhage: implications for surveillance and screening. In: Sanyal AJ, Shah VH, eds. *Portal Hypertension: Pathobiology, Evaluation and Treatment.* Totowa, NJ: Humana Press; 2005: 167–182.

Akriviadis E, Botla R, Briggs W, et al. Pentoxifylline improves short-term survival in severe acute alcoholic hepatitis: a double-blind, placebo-controlled trial. *Gastroenterology* 2000;119:1637–1648.

Alam I, Bass NM, Bacchetti P, et al. Hepatic tissue endothelin-1 levels in chronic liver disease correlate with disease severity and ascites. *Am J Gastroenterol* 2000;95: 199–203.

Als-Nielsen B, Gluud LL, Gluud C. Nonabsorbable disaccharides for hepatic encephalopathy. *Cochrane Database Syst Rev* 2004;2. Art. No.: CD003044. DOI: 10.1002/ 14651858.CD003044.pub2.

Anthony PP, Ishak NG, Nayak NC, et al. The morphology of cirrhosis: recommendations on definition, nomenclature, and classification by a working group sponsored by the World Health Organization. *J Clin Pathol* 1978;31:395–414.

Arroyo V, Terra C, Gines P. New treatments of hepatorenal syndrome. *Semin Liver Dis* 2006;26:254–264.

Bataller R Gines P. Cirrhosis of the liver. In: Federman DD, Dale DC, Feldman M, et al., eds. *ACP Medicine.* WebMD Corporation, 2007. Accessed July 15, 2007.

Bernard B, Grange JD, Khac EN, et al. Antibiotic prophylaxis for the prevention of bacterial infections in cirrhotic patients with gastrointestinal bleeding: a meta-analysis. *Hepatology* 1999;29:1655–1661.

Bruix J, Sherman M; Practice Guidelines Committee, American Association for the Study of Liver Diseases. Management of hepatocellular carcinoma. *Hepatology* 2005;42: 1208–1236.

Cardenas A Arroyo V. Management of ascites and hepatic hydrothorax. *Best Pract Res Clin Gastroenterol* 2007;21:55–75.

Cardenas A Gines P. Mechanisms of sodium retention, ascites formation and renal dysfunction in cirrhosis. In: Sanyal AJ, Shah VH, eds. *Portal Hypertension: Pathobiology, Evaluation and Treatment.* Totowa, NJ: Humana Press; 2005:65–84.

Chung RT, Podolsky DK. Cirrhosis and its complications. In: Kasper DL, Fauci AS, Longo DL, et al., eds. *Harrison's Principle of Internal Medicine.* 16th ed. New York: McGraw-Hill; 2005:1858–1868.

Crawford JM. Liver and biliary tract. In: Vinay KV, Abbas AA, Fausto N, eds. *Robbins and Cotran Pathologic Basis of Disease.* 7th ed. Philadelphia: Elsevier Saunders; 2005: 877–927.

D'Amico G, Pagliaro L, Bosch J. Pharmacological treatment of portal hypertension: an evidence-based approach. *Semin Liver Dis* 1999;19:475–505.

De la Pena J, Brullet E, Sanchez-Hernandez E, et al. Variceal ligation plus nadolol compared with ligation for prophylaxis of variceal rebleeding: a multicenter trial. *Hepatology* 2005;4:572–578.

El-Serag HB, Mason AC, Key C. Trends in survival of patients with hepatocellular carcinoma between 1977 and 1996 in the United States. *Hepatology* 2001;33(1): 62–65.

Felisart J, Rimola A, Arroyo V, et al. Cefotaxime is more effective than is ampicillin-tobramycin in cirrhotics with severe infections. *Hepatology* 1985;5:457–462.

Francoz C, Belghiti J, Durand F. Indications for liver transplantation in patients with complications of cirrhosis. *Best Pract Res Clin Gastroenterol* 2007;21: 175–190.

Ghassemi S, Garcia-Tsao G. Prevention and treatment of infections in patients with cirrhosis. *Best Pract Res Clin Gastroenterol* 2007;21:77–93.

Gines P, Rimola A, Planas R, et al. Norfloxacin prevents spontaneous bacterial peritonitis recurrence in cirrhosis: results of a double-blind, placebo-controlled trial. *Hepatology* 1990;12:716–724.

Gines P, Tito L, Arroyo V, et al. Randomized comparative study of therapeutic paracentesis with and without intravenous albumin in cirrhosis. *Gastroenterology* 1988;94: 1493–1502.

Graham DY, Smith JL. The course of patients after variceal hemorrhage. *Gastroenterology* 1981;80:800–809.

Groszmann RJ, Garcia-Tsao G, Bosch J, et al. Beta-blockers to prevent gastroesophageal varices in patients with cirrhosis. *N Engl J Med* 2005;353:2254–2261.

Kamath PS, Kim WR; Advanced Liver Disease Study Group. The model for end-stage liver disease (MELD). *Hepatology* 2007;45:797–805.

Mandell MS. The diagnosis and treatment of hepatopulmonary syndrome. *Clin Liver Dis* 2006;10:387–405.

Moreau R, Lebrec D. Diagnosis and treatment of acute renal failure in patients with cirrhosis. *Best Pract Res Clin Gastroenterol* 2007;21:111–123.

Pagliaro L, D'Amico G, Sorensen TI, et al. Prevention of first bleeding in cirrhosis: a meta-analysis of randomized trials of nonsurgical treatment. *Ann Intern Med* 1992; 117:59–70.

Pinzani M, Vizzutti F. Anatomy and vascular biology of the cells in the portal circulation. In: Sanyal AJ, Shah VH, eds. *Portal Hypertension: Pathobiology, Evaluation, and Treatment.* Totowa, NJ: Humana Press; 2005:15–36.

Poynard T, Calès P, Pasta L, et al. Beta-adrenergic-antagonist drugs in the prevention of gastrointestinal bleeding in patients with cirrhosis and esophageal varices. An analysis of data and prognostic factors in 589 patients from four randomized clinical trials. Franco-Italian Multicenter Study Group. *N Engl J Med* 1991;324: 1532–1538.

Rockey DC. Cell and molecular mechanisms of increased intrahepatic resistance and hemodynamic correlates. In: Sanyal AJ, Shah VH, eds. *Portal Hypertension: Pathobiology, Evaluation, and Treatment.* Totowa, NJ: Humana Press; 2005: 37–50.

Russo MW, Sood A, Jacobson IM, et al. Transjugular intrahepatic portosystemic shunt for refractory ascites: an analysis of the literature on efficacy, morbidity, and mortality. *Am J Gastroenterol* 2003;98:2521–2527.

Saab S, Nieto JM, Lewis SK, Runyon BA. TIPS versus paracentesis for cirrhotic patients with refractory ascites. *Cochrane Database Syst Rev* 2006;4. Art. No.: CD004889. DOI: 10.1002/14651858.CD004889.pub2.

Sanyal AJ, Shah VH, eds. *Portal Hypertension: Pathobiology, Evaluation, and Treatment.* Totowa, NJ: Humana Press; 2005.

Schmidt LE, Ring-Larsen H. Vasoconstrictor therapy for hepatorenal syndrome in liver cirrhosis. *Curr Pharm Des* 2006;12:4637–4647.

Schrier RW, Arroyo V, Bernardi M, et al. Peripheral arterial vasodilation hypothesis: a proposal for the initiation of renal sodium and water retention in cirrhosis. *Hepatology* 1988;8:1151–1157.

Senzolo M, Cholongitas E, Tibballs J, et al. Transjugular intrahepatic portosystemic shunt in the management of ascites and hepatorenal syndrome. *Eur J Gastroenterol Hepatol* 2006;18:1143–1150.

Sort P, Navasa M, Arroyo V, et al. Effect of intravenous albumin on renal impairment and mortality in patients with cirrhosis and spontaneous bacterial peritonitis. *N Engl J Med* 1999;341:403–409.

Tito L, Rimola A, Gines P, et al. Recurrence of spontaneous bacterial peritonitis in cirrhosis: frequency and predictive factors. *Hepatology* 1988;8:27–31.

Vong S, Bell BP. Chronic liver disease mortality in the United States, 1990–1998. *Hepatology* 2004;39:476–483.

Wright G, Jalan R. Management of hepatic encephalopathy in patients with cirrhosis. *Best Pract Res Clin Gastroenterol* 2007;21:95–110.

Pancreatic Disorders

Daniel A. Ringold and Sreenivasa Jonnalagadda

INTRODUCTION

The pancreas is a mixed endocrine and exocrine gland consisting of lobular subunits composed of acini. The exocrine pancreas consists of acinar, centroacinar, and ductal cells. The acinar cells secrete approximately 20 digestive enzymes (in zymogen granules) into the central ductule of the acinus, which then connects with the intralobular ducts to form the interlobular ducts; these ducts, in turn, join to form the main pancreatic duct. The pancreatic duct then empties into the duodenum through the ampulla of Vater.

The pancreas lies in the retroperitoneal space of the upper abdomen. Because of its location, pancreatic disorders are generally more difficult to manage medically and surgically than those of other abdominal viscera. The central position of the pancreas provides for lymphatic drainage along several major routes (splenic, hepatic, and superior mesenteric nodal systems as well as the aortocaval and other posterior abdominal wall lymphatic vessels). The association with vital major vessels of the epigastrium also makes diseases of the pancreas difficult to treat. When a tumor spreads a short distance to involve the superior mesenteric vein, the portal vein, or the celiac axis, it usually considered incurable. If the gland is removed, the need to excise the vessels and lymph nodes associated with it often makes it necessary to remove the duodenum, gallbladder, distal bile duct, spleen, upper jejunum, and part of the stomach. Finally, the vascular nature of the pancreas and the adjacent organs makes hemorrhage the most common postoperative complication of pancreatic resection.

ACUTE PANCREATITIS

Causes

Pathophysiology

- The incidence of acute pancreatitis ranges from 1 to 5 per 10,000 per year. Two histologic forms of acute pancreatitis are recognized: interstitial and hemorrhagic. In interstitial pancreatitis, the gland is edematous, but its gross architecture is preserved, and hemorrhage is absent. In the hemorrhagic form, marked tissue necrosis and hemorrhage are apparent. Surrounding areas of fat necrosis are also prominent. Large hematomas often occur in the retroperitoneal space, and vascular inflammation or thrombosis is common. Mortality is more likely to occur with the hemorrhagic form. Clinically, pancreatitis is divided into non-necrotizing and necrotizing forms.
- Processes that contribute to the initiation of pancreatitis include pancreatic duct obstruction, pancreatic ischemia, and the premature activation of zymogens within

the pancreatic acinar cells. Acute pancreatitis is an autodigestive process that occurs when the proteolytic enzymes are prematurely activated within the pancreas rather than in the intestinal lumen. The active enzymes digest membranes within the pancreas, leading to edema, vascular damage, cellular injury, and death. This, in turn, leads to the further release of inflammatory cytokines (tumor necrosis factor, interleukin-1, platelet-activating factor) that recruit inflammatory cells and further increase vascular permeability. Eventually, this cascade of events leads to the development of acute pancreatitis and its systemic manifestations. Most cases of mild, acute pancreatitis are self-limited, with a mortality rate of 1%. Necrotizing pancreatitis occurs when areas of the pancreas become devitalized, predisposing patients to septic complications. Despite advances in intensive care medicine, severe necrotizing pancreatitis often has a complicated course, with a mortality rate approaching 30%.

Differential Diagnosis

Gallstones

Gallstone disease and excessive alcohol use account for 70% to 80% of cases of acute pancreatitis in western countries. Although gallstones are etiologically linked to pancreatitis, this condition develops in only a small percentage of patients with gallstones. While the precise pathogenesis is unclear, gallstones are thought to cause pancreatitis by mechanically obstructing the pancreatic duct where it joins the common bile duct leading to pancreatic ductal hypertension or by allowing the reflux of bile or duodenal contents into the pancreatic duct after passage across the sphincter of Oddi, thereby initiating the cascade of events described above.

Alcohol

A single binge use of alcohol rarely, if ever, causes pancreatitis. Alcohol-induced pancreatitis occurs in persons with long-standing alcohol use. Because only approximately 5% of chronic heavy alcohol users develop pancreatitis, other hereditary or environmental risk factors including smoking likely play a role.

Drugs

Drugs commonly implicated include pancreatitis include azathioprine, 6-mercaptopurine, L-asparaginase, pentamidine, didanosine, valproic acid, furosemide, sulfonamides, tetracyclines, estrogens, metronidazole, and erythromycin.

Trauma

Acute pancreatitis can be seen after blunt or penetrating abdominal trauma. Iatrogenic causes include endoscopic retrograde cholangiopancreatography (ERCP), pancreaticobiliary surgery, or cardiopulmonary bypass.

Hypertriglyceridemia

The breakdown products of triglycerides are responsible for inducing pancreatitis. When lipase in the pancreatic capillary bed acts on the high levels of triglycerides in the serum, toxic free fatty acids are generated. Although triglyceride levels >2000 to 3000 mg/dL usually are required for pancreatitis to develop, it can occur when serum levels are only 500 mg/dL. In general, a level of >1000 mg/dL suggests hypertriglyceridemia as a cause of the pancreatitis. Pancreatitis itself can elevate triglycerides in a few patients. Additionally, the typical hypocaloric regimen recommended during a pancreatitis episode (nil by mouth) results in rapid decline in triglyceride levels. Fasting triglyceride levels should be measured after discharge from the hospital to ascertain if hypertriglyceridemia is the cause of pancreatitis.

Infections

Infections are thought to be rare causes of pancreatitis. The most common viral infections that involve the pancreas are mumps, cytomegalovirus, and coxsackie B virus. Viral hepatitis, especially hepatitis B, has also been associated with pancreatitis. Patients with human immunodeficiency virus (HIV) develop pancreatitis at a higher rate than the general population. The virus itself appears to be the cause in some cases, but other factors (antiretroviral medications, alcohol abuse, dyslipidemia) also may play a role. Interestingly, asymptomatic hyperamylasemia and hyperlipasemia have been reported in up to 40% of patients with acquired immunodeficiency syndrome (AIDS). Bacteria associated with acute pancreatitis include *Salmonella, Shigella, Campylobacter,* hemorrhagic *Escherichia coli, Legionella, Leptospira,* and *Brucella* species. Pancreatitis associated with these infections is most likely toxin mediated and improves with clearance of the organisms.

Miscellaneous Causes
Other less common causes of pancreatitis include tumors (both benign and malignant), autoimmune disorders, hypercalcemia, hereditary pancreatitis, pancreas divisum, and papillary stenosis (sphincter of Oddi dysfunction).

Idiopathic
Despite an extensive workup, the cause will not be identifiable in 30% of cases of acute pancreatitis.

Presentation

History and Physical Examination
The hallmark of acute pancreatitis is abdominal pain located in the epigastric and periumbilical areas, radiating to the back. The pain typically is more intense when the patient is supine and may be relieved if the patient leans forward or assumes a fetal position. The pain worsens with food and alcohol ingestion. Nausea, emesis, and abdominal distention are also frequently reported. Hematemesis, melena, and diarrhea are infrequent. On physical examination, abdominal tenderness ranges from mild epigastric tenderness to rigidity with rebound tenderness. Scleral icterus may be seen because of biliary obstruction or accompanying liver disease. A faint bluish discoloration around the umbilicus (Cullen's sign) or flank (Turner's sign) is rarely seen.

Management

Diagnostic Evaluation
    Blood Tests. **Amylase** and **lipase** are enzymes released from the pancreas during acute pancreatitis. Amylase and lipase elevations at least twice the upper limit of normal are required to establish conclusively a diagnosis of pancreatitis. Lipase has slightly superior sensitivity and specificity than amylase. Plasma levels of both enzymes peak at 24 hours of symptoms, but amylase has a shorter half-life.
    Abdominal Imaging. Abdominal **ultrasonography** is of limited utility in visualizing the pancreas, but is very useful in establishing gallstones as the cause and should be the initial imaging modality in patients presenting with acute pancreatitis. Patients with typical symptoms and corresponding elevations of pancreatic enzymes do not necessarily require cross-sectional imaging with **computed tomography** (CT) for the initial diagnosis of pancreatitis. The CT scan may be normal in up to 30% of patients with mild pancreatitis, but it is almost always abnormal in patients with moderate or severe disease. CT scans should be obtained if the diagnosis is in doubt, patients do not improve within a few days, or if initial clinical response was followed by sudden clinical deterioration. Diagnostic CT should be performed using a pancreatic protocol, which involves thin slices through the pancreas during several contrast phases. Disruption of the pancreatic microcirculation results in necrosis of the pancreatic tissue and can be demonstrated on a CT scan. The severity of pancreatitis can also be staged based on these findings. Important findings include pancreatic

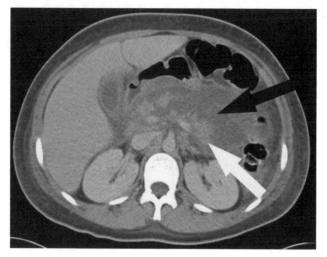

FIGURE 21-1. Computed tomography scan demonstrating pancreatic edema and necrosis in an 18-year-old man with gallstone-pancreatitis. Note the large areas of low-attenuation (*dark gray*) within the pancreatic bed (*black arrow*) compared with the areas with relatively preserved blood flow (*white arrow*). Normally, the pancreas has similar attenuation as the adjacent liver.

swelling, peripancreatic infiltrates, peripancreatic fluid collections, vascular thrombosis, and areas of nonenhancement because of necrosis (Fig. 21-1). **Magnetic resonance imaging (MRI)** has also emerged as an effective modality for evaluating pancreatitis. It is useful when renal insufficiency or dye allergies preclude the use of CT, but is also not routinely required.

Predictors of Severity

Because the severity of pancreatitis correlates with the prognosis, stratifying patients early during the hospital course is important. Several approaches have been used to differentiate those patients who have a mild course from those with a more serious illness. These rating schemes include Ranson's criteria, modified Glasgow criteria, Acute Physiologic and Chronic Health Evaluation (APACHE) II score, and the CT Severity Index (Table 21-1). When compared at 48 hours after admission, the systems are similar. The disadvantage of Ranson's criteria is that patients must be scored on admission and at 48 hours to obtain a completed score. The modified Glasgow criteria and the APACHE II scoring system can be calculated anytime during the hospital stay. The CT Severity Index does not use any clinical or laboratory parameters and only uses findings seen at imaging. This system is accurate in differentiating mild from severe pancreatitis.

Treatment

Mild Acute Pancreatitis. Treatment is supportive with bed rest, no oral intake, intravenous hydration, electrolyte replacement, antiemetics, and analgesics (meperidine or morphine). Nasogastric suction may be useful to alleviate the symptoms of nausea, emesis, and abdominal distention. The patient can be cautiously fed once the abdominal pain resolves.

TABLE 21-1 COMPARISON OF SEVERITY SCORING SYSTEMS FOR ACUTE PANCREATITIS

Ranson's Criteria[a]		Glasgow Criteria	Computerized Tomography (CT) Scoring Criteria	
On Admission	**Within 48 hrs**		**Score**	**CT Findings**
WBC >16,000/mm^3	Hematocrit decrease by 10%	WBC >15,000/mm^3	0	Normal pancreas
Age >55 yrs	BUN increase by >5mg/dL	BUN >45mg/dL without response to fluids	1	Focal or diffuse pancreatic enlargement
	Calcium <8 mg/dL	Calcium <8 mg/dL	2	Peripancreatic inflammation with intrinsic pancreatic abnormalities
	Arterial pO$_2$ <60 mm Hg	Arterial pO$_2$ <60 mm Hg	3	Presence of single fluid collection
AST >250 IU/L	Base deficit >4 mEq/L	AST >200 U/L	4	Presence of two or more fluid collections or gas in the pancreas and/or retroperitoneum
LDH >350 IU/L	Fluid sequestration >6 L	LDH >600 U/L	**Score**	**Necrosis (%)**
Glucose >200 mg/dL		Glucose >180 mg/dL without diabetes	0	0
		Albumin <3.2 g/dL	2	<33
			4	33–50
			6	≥50
Mortality rate of fewer than or equal to four criteria is <15% and considered mild disease. Mortality rate rises greatly with more than four criteria.		Severe pancreatitis is defined as the presence of three or more of the above criteria within 48 hrs of evaluation.	CT severity index is defined as the sum of the CT findings score and the pancreatic necrosis score. The maximum is 10 and >6 predicts sever disease. A severity score of 7–10 had a 92% complication rate and a 17% mortality rate, whereas a score of 0 or 1 had zero morbidity or mortality.	

AST, aspartate aminotransferase; BUN, blood urea nitrogen; LDH, lactate dehydrogenase; WBC, white blood cell count.

[a]Applies to nonbiliary causes of pancreatitis. Criteria are adjusted with biliary pancreatitis.

Adapted from Ranson JHC, Rifkind KM, Roses DF, et al. *Surg Gynecol Obstet* 1974;139:69; Corfield AP, Williamson RCN, McMahon MJ, et al. *Lancet* 1985;24:403; and Balthazar EJ, Robinson DL, Megibow AJ, et al. *Radiology* 1990;174:331, with permission.

Severe Acute Pancreatitis. The treatment of severe pancreatitis, like milder forms, is primarily supportive, with the exception that patients require more vigorous fluid resuscitation. Patients typically require close monitoring in the intensive care unit. A patient-controlled analgesic pump is often required to achieve adequate levels of pain control. Other treatment modalities are discussed below. Patients should be monitored closely for signs of clinical deterioration from multisystem organ failure (renal, respiratory, cardiovascular, or sepsis).

Antibiotics. The issue of prophylactic antibiotics in pancreatitis is contentious. In general, prophylactic antibiotics are recommended in cases of severe necrotizing pancreatitis or suspected biliary pancreatitis with cholangitis, whereas they are not recommended for mild pancreatitis. Appropriate antibiotics should be active against a wide variety of organisms—in particular, gram-negative bacilli. The most commonly used regimens include imipenem, meropenem, or a combination of a fluoroquinolone and metronidazole. The optimal length of treatment is not known, but antibiotics are usually continued for 10 to 14 days or until clinical improvement is seen. Caution should be exercised, because prolonged use of broad-spectrum antibiotics is associated with resistant bacterial and disseminated fungal infections.

Endoscopic Retrograde Cholangiopancreatography. ERCP should be performed in patients with presumed gallstone pancreatitis with suspected residual common bile duct stones as suggested by persistently elevated liver enzymes or bilirubin, dilated common bile duct, or obvious choledocholithiasis seen during ultrasonography or other imaging and in those with findings suggestive of cholangitis (right upper quadrant abdominal pain and tenderness, fever >39°C, leukocyte count >20,000). ERCP with sphincterotomy has been shown to reduce length of hospital stay and mortality in patients with suspected residual bile duct stones when performed 24 to 72 hours after presentation.

Nutrition. Pancreatitis creates a hypermetabolic state for which the body has limited ability to cope beyond a short time period. If the pancreatitis is severe, it may require weeks or months before oral feedings are reintroduced. If symptoms do not resolve and an oral diet cannot be resumed in 5 to 7 days, other avenues for nutritional support have to be considered. Enteral tube feeding delivered to the jejunum (beyond the ligament of Treitz) is the safest manner in which to deliver nutrition. In bypassing the stomach and duodenum, jejunal feedings theoretically avoid the meal-driven pancreatic stimulation that can lead to abdominal pain or recurrent attacks of pancreatitis. Further, enteral feedings are thought to maintain the health and barrier function of the bowel itself. This is important because the superinfection of pancreatic fluid collections is thought to occur through bacterial translocation. For this reason, total parental nutrition (TPN) should be considered as a second option in feeding patients with moderate to severe pancreatitis. Although TPN is effective in delivering calories, minerals, and micronutrients, it requires central venous access and monitoring of key metabolic parameters, and it carries a significant risk of line sepsis and is costly.

Management of Fluid Collections

Pseudocysts develop in 15% of patients with pancreatitis. Previously, any pseudocyst larger than 6 cm persisting for 6 weeks was managed with a drainage procedure. It now clear, however, that some of these pseudocysts that are not enlarging or causing symptoms will resolve without intervention and can be monitored with serial CT scans. In patients with enlarging or symptomatic, noninfected pseudocysts, endoscopic or radiological drainage is an attractive method. Radiologic placement of drainage catheters is successful, but it can result in pancreatocutaneous fistulas. In recent years, transluminal endoscopic approaches have been increasingly adopted to treat symptomatic fluid collections. For endoscopic drainage to be successful, the fluid collection should not be multiloculated and should not contain excessive amounts of debris or necrotic material. The absence of pseudoaneruysms in the wall of the cyst should be confirmed with CT scan before attempting endoscopic drainage. After identifying the site in the stomach or duodenum for puncture with or without endoscopic ultrasonography (EUS) guidance to locate an area devoid of blood vessels, a guidewire is passed into the cavity, the tract dilated with a balloon, and "pigtail" stents or nasocystic drains are placed within. This allows for decompression and drainage of the pseudocyst contents directly into the bowel through the cystenterostomy (Fig. 21-2). Patients are followed with serial imaging studies to document resolution of the pseudocyst. Once the pseudocyst has resolved, the stents or drains may be removed.

Occasionally, bacterial colonization of a pseudocyst or inflammatory mass occurs, resulting in an infected pancreatic necrosis or abscess. The clinical manifestations include worsening pain, fever, septic physiology, and an elevated white blood cell count. Aspiration of any low-density areas or fluid collections under CT or ultrasound guidance can guide further interventions. If organisms or polymorphonuclear neutrophils are seen, the patient should undergo percutaneous drainage or surgical débridement. The typically viscous and loculated nature of infected fluid collections tends to render endoscopic drainage ineffective. In rare instances, however, direct endoscopic débridement through a cystenterostomy and irrigation of the cyst for several days via a nasocystic drain have been successfully performed in poor surgical candidates with solitary infected fluid collections.

CHRONIC PANCREATITIS

Causes

Pathophysiology

Chronic pancreatitis is an inflammatory disease of the pancreas characterized by irreversible damage of the pancreatic architecture. This includes irregular fibrosis, acinar cell loss, islet cell loss, and inflammatory cell infiltrates. The incidence of chronic pancreatitis is approximately 4 of 100,000 per year, whereas the prevalence is approximately 13 of 100,000. Alcohol in Western societies (70%–80%) and malnutrition worldwide are the major causes of chronic pancreatitis. In general, prolonged alcohol intake (6–12 years) is required to produce symptomatic chronic pancreatitis. (See Table 21-2 for the TIGAR-O classification system for etiologic risk factors for chronic pancreatitis.)

Presentation

Clinical Presentation

Abdominal Pain. The presenting symptom of most patients with chronic pancreatitis is dull and constant epigastric or periumbilical pain. The pain may radiate directly to the back. Pain could occur periodically, lasting several days, or occasionally be constant. The aggravation of pain by eating is common in chronic pancreatitis, however, other medical conditions (e.g., mesenteric ischemia and irritable bowel syndrome) can also result in a similar presentation. Pain in chronic pancreatitis can continue, diminish, or disappear completely in the most advanced stages. Chronic pancreatitis is painless in approximately 15% of patients. Idiopathic pancreatitis is more likely to be painless than is the alcoholic variety.

Weight Loss. Nausea, vomiting, anorexia, and weight loss are common in chronic pancreatitis. Malabsorption, sitophobia , pancreatic malignancy, or uncontrolled diabetes may contribute to weight loss.

Malabsorption. When <10% of the normal exocrine secretion of pancreatic enzymes remains in a patient with chronic pancreatitis, diarrhea, steatorrhea, and azotorrhea

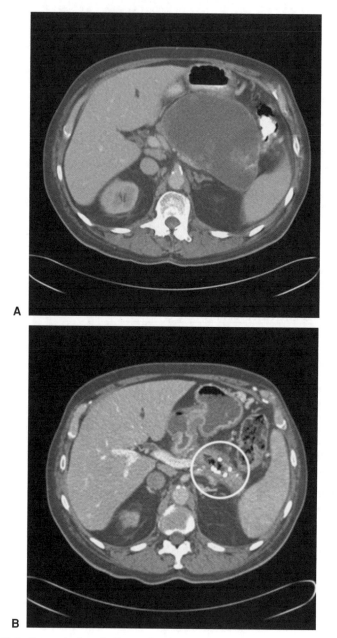

FIGURE 21-2. Demonstration of efficacy of endoscopic pancreatic pseudocyst drainage in a 58-year-old man with severe pancreatitis who developed a large pseudocyst as seen on computed tomography (**A**). He was symptomatic with abdominal pain, early satiety, and nausea. Therefore multiple "pigtail" stents were endoscopically placed from the stomach into the cavity, and the cyst resolved over a period of 4 months (*white circle*) (**B**).

TABLE 21-2	TIGAR-O CLASSIFICATION SYSTEM OF CHRONIC PANCREATITIS
Toxic-metabolic	Alcohol, tobacco, hypercalcemia, hyperlipidemia, chronic renal failure, medications (phenacetin abuse)
Idiopathic	Early onset, late onset, tropical
Genetic	Cationic trypsinogen, cystic fibrosis transmembrane conductance regulator mutations
Autoimmune	Sjögren's syndrome, inflammatory bowel disease, primary biliary cirrhosis
Recurrent and severe acute pancreatitis	Postnecrotic, recurrent acute pancreatitis, vascular disease, postirradiation
Obstructive	Pancreas divisum, duct obstruction (tumor), posttraumatic pancreatic duct scars, preampullary duodenal wall cysts

Adapted from: Etemad B, Whitcomb DC. Chronic pancreatitis: diagnosis, classification, and new genetic developments. *Gastroenterology* 2001;120:682–707, with permission.

(protein malabsorption) can occur. These symptoms tend to occur relatively late in the course of chronic pancreatitis. Fecal weight tends to be less in pancreatic malabsorption than in other conditions with comparable steatorrhea. Patients may pass bulky, formed stool as opposed to the frank watery diarrhea observed in other conditions.

Pancreatic Diabetes. Clinically evident diabetes, which occurs relatively late in the disease, is seen in up to 60% of patients with chronic pancreatitis. Diabetic ketoacidosis and diabetic nephropathy are relatively uncommon in this form of diabetes.

Other Clinical Features. Less common manifestations of chronic pancreatitis include jaundice (extrinsic bile duct obstruction or stricture), ascites, pleural effusion, painful subcutaneous nodules (pancreatic panniculitis), and polyarthritis of the small joints of the hands.

Physical Examination

The physical examination usually is of limited assistance in the diagnosis of chronic pancreatitis because the intensity of the patient's complaint tends to be out of proportion to the physical signs. Epigastric tenderness may be present during the painful episodes as well as during periods of remission. Complications of chronic pancreatitis (large pseudocysts, ascites, or pleural effusions) may be detected on physical examination.

Management

Diagnostic Evaluation

The diagnosis of chronic pancreatitis often can be made based on the history and relatively simple radiographic tests. Routine blood studies usually are not helpful in making the diagnosis of chronic pancreatitis. Leukocytosis may be observed during acute exacerbations. Anemia and fat-soluble vitamin deficiency states (hypocalcemia, hypoprothrombinemia, night blindness) are seldom seen in association with the steatorrhea of chronic pancreatitis. Varying degrees of cholestasis can be seen secondary to involvement of the common bile duct by pancreatic fibrosis. This can cause elevations in serum alkaline phosphatase, and jaundice can result from more severe involvement.

Amylase and Lipase

In contrast to attacks of acute pancreatitis, in which the serum level of pancreatic enzymes is usually elevated, serum enzyme levels may be elevated, normal, or low in chronic pancreatitis.

Direct Tests of Pancreatic Exocrine Secretion

Pancreatic exocrine output is directly measured by two similar methods employing pancreatic stimlation with secretin, cholecystikin, or both. These tests measure peak bicarbonate concentrations or enzyme activity after hormonal stimulation. If the levels are subnormal, chronic pancreatitis is suggested. One method relies on the placement of a multilumen aspiration catheter in the distal duodenum, whereas the other uses endoscopic fluid aspiration. A third method of direct testing for chronic pancreatitis is the measurement of pancreatic polypeptide. A subnormal rise in plasma pancreatic polypeptide after stimulation with a protein-rich meal or secretin infusion is an indicator of chronic pancreatitis. These tests are seldomly used in clinical practice.

Indirect Tests of Pancreatic Exocrine Secretion

Indirect tests of pancreatic exocrine secretion measure either pancreatic enzymes or the absorption of some compound first requiring digestion by pancreatic enzymes. Because clinically detectable nutrient malabsorption does not occur until pancreatic enzyme secretion has diminished to <10% of normal, tests of pancreatic function are unable to detect early chronic pancreatitis. The **bentiromide test** involves ingestion of N-benzoyl-L-tyrosyl-p-aminobenzoic acid (NBT-PABA), a tripeptide that is digested by chymotrypsin with the release of paraaminobenzoic acid (PABA). Free PABA is absorbed in the small bowel and excreted by the kidney. The quantity excreted in urine is used as a measure of pancreatic exocrine function. The diagnosis of pancreatic insufficiency by way of measurements of **fecal chymotrypsin activity** is rapid and simple, but the sensitivity of this test is considered too low to be recommended in clinical practice. In contrast, **fecal elastase measurements** appear to be much more sensitive and specific in the diagnosis of moderate to severe pancreatic insufficiency.

Imaging Studies

Abdominal Plain Films. The evaluation should begin with a plain film of the abdomen. The demonstration of **diffuse, speckled calcification of the pancreas on a plain film of the abdomen** is diagnostic of chronic pancreatitis. Although often seen in patients with advanced pancreatitis, the presence of pancreatic calcifications does not correlate with disease severity.

Ultrasound. Findings on ultrasonography that correlate with marked pancreatic changes on ERCP include dilation of the main pancreatic duct to >4 mm (>1 cm) cavities, and calcifications. When a satisfactory examination is obtained, the reported sensitivity of this test for chronic pancreatitis is approximately 70%, and the specificity is 90%.

CT Scan. CT is more sensitive than ultrasonography for the diagnosis of chronic pancreatitis. Besides being significantly more expensive, CT carries the additional risks of contrast reactions and radiation exposure. The most common diagnostic findings of chronic pancreatitis on CT include duct dilation, calcifications, and cystic lesions. Less common diagnostic findings include enlargement or atrophy of the pancreas and heterogeneous density of the parenchyma.

Magnetic Resonance Cholangiopancreatography. Magnetic resonance cholangiopancreatography (MRCP) is useful in the evaluation of chronic pancreatitis. MRCP allows for accurate delineation of the pancreatic duct (presence of dilation, stones, or strictures), evaluation of pancreatic parenchyma as well as the detection of subtle solid and cystic lesions. Additionally, MRCP may be more desirable than CT in that it avoids the exposure to ionizing radiation and iodinated intravenous contrast.

Endoscopic Retrograde Cholangiopancreatography. ERCP is a sensitive and specific imaging tool for the diagnosis of chronic pancreatitis. In mild pancreatitis, the changes are limited to the side-branch ducts, which show dilation and irregularity. Moderate pancreatitis is characterized by the additional findings of dilation and tortuosity of the main pancreatic duct. Advanced pancreatitis has the additional findings of ductal stenosis, stone formation, cyst formation, or atrophy of the pancreas. The widespread availability of EUS and MRCP has largely supplanted the use of ERCP for diagnostic pancreatography. ERCP is typically performed with intent to deliver therapy as directed by other imaging modalities rather than purely as a diagnostic procedure.

Endoscopic Ultrasonography. EUS provides more detailed structural information of the pancreas compared with routine ultrasonosgraphy and CT scan and does not carry the same risk of complications as ERCP. EUS allows for evaluation of ductal and parenchymal changes, such as echotexture of the gland, calcifications, lobulations, and bands of fibrosis. It also allows for direct tissue sampling by fine needle aspiration (FNA) if indicated.

Treatment of Pain
Avoidance of Alcohol. Avoiding alcohol consumption decreases the frequency and severity of abdominal pain in chronic alcoholic pancreatitis. All patients with excessive alcohol consumption should be referred to an appropriate treatment program. In patients who maintain significant exocrine secretory function, pain may be provoked by alcohol, which acts as a pancreatic secretagogue. In patients whose exocrine secretion is drastically reduced, alcohol may play a lesser role in the mechanism of pain. Further studies are needed to clarify the role of alcohol in pain production.

Analgesics. Analgesics remain the main method for pain control in chronic pancreatitis. Initially, non-narcotic analgesics, such as salicylates or acetaminophen, should be used. As pain severity increases, the dose or frequency of these simpler analgesics should be increased before switching to narcotics. In severe cases, however, opiate analgesics are required. Because many of these patients have addictive personalities, opiate dependence is a frequent problem, and the participation of a pain management specialist is helpful.

Celiac Plexus Block. Celiac ganglion injections have been used for control of pancreatic pain. This procedure can be performed either by radiologists using fluoroscopy or gastroenterologists using EUS guidance. Typically, absolute alcohol is injected into the area where the celiac plexus lies. In small, uncontrolled series of patients with chronic pancreatitis with debilitating pain, this procedure has produced mixed results. The occasional benefits almost never last for more than a few months, and repeated treatment may not be as effective.

Enzyme Therapy. Several groups of investigators confirmed that intestinal administration of trypsin or chymotrypsin inhibits pancreatic enzyme secretion. Decreased enzyme secretion can result in hyperstimulation of the pancreas (secondary to elevated plasma cholecystokinin levels), resulting in pain. It is therefore theorized that effective enzyme replacement therapy should reduce pancreatic stimulation, decrease intraductal pressure, and diminish pain. In most patients, a trial of high-dose, nonenteric-coated pancreatic enzymes is prescribed with meals for several weeks in any patient with painful chronic pancreatitis. Typically, a starting dose of at least 48,000 units of lipase, 90,000 units of amylase and 90,000 units of protease are taken with each meal. It is also recommended that patients take a histamine-2 receptor antagonist or proton-pump inhibitor to diminish enzyme degradation by gastric acid. The best results are seen in pancreatitis of nonalcoholic etiology, with symptoms of constant, rather than recurrent, pain and only mild to moderate pancreatic insufficiency.

Octreotide. Somatostatin is a naturally occurring hormone that has been shown to inhibit pancreatic secretion. Octreotide is a synthetic long-acting analog of somatostatin that has been shown to inhibit cholecystokinin (CCK) release and both basal and neurally stimulated pancreatic secretion. Randomized studies of patients with advanced chronic pancreatitis and severe pain suggest (without reaching statistical significance), that 200 μg of octreotide administered subcutaneously three times per day produced the greatest pain relief (65% vs. 35% of patients with placebo), especially in patients with constant as opposed to intermittent pain. Additional studies are needed to further clarify the role of octreotide in the management of chronic pancreatitis pain.

Endoscopic Therapy. Endoscopic therapy has been used for control of pain in chronic pancreatitis, with the aim of alleviating obstruction of flow caused by ductal strictures, stones, or papillary stenosis. Ductal strictures are sometimes treated by balloon dilation and, in most cases, then followed by stent placement across the stricture. Endoscopic techniques also have been used for the removal of pancreatic stones in chronic pancreatitis. In the cases of large stones, extracorporeal shockwave lithotripsy is used in conjunction with ERCP to fragment and then remove stones. Papillary stenosis is treated with pancreatic sphincterotomy.

Surgical Treatment. A growing body of evidence suggests that surgical therapies for chronic pancreatitis are superior to endoscopic management in the ability to provide long-lasting pain relief. The type of surgery is selected according to the perceived mechanism for the pain, the severity of pain, ductal morphology, and the extent of parenchymal disease. Patients who have ductal dilation have a 70% to 80% chance of obtaining pain relief with either a partial resection with pancreaticojejunostomy or lateral pancreaticojejunostomy. Other options include partial pancreatectomy or near total pancreatectomy with islet cell transplantation. Distal pancreatectomy can also be considered in those with focal changes limited to the tail of the pancreas.

Treatment of Pancreatic Exocrine Insufficiency

Although it is not common to see complete correction of steatorrhea in patients with chronic pancreatitis, it is possible to bring the steatorrhea under control. Porcine pancreatic enzymes are the cornerstone of therapy of malabsorption in patients with chronic pancreatic. It is critical that sufficient amounts of enzyme are delivered to the small bowel to abolish azotorrhea and significantly reduce steatorrhea. Generally, 30,000 units of pancreatic lipase taken with each meal is adequate to reduce steatorrhea and prevent further weight loss. The addition of acid-suppressive agents reduces degradation in the stomach and increases the amount of pancreatic enzymes available in the small bowel to assist in fat digestion. The dosage of the pancreatic enzyme supplements can be titrated to treat the patient's symptoms and malabsorption adequately.

PANCREATIC CANCER

Approximately 28,000 new cases of pancreatic cancer occur every year in the United States, and nearly all of these patients eventually die from the disease. Although surgical resection of the tumor offers the only chance for cure, patients having "curative resections" have median and 5-year survivals of only 18 to 20 months and 10%, respectively. The peak incidence of pancreatic carcinoma occurs in the seventh decade of life, and there is a slight male predominance. The overall incidence of the disease is 30% to 40% higher in blacks than in whites. Risk factors related to pancreatic cancer are listed below.

Causes

Pathophysiology

Ductal adenocarcinoma and its variants make up >90% of all malignant exocrine pancreatic tumors. Approximately two-thirds of ductal adenocarcinomas occur in the head of the gland, with the rest in the body or tail. Tumors of the head of the pancreas are usually

≥2 cm in diameter, and 70% to 80% have metastasized to regional lymph nodes by the time they are discovered. Tumors of the body and tail commonly are more advanced and larger (5–7 cm) when discovered, because they do not produce symptoms as early as pancreatic head tumors. The symptoms from tumors in the body and tail are usually caused by malignant infiltration of the retroperitoneal structures, which produces pain. By the time of diagnosis, almost all are unresectable. The best outcome is seen in patients who have well-differentiated neoplasms, without retroperitoneal invasion or lymph node metastases. Because pancreatic cancer has usually spread to lymph nodes or vascular structures at the time of diagnosis, most patients have at least stage III disease. Patients with stage IV disease (distant metastases) cannot be cured and their tumors are considered unresectable.

Presentation

Risk Factors

Smoking. Around the world, the risk factor most strongly linked to pancreatic cancer is cigarette smoking. It approximately doubles the chance of developing the disease. The risk of pancreatic cancer rapidly decreases when individuals discontinue cigarette use. The relative risk falls to approximately 1 10 to 15 years after quitting smoking.

Chronic Pancreatitis. Epidemiologic studies suggest that the relative risk of developing pancreatic cancer in patients with chronic pancreatitis is increased by up to 15 times when compared with control populations. This suggests that changes associated with chronic inflammation and fibrosis in the pancreas are important in the development of cancer. This increased risk of pancreatic cancer is seen in hereditary chronic pancreatitis, kindreds with multiple tumor suppressor-1 gene mutations, and other familial cancer syndromes, such as Peutz-Jeghers syndrome as well as tropical chronic pancreatitis. Chronic pancreatitis, however, accounts for only a small fraction of patients who have pancreatic cancer.

Surgery. Patients who have had a partial gastrectomy have a three- to sevenfold greater risk of developing pancreatic cancer. The apparent increase in incidence may be related to altered metabolism of ingested carcinogens by the remaining stomach and small intestine after surgery.

Diet. Meats and foods of animal origin increase the risk of pancreatic cancer, whereas foods of plant origin and dietary fiber appear to be protective.

Obesity. A body mass index of >30 kg/m^2 is also reported to be associated with increased cancer risk.

Clinical Presentation

Jaundice. Jaundice, accompanied by pain, is the presenting symptom in 80% to 90% of patients with cancer of the head of the pancreas.

Abdominal Pain. Epigastric or right upper quadrant abdominal pain can occur owing to biliary tree obstruction. Similar pain or discomfort in the left upper quadrant, back, or periumbilical areas could also result from pancreatic duct distention associated with pancreatic duct obstruction, or invasion of retroperitoneal or somatic nerves.

Weight Loss. By the time of diagnosis, weight loss of $>10\%$ of ideal body weight is common. Pain associated with the tumor produces anorexia, and the decreased food intake leads to weight loss. Proinflammatory cytokines, especially tumor necrosis factor-α, play a prominent role in the pathogenesis of pancreatic cancer cachexia. Malabsorption from pancreatic insufficiency can also contribute to weight loss.

Diabetes Mellitus. Diabetes sometimes appears as an early manifestation of pancreatic cancer, occurring many months before the tumor becomes evident.

Other Clinical Features. Light-colored stools and dark urine are seen if obstructive jaundice exists. Other symptoms include pruritus, nausea, emesis, and weakness. Emesis may be caused by duodenal or gastric outlet obstruction from tumor invasion. Gastrointestinal

(GI) bleeding can occur from direct invasion of the tumor into the duodenum, stomach, or colon. Migratory thrombophlebitis (Trousseau's sign) is reported in approximately 10% of patients and may be the earliest presenting sign. There is also a poorly understood association of pancreatic malignancy with major depression.

Management

Diagnostic Evaluation

The two main goals in the workup of a patient with presumed pancreatic cancer are (a) Establish the diagnosis with certainty and (b) determine if the patient should undergo a surgical procedure to resect or palliate the disease.

Carbohydrate Antigen 19-9 Levels. Carbohydrate antigen (CA) 19-9 is the most sensitive (80%) and specific (90%) tumor marker for pancreatic cancer; however, it is almost never positive with small tumors (<1 cm). CA 19-9 values also may be abnormal with other cancers (gastric, colorectal cancer) and with some benign conditions (cholangitis, biliary obstruction). Determination of serum CA 19-9 levels may be useful to provide some assurance that the tumor has been resected in its entirety, to signal the presence of recurrent disease after resection, and to determine the response to adjuvant therapy.

Ultrasound. Ultrasonography may be useful in patients with jaundice to distinguish between intrahepatic and extrahepatic causes. Extrahepatic obstruction from a pancreatic (or periampullary) cancer is expected to show dilated intrahepatic and extrahepatic biliary ducts. Although the specificity of ultrasonography to diagnose pancreatic cancer ranges from 90% to 99%, the sensitivity is as low as 75%. Usually additional imaging, as described below, is required when a pancreatic malignancy is suspected.

CT Scan. Triple phase CT is an excellent tool for the preoperative staging of pancreatic cancer. It provides information about site of the lesion, its resectability (e.g., presence of hepatic metastases, vascular invasion) and its vascular anatomy. CT scan is able to detect tumors approximately ≥2 cm in diameter, which appear as low-attenuating areas, because they are poorly perfused as compared with the adjacent pancreatic tissue. Metastatic cancer in lymph nodes and small hepatic metastases may be not appreciated by CT.

MRI. In patients who cannot undergo a CT scan, an MRI is a reasonable alternative for cross-sectional imaging. MRI does not typically provide information in addition to that obtained from CT.

Endoscopic Retrograde Cholangiopancreatography. ERCP has a sensitivity of 95% and a specificity of 85% for the diagnosis of pancreatic cancer. Performed successfully in more than 90% of patients, ERCP occasionally detects tumors not seen on imaging studies. At the time of ERCP, cytology brushings from the bile duct can be obtained, which have a sensitivity between 20% and 60% in confirming the diagnosis of malignancy. A stent can also be placed into the obstructed common bile duct to palliate patients who are not surgical candidates. In addition, some surgeons and oncologists may want the stent placed in the bile duct to ensure adequate biliary drainage before initiation of chemotherapy. This may decrease the risk of, and allow for monitoring for, hepatotoxic adverse events related to chemotherapy. In these cases, endoscopists can place either a plastic or a short metal stent. Despite its value, ERCP is not required in all patients with pancreatic cancer. If a patient has a history typical for pancreatic cancer (e.g., pain, jaundice, weight loss) and a mass in the head of the pancreas evident on CT scan, then the patient could potentially undergo surgical exploration without need for a preoperative ERCP. An ERCP for drainage of the biliary tree and cytological sampling can be performed if the bilirubin is markedly elevated, nutritional status is poor, and delays in surgical intervention are anticipated. The *only* absolute indications for an ERCP are cholangitis, intractable pruritus, and hyperbilirubinemia that has to be treated before the initiation of chemotherapy.

Endoscopic Ultrasound. EUS is a highly sensitive tool for local and regional staging. It is complementary to cross-sectional imaging because it does not provide information about distant metastatic disease. EUS provides reliable information about major vascular involvement and lymph node enlargement. FNA of the primary pancreatic lesion or potential lymph node metastasis can be performed during EUS. Additionally, EUS with FNA is used to establish the diagnosis when cross-sectional imaging is equivocal regarding the presence of a mass.

Fine-Needle Aspiration. FNA for cytology is obtained either percutaneously under CT or ultrasound guidance or endoscopically by EUS. Tissue sampling should be pursued when cytologic proof of malignancy alters management, for instance as a prerequisite for chemotherapy, radiation therapy, or palliative stenting with a permanent metal stent. Seeding of the peritoneal cavity, as has been described following percutaneous sampling, can be avoided with the endoscopic technique.

Staging Laparoscopy

Because of the aggressive nature of pancreatic cancer, metastatic disease at the time of presentation is common. Some of these metastases may be small or diffuse (hepatic or peritoneal implants) and remain unrecognized in the initial diagnostic evaluation. A number of case series have demonstrated that 10% to 40% of tumors thought to be resectable actually had distant or local spread that would have precluded resection. A staging laparoscopy complements the noninvasive staging and helps the surgeon decide tumor resectability. In addition to inspecting the abdominal cavity for frank metastasis, peritoneal washings are taken for cytology, peritoneal nodules or lymph nodes are sampled, and probe ultrasound of the pancreas or liver can be performed. Because pancreatic tumors in the body and tail commonly metastasize to the peritoneum and liver, staging laparoscopy may be particularly useful in these patients.

Treatment

Surgery. Pancreatic cancer surgery is performed with curative intent only if no evidence of metastatic disease is seen on the preoperative imaging studies and staging laparoscopy. The type of surgery performed for pancreatic cancer mainly depends on the location of the tumor. A pancreaticoduodenectomy (Whipple or pylorus-sparing Whipple resection) is typically performed for tumors involving the pancreatic head. The classic Whipple resection involves a partial gastrectomy (antrectomy), cholecystectomy, and removal of the distal common bile duct, head of the pancreas, duodenum, proximal jejunum, and regional lymph nodes. Reconstruction requires a pancreaticojejunostomy, hepaticojejunostomy, and a gastrojejunostomy. For tumors involving the body or tail of the pancreas, a distal pancreatectomy and splenectomy are performed. Rarely, patients are offered a total pancreatectomy for large or multifocal tumors.

Surgical Palliation. When resection of the primary tumor is not possible, palliative procedures are performed. An anastomosis between the common bile duct and jejunum (choledochojejunostomy) serves to bypass the bile duct obstruction. Fifteen to 20% of these patients eventually develop duodenal obstruction and a gastrojejunostomy is often performed during the initial surgery if a curative resection is not feasible.

Nonsurgical Palliation. Endoscopically placed metal or polyethylene stents are commonly used to relieve biliary obstructions. Polyethylene stents need to be replaced every 3–4 months due to their occlusion from bacterial biofilm and precipitated debris from the bile duct. Metal stents may be covered or uncovered and typically cannot be removed after placement (Fig. 21-3). They maintain patency longer and improve both quality of life and mortality compared with plastic stents. Metal stents are placed with the expectation that they will remain patent for the life of the patient. Tumor ingrowth can result in stent occlusion, however, and a new stent can be placed within the old

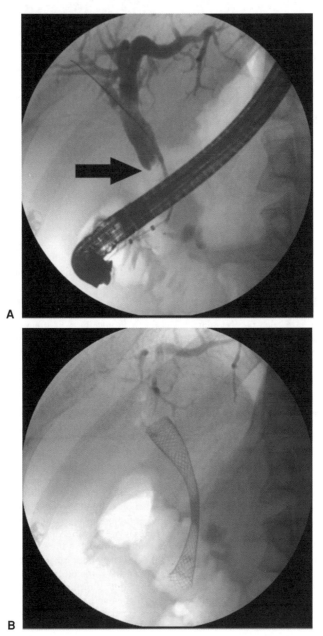

FIGURE 21-3. Endoscopic palliation of pancreatic cancer. A 69-year-old man developed jaundice and a pancreatic mass was found that had metastasized to the liver. The decision was to administer palliative chemotherapy and place a metal biliary stent. The initial fluoroscopic cholangiogram demonstrates markedly dilated proximal and intrahepatic bile ducts with a "cut-off" (*arrow*) in the distal bile duct resulting from a malignant stricture (**A**). Fluoroscopic image demonstrates successful placement of a metallic self-expanding biliary stent across the malignant stricture (**B**).

stent to relieve the obstruction. Gastric outlet obstruction can also be palliated effectively by endoscopic placement of expandable metal stents.

Adjuvant and Neoadjuvant Treatment. 5-Fluorouracil, combined with radiation therapy, confers a modest prolongation of survival in patients with locally advanced pancreatic cancer. Gemcitabine has been shown to increase the quality of life in patients with advanced pancreatic cancer, but survival is only modestly improved. Neoadjuvant chemotherapy is given to some patients in the hope of downstaging locally advanced tumors to improve resection rates. Studies have not yet clearly demonstrated prolonged survival, however.

KEY POINTS TO REMEMBER

- Gallstone disease and excessive alcohol use account for 70% to 80% of cases of acute pancreatitis in industrialized countries.
- The hallmark of acute pancreatitis is abdominal pain that is typically located in the epigastrium and periumbilical area and radiates to the back.
- Treatment of acute pancreatitis is supportive with bed rest, no oral intake, IV hydration, electrolyte replacement, and analgesia.
- Alcohol in Western societies (70%–80%) and malnutrition worldwide are the major causes of chronic pancreatitis.
- Endoscopic drainage has emerged as an effective alternative for symptomatic, noninfected pancreatic fluid collections.
- When exocrine secretion of pancreatic enzymes is reduced to <10%, diarrhea, steatorrhea, and azotorrhea can occur. These symptoms tend to occur relatively late in the course of chronic pancreatitis.
- Avoiding alcohol consumption decreases the frequency and severity of abdominal pain in chronic alcoholic pancreatitis.
- The median duration of survival for pancreatic cancer is only 18 to 20 months, and the 5-year survival rate is 10%.
- A Whipple procedure, only performed with pancreatic cancer if no evidence of metastatic disease exists, is done with curative intent.

REFERENCES AND SUGGESTED READINGS

Balthazar EJ, Robinson DL, Megibow AJ, Ranson JH. Acute pancreatitis: value of CT in establishing prognosis. *Radiology* 1990;174:331–336.

Corfield AP, Williamson RCN, McMahon MJ, et al. Prediction of severity in acute pancreatitis: prospective comparison of three prognostic indices. *Lancet* 1985;24:403–407.

Dominguez-Munoz JE, ed. *Clinical Pancreatology for Practicing Gastroenterologists and Surgeons.* Malden, Massachusetts: Blackwell; 2005.

Etemad B, Whitcomb DC. Chronic pancreatitis: diagnosis, classification, and new genetic developments. *Gastroenterology* 2001;120:682–707.

Fauci AS, Braunwald E, Isselbacher KJ, et al., eds. *Harrison's Principles of Internal Medicine.* 14th ed. New York: McGraw-Hill; 1998.

Grendall JH. Acute pancreatitis. *Clin Perspect Gastroenterol* 2000;3(6):327–333.

Mergener K, Baillie J. Acute pancreatitis. *BMJ* 1998;316:44–48.

Nunes QM, Lobo DL. Pancreatic cancer. *Surgery (Oxford)* 2007;25(3):87–94.

Ranson JHC, Rifkind KM, Roses DF, et al. Prognostic signs and the role of operative management in acute pancreatitis. *Surg Gynecol Obstet* 1974;139:69–81.

Yamada T. *Textbook and Atlas of Gastroenterology on CD-ROM.* Philadelphia: Lippincott Williams & Wilkins; 1999.

Biliary Tract Disorders

Somal S. Shah and Riad Azar

BACKGROUND

Diseases of the biliary tract are frequently encountered in both primary care and specialty settings. They represent a broad spectrum of diseases, ranging from benign gallstone disease to life-threatening cholangitis and cancers. Because these disorders are widely prevalent, all physicians need to become familiar with the diagnosis and management of biliary tract disorders.

DISORDERS OF THE GALLBLADDER

Cholelithiasis

Introduction
- **Cholelithiasis** is defined as the presence of concretions (gallstones) in the gallbladder or bile ducts. Gallstones are typically formed when supersaturation of cholesterol occurs in bile. Black pigment stones develop in conditions associated with chronic hemolysis, especially sickle cell disease and hereditary spherocytosis. Black stones may also be seen in cirrhotics. In contrast, brown pigment stones are formed when bacteria within the biliary tree cause bilirubin to deconjugate and combine with calcium, forming the insoluble calcium bilirubinate.
- Cholelithiasis is an extremely common disorder, particularly in women and the obese. The prevalence ranges from 10% to 15% in 40-year-old white women to as high as 70% in female Pima Indians. Cholesterol stones, which account for 75% to 90% of gallstones, are seen with increased frequency in female patients, multiparity, pregnancy, obesity, Crohn's disease, total parenteral nutrition, and Native Americans.

Causes
Clinical presentation results when gallstones occlude the cystic duct, pass into the common bile duct, or erode through the wall of the gallbladder. Therefore, presentation of gallstone disease includes biliary pain (also called biliary colic), acute cholecystitis, choledocholithiasis, acute cholangitis, gallstone pancreatitis, and gallstone ileus.

Natural History
Although cholelithiasis is common, most patients with gallstones are asymptomatic. Approximately 80% of patients with gallstones never develop symptoms. The risk of developing biliary pain is 1% to 2% per year. After the first episode of biliary pain, a 1% per year risk exists of developing a severe complication such as acute pancreatitis.

Presentation
   Biliary Pain.   The term classically used to describe biliary pain is **biliary colic**, but this is a misnomer because the pain is typically not colicky. Patients with biliary pain describe

episodes of epigastric or right upper quadrant pain—usually after eating—that may radiate to the right scapula or shoulder. The pain gradually increases over 30 minutes and then plateaus for 1 hour or longer before subsiding. Associated dyspeptic symptoms may occur, including bloating, nausea, or vomiting. The interval between attacks is variable, and weeks or months may pass between episodes. The pain is caused by transient occlusion of the cystic duct neck by a gallstone. Physical examination is generally unhelpful, but right upper quadrant tenderness can be present.

Clinical judgment is required to determine whether gallstones are causing pain or dyspeptic symptoms. Laparoscopic cholecystectomy is the treatment of choice, associated with a significantly shorter hospital stay and quicker convalescence compared with open cholecystectomy. Complications include bile duct injuries and bile leakage from the cystic duct remnant. For patients who are poor surgical candidates, oral dissolution therapy with ursodiol or chenodiol can be attempted; however, this is a slow process and rarely results in complete resolution of stones especially those that are >5 mm in size. In addition, gallstones can be removed through a cholecystostomy, but this requires multiple procedures, and the potential for gallstone recurrence remains.

Management

Asymptomatic Cholelithiasis. Gallstones are often found incidentally during evaluation for other conditions. Ultrasound remains the best investigative study, with 95% sensitivity and specificity for gallbladder stones. The yield is highest after fasting, and stones are identified by the presence of mobile echogenic objects that produce acoustic shadowing. Gallbladder sludge may also be seen as echogenic material that layers but does not produce acoustic shadowing. Cholelithiasis may also be identified with computed tomography (CT) scanning, although the sensitivity is lower than that of ultrasound. In addition, CT has the additional drawbacks of radiation exposure and expense. Because 80% of patients remain asymptomatic, the consensus is that prophylactic cholecystectomy is not indicated. Important exceptions are patients with a calcified or "porcelain" gallbladder and Native Americans with gallstones. Because these patients are at very high risk for gallbladder cancer, cholecystectomy should be performed even in the absence of symptoms. Also, patients with chronic medical conditions that can be adversely affected by an episode of cholecystitis or pancreatitis (e.g., brittle Type 1 diabetes mellitus) may benefit from elective cholecystectomy.

Acute Cholecystitis

Introduction

Acute cholecystitis is defined as inflammation or hemorrhagic necrosis, with variable infection, ulceration, and neutrophilic infiltration of the gallbladder wall, usually resulting from impaction of a stone in the cystic duct. In contrast, acalculous cholecystitis is an acute inflammatory disease of the gallbladder not associated with gallstones, but associated with bile stasis in the gallbladder because of impaired gallbladder motility, usually in the setting of significant comorbid illnesses.

Causes

Cystic duct occlusion results in bile stasis, gallbladder wall edema, gallbladder distention, inflammatory exudate, and finally bacterial infection. **Acalculous cholecystitis** is defined as cholecystitis in the absence of gallstones. This condition, which is most often seen in critically ill patients, is caused by gallbladder ischemia resulting in bile stasis and gallbladder distention.

Presentation

Patients typically present with steady upper abdominal pain that lasts hours, with associated nausea, vomiting, and fever. The presentation may be more subtle in the elderly. If bacteremic, patients may present with high fever, rigors, and severe abdominal tenderness. Examination often reveals right upper quadrant tenderness or a positive Murphy's sign (pain with palpation of the right upper quadrant during inspiration with subsequent inhibition of inspiration). Most patients have a modest leukocytosis and normal or only slightly increased transaminases and bilirubin. **Significantly increased transaminases or bilirubin should raise suspicion of a common bile duct stone.**

Management
- Patients with suspected acute cholecystitis should undergo ultrasonography. Important findings include gallstones, sonographic Murphy's sign, gallbladder wall thickening, and pericholecystic fluid. If the diagnosis remains in doubt, cholescintigraphy (hepatoiminodiacetic acid [HIDA], paraisopropyliminodiacetic acid [PIPIDA], or diisopropyl iminodiacetic acid [DISIDA] scan) should be performed. Radiolabeled iminodiacetic acid derivatives are administered, which are rapidly extracted by the liver and then excreted into bile. A normal study shows radioactivity in the gallbladder, common bile duct, and small intestine within 60 minutes. In acute cholecystitis, there is delayed filling of the gallbladder because of cystic duct obstruction.
- Patients with acute cholecystitis are made NPO but are given intravenous (IV) fluids and broad-spectrum antibiotics to treat secondary infection. Nasogastric suction is performed if the abdomen is distended or if the patient is vomiting. Prompt surgical consultation should be obtained.
- Definitive management is laparoscopic or open cholecystectomy. Most clinicians recommend waiting 24 to 48 hours until the patient has clinically stabilized, but surgery should be performed more urgently if the condition deteriorates. Patients who are poor surgical candidates should have percutaneous cholecystostomy or transpapillary endoscopic drainage of the gallbladder.
- Complications of acute cholecystitis include gallbladder perforation, emphysematous cholecystitis caused by gas-forming bacteria, and gallstone ileus.

Gallstone Pancreatitis

Gallstone pancreatitis is discussed in detail in Chapter 21, *Pancreatic Disorders*.

Gallstone Ileus

Gallstone ileus consists of mechanical intestinal obstruction resulting from the passage of a large gallstone into the bowel lumen. Gallstones can erode through the wall of the gallbladder into the small intestine. The stones can then cause obstruction, usually at the terminal ileum. Patients present with acute partial small bowel obstruction. This condition is seen more commonly in the elderly and in women. The diagnosis is suggested by the findings of air in the biliary tree with dilated loops of bowel and air fluid levels on an x-ray study. Abdominal ultrasound is useful in detecting biliary stones, and barium upper gastrointestinal (GI) series x-ray study may be needed to detect a duodenal–biliary fistula. Treatment is surgical enterotomy with removal of the stones. Most cases of gallstone ileus are caused by rare large stones and, therefore, recurrent obstruction is uncommon. Because cholecystectomy and surgical closure of the fistula are associated with high morbidity and mortality, these procedures should be pursued only in patients in excellent general health.

Gallbladder Carcinoma

Introduction
Gallbladder cancer represents the most common biliary tract malignancy. It is predominantly seen in elderly women. Up to 80% have a history of gallstones, and there is a higher

incidence with longer duration of gallstones, p53 or K-ras mutations. It is the most common GI malignancy in Native Americans. Approximately 90% of patients are diagnosed after the disease has spread beyond the gallbladder. Patients who have a calcified or "porcelain" gallbladder are at very high risk of gallbladder cancer and should undergo cholecystectomy even if asymptomatic.

Presentation

Patients typically present with prolonged abdominal pain, which may be difficult to differentiate from biliary pain, or acute cholecystitis. Other common symptoms include nausea, vomiting, weight loss, and jaundice.

Management

- Ultrasonography often detects masses within the gallbladder lumen or irregular gallbladder wall thickening. A normal ultrasound does not rule out gallbladder cancer, however. CT scanning demonstrates masses and gallbladder thickening and provides additional evidence for extent of disease. Fine-needle aspiration during endoscopic ultrasound has also been used to evaluate peripancreatic and periportal lymphadenopathy. Endoscopic retrograde cholangiopancreatography (ERCP) or percutaneous transhepatic cholangiography is indicated in patients with evidence of biliary obstruction. Cholangiography may also permit stent placement for biliary decompression. Histologic diagnosis for tumors that appear unresectable can be accomplished with percutaneous biopsy or ERCP. If resection is planned, preoperative tissue diagnosis is unnecessary. Carcinoembryonic antigen and carbohydrate antigen 19-9 (CA19-9) are both often elevated. Increases in serum bilirubin and alkaline phosphatase generally indicate the presence of advanced disease.
- Most patients present with advanced unresectable disease. The overall 5-year survival rate is <5%, but patients with advanced cancer have a median survival of only 45 to 127 days. Patients with unresectable disease may be given chemotherapy with agents such as 5-fluorouracil (5-FU), adriamycin, gemcitabine, and nitro ureases, but results are not encouraging. Most patients with unresectable disease will need palliative treatments, such as endoscopic stent placement or percutaneous biliary drainage. Patients whose cancers are staged between I and III have potentially resectable tumors. Depending on the extent of spread, surgery may be as simple as cholecystectomy or require extensive hepatic, pancreatic, and duodenal resection.

BILE DUCT DISORDERS

Choledocholithiasis

Introduction

Choledocholithiasis consists of stones in the bile ducts. Stones may pass from the gallbladder into the common bile duct or form *de novo* in the bile ducts. Retained common bile duct stones may be present for years after cholecystectomy before causing any problems. They can be identified during a cholecystectomy through intraoperative cholangiography.

Presentation

Patients with choledocholithiasis may be asymptomatic or present with a broad range of syndromes, depending on the location of the stone. Symptoms include pain, jaundice or abnormal liver function tests, cholangitis, and occasionally pancreatitis. One unusual presentation is **Mirizzi syndrome**, defined as a stone impacted in the cystic duct or neck of the gallbladder that causes external compression of the common bile duct.

Management

Usual laboratory abnormalities seen with choledocholithiasis include elevated transaminases, alkaline phosphatase, bilirubin, and, if complicated with pancreatitis, elevations in amylase and lipase. The best initial diagnostic study is abdominal ultrasound, which is very sensitive for dilated bile ducts but less sensitive (30%–50%) for common bile duct stones. *Absence of ductal dilatation does not exclude choledocholithiasis*, however. CT scanning may also be useful but also has lower sensitivity for common bile duct stones. Management of choledocholithiasis includes nonsurgical treatments (e.g., endoscopic papillotomy with balloon extraction, mechanical lithotripsy), and surgical approaches, including cholecystectomy with laparoscopic stone removal. ERCP allows the diagnosis and extraction of bile duct stones. Thus, in patients with high clinical suspicion of choledocholithiasis, especially in the presence of ductal dilatation on imaging and liver function test (LFT) abnormalities, an ERCP should be performed even if both ultrasound and a CT do not demonstrate choledocholithiasis. In patients in whom clinical suspicion is lower, a magnetic resonance cholangiopancreatography (MRCP) or endoscopic ultrasound can be used as further diagnostic modalities. Both imaging techniques have been shown to have similar sensitivities and specificities in diagnosing choledocholithiasis. The decision to perform MRCP versus endoscopic ultrasound is primarily based on availability and a patient's ability to tolerate one test over another. Endoscopic ultrasound does offer a distinct advantage in that if it is positive, a therapeutic ERCP can be performed while the patient is still under sedation. Although improved experience with ERCP has led to improved outcomes, risk of major complications remains, including pancreatitis, bleeding, perforation, and sepsis. For patients found to have choledocholithiasis during laparoscopic cholecystectomy, surgeons can remove the stones through laparoscopic or open common bile duct exploration. An alternative approach is ERCP with stone extraction.

Acute Cholangitis

Introduction

Acute cholangitis is defined as sudden onset of inflammation of the bile duct, typically from bacterial infection complicating an obstructed duct. Choledocholithiasis causes most cases of cholangitis, although patients with biliary neoplasms or inflammatory biliary strictures caused by primary sclerosing cholangitis (PSC) can develop cholangitis if they have undergone prior biliary interventions (e.g., ERCP).

Presentation

Approximately 70% of patients present with all three components of Charcot's triad: pain, jaundice, and fever. If suppurative cholangitis develops, patients will additionally present with mental status changes and hypotension (Reynold's pentad). Leukocytosis and markedly increased bilirubin and alkaline phosphatase are usually present. Blood cultures are frequently positive if gram-negative bacteria are the cause of the infection, especially in cases of suppurative cholangitis. The most common organisms isolated are gram-negative rods such as *Escherichia coli*, enterococci, and anaerobes, particularly in the elderly.

Management

Broad-spectrum antibiotics and aggressive fluid resuscitation should be immediately started if cholangitis is suspected. Typically, ureidopenicillins, fourth generation cephalosporins, or the carbapenems are the empiric antibiotics of choice. The diagnosis must then be made quickly, as patients are at risk of developing severe sepsis. Ultrasound or abdominal CT should be performed, looking for ductal dilatation or common bile duct stones. A negative study finding, however, does not rule out cholangitis, because the common duct may not be dilated early in the course of disease, and common duct stones may be missed. ERCP must be performed emergently in suspected cases of cholangitis, especially if the patient is clinically deteriorating. Therefore, the ERCP team should be notified immediately in any case of suspected acute cholangitis. ERCP identifies common duct stones or strictures and allows therapeutic interventions, such as sphincterotomy, biliary drainage, stone extraction, and biliary stent placement. If ERCP is unsuccessful or cannot be performed, then percutaneous transhepatic cholangiography (PTC) or surgical decompression should be pursued. Both of these procedures, however, have an increase in mortality and morbidity rates compared with ERCP. Antibiotics are usually given for a total of 7 to 10 days, but they can be stopped earlier if good biliary drainage is established. For patients who have their gallbladders, resolution of cholangitis should lead to prompt laparoscopic cholecystectomy.

Bile Peritonitis

Introduction
Bile peritonitis occurs when bile leaks into the peritoneal cavity leading to acute peritoneal inflammation. Bile leaks after cholecystectomy or hepatic surgery are common inciting events. Most bile leaks after a cholecystectomy occur at the cystic duct stump or duct of Luschka, with bile spillage into the peritoneal cavity resulting in bile peritonitis and severe abdominal pain. Occasionally, large collections of bile (bilomas) can form around the biliary tree, resulting in pain and leading to bacterial infections.

Presentation and Management
Patients usually present shortly after surgery with abdominal pain. Abdominal CT scan usually reveals fluid or a biloma centered around the biliary tree. A HIDA scan confirms the diagnosis by revealing spillage of radio tracer into the abdominal cavity. Large bilomas usually require percutaneous drainage, especially if they are infected. ERCP is often used to place biliary stents to encourage preferential flow of bile into the duodenum, which allows the leak site to heal. If bile duct stones are seen, a biliary sphincterotomy with stone extraction is usually performed before stent placement. Most leaks close within 6 weeks. For leaks that persist after stent placement, repeat ERCP with multiple stent placements can be reattempted. Repeat laparoscopy is an alternate option to drain bile from the peritoneal cavity, to reestablish biliary drainage, or as a last resort if ERCP with stent placement fails.

Primary Sclerosing Cholangitis

Introduction
Primary sclerosing cholangitis is defined as inflammation of the intrahepatic and extrahepatic bile ducts from an autoimmune mechanism. This disease typically leads to cholestasis, jaundice, and eventually liver failure. Of patients, 75% are male, and the average age at diagnosis is 40 years, although the disease can often be diagnosed in childhood.

Causes
- Up to 70% of PSC occurs in the setting of inflammatory bowel disease (IBD), with ulcerative colitis accounting for 90% of those cases. No relationship exists between the duration and severity of IBD and the development of PSC. Although colectomy is curative for colonic disease in ulcerative colitis, it does not eliminate the risk of PSC.
- The etiology of PSC is unknown. Animal and in vitro models have identified infections, autoimmunity, cytokines, and bile acid transporter or ion channel abnormalities as underlying causes for PSC. Both intrahepatic and extrahepatic bile ducts are involved with strictures. The disease process is usually diffuse, with obliterative fibrosis distributed throughout the biliary system.

Presentation
Tight strictures predispose the patient to intermittent obstruction of biliary flow with subsequent bacterial cholangitis. Obstruction of biliary flow causes reflux of bile into the

hepatocytes. The onset of disease is often insidious, with the gradual onset of fatigue, pruritus, and jaundice. Pruritus caused by deposition of bile acids in the skin can be severe. If advanced liver disease has already developed, some patients present with variceal bleeding, encephalopathy, or ascites. Steatorrhea and malabsorption of fat-soluble vitamins may develop late in disease because of decreased secretion of bile acids. Metabolic bone disease, most commonly osteoporosis, occurs frequently in PSC for unclear reasons. PSC follows a slowly progressive course, with a median survival of approximately 10 years from diagnosis.

Management

- Approximately 25% of patients are diagnosed from abnormal laboratory tests before symptoms have developed. Most have significantly elevated alkaline phosphatase, γ-glutamyltransferase, and bilirubin. The transaminases are elevated to a lesser degree. In addition, many patients will have positive antinuclear antibodies and antineutrophil cytoplasmic antibodies (p-ANCA) levels, suggesting that PSC is immune mediated. Patients with IBD who present with **elevated alkaline phosphatase** should have an aggressive evaluation to look for PSC. Definitive diagnosis is made by imaging of the biliary tree with either ERCP or PTC. MRCP is increasingly being used as a noninvasive option. The classic finding is multifocal stricturing of the intrahepatic and extrahepatic bile ducts with intervening normal or dilated segments. This is often described as a "*string of beads*" appearance. Secondary causes of strictures, including trauma, ischemia, tumors, and certain infections (cytomegalovirus, cryptosporidium), need to be excluded. A minority of patients who do not have the classic cholangiographic findings demonstrate small duct cholangitis on liver biopsy.
- Various medical therapies, such as immunosuppressants, corticosteroids, and antibiotics, have not been proved successful in slowing progression of disease, although ursodeoxycholic acid improves biochemical abnormalities. Management is therefore primarily supportive until end-stage liver disease (ESLD) develops, at which point liver transplantation is offered. Indications for transplantation include refractory ascites, recurrent bacterial cholangitis, encephalopathy, and variceal bleeding. The survival rate 10 years after transplantation is approximately 79%, although patients with PSC have a higher retransplantation rate than all other patients with ESLD caused by recurrent disease.

The specific complications are managed as follows:

Pruritus. Pruritus can be particularly severe in PSC and can be difficult to manage. The exact mechanism remains unknown, but may involve the accumulation of pruritogenic substances secondary to decreased bile excretion or increased opioidergic tone. Symptoms often respond to bile acid-binding resins, such as cholestyramine at a dose of 4 g PO BID to QID. Other medical options include colestipol, ursodiol, rifampicin, odansetron, and immunosuppressants. Antihistamines seem to have no effect on pruritus beyond possible sedation effects. Nonpharmacologic therapies that have shown promise include photodynamic therapy and, in extreme cases, liver transplantation. Other supportive therapies, such as emollients, lotions, or cold compressives, have not proved efficacy in PSC.

Bacterial Cholangitis. Bacterial cholangitis is more frequent in patients who have had manipulation of the biliary tract or have developed a dominant stricture. Cholelithiasis or choledocholithiasis can also contribute to the development of bacterial cholangitis. Patients typically present with fever and worsening jaundice, and often have recurrent episodes. After empiric antibiotics are started, treatment is directed at relieving the obstruction, usually endoscopically. ERCP allows dilation of large strictures, biliary decompression, and removal of stones. Prospective studies have not shown any benefit in placing endoprostheses across strictures. Furthermore, stent occlusion and cholangitis frequently occur with stent placement. Long-term prophylactic antibiotics have not been shown to have any benefit in preventing cholangitis.

Dominant Stricture. Approximately 20% of patients develop a dominant stricture. Cholangiography demonstrates the dominant stricture and balloon dilatation with stent placement can be performed. It is often very difficult to differentiate a dominant stricture from cholangiocarcinoma. Tumor markers, such as CA19-9, carcinoembryonic antigen (CEA), and cytologic brushings, may be of some value in identifying patients with cholangiocarcinoma. A recently developed technology called "spyglass" allows direct visualization of the bile duct during ERCP through fiberoptics. Direct biopsy of the strictures can also be obtained, potentially improving the detection of early cholangiocarcinomas.

Cholangiocarcinoma. Patients with PSC have a 10% to 30% chance of developing bile duct cancer. This is often very difficult to diagnose in the setting of PSC. Despite knowing that patients with PSC are at high risk for cholangiocarcinoma, no affective way has been found to screen for cholangiocarcinoma. Patients with PSC with concomitant IBD also have an increased risk of colon cancer, but preliminary reports suggest that this risk may be decreased with the use of ursodeoxycholic acid (UDCA).

Portal Hypertension. Advanced PSC eventually leads to ESLD, with the subsequent development of portal hypertension. Variceal bleeding, portosystemic encephalopathy, and ascites are managed as with other types of ESLD. Liver transplantation is the treatment of choice in patients with ESLD from PSC.

Cholangiocarcinoma

Introduction

Bile duct cancer is a relatively rare tumor seen primarily in middle-aged men with a reported incidence of 8 per million in the United States. The strongest association is with PSC, but it is also seen with chronic liver disease, ulcerative colitis, parasitic biliary disease, choledochal cysts, hepatitis C, and smoking.

Causes

The pathophysiologic mechanism for cancer development is unknown, but chronic biliary inflammation is thought to contribute to cancer formation.

Presentation

Patients typically present with anorexia, weight loss, acholic stool, abdominal pain, pruritus, and jaundice when the tumor causes significant obstruction. A Klatskin tumor is a bile duct cancer with involvement of the hilum of the right and left hepatic ducts. Some bile duct tumors spread diffusely throughout the liver, making it difficult to distinguish from PSC. Most tumors are locally invasive and do not metastasize. Prognosis is grim, with rare patient survival more than 1 year.

Management

- Most patients have elevated alkaline phosphatase and bilirubin. Ultrasonography and abdominal CT scan are useful in identifying intrahepatic or extrahepatic ductal dilation, but the primary tumors are often difficult to visualize. Magnetic resonance imaging (MRI) or MRCP may be more sensitive in identifying the primary tumor. ERCP or PTC provides direct imaging of the biliary system and can define the extent of tumor spread. During ERCP, tissue diagnosis can be made using bile cytology, cytologic brushings, or cholangioscopic biopsies. Biopsies obtained through percutaneous or transluminal means are not recommended because of the danger of tumor seeding. Regional lymph node sampling can also be done via endoscopic ultrasound (EUS) in early disease to evaluate for surgical resection or liver transplantation. EUS can also be used to obtain fine-needle aspirations in patients with unsuccessful ERCP or those who have had negative cytology results. The histologic diagnosis of cholangiocarcinoma may be challenging, because many tumors are well-differentiated and occur in the setting of PSC. Elevations in CA19-9 are the most sensitive and specific tumor marker in cholangiocarcinoma, but this marker is also elevated many times in concomitant bacterial cholangitis.

- Surgical resection represents the only option for long-term survival. Distal extrahepatic and intrahepatic tumors are more likely to be resectable than proximal extrahepatic tumors. Median survival for resectable tumors is 3 years, but only 1 year if unresectable. A high recurrence rate is seen for patients after resection, and adjuvant chemoradiation has not been shown to improve survival. Liver transplantation combined with neoadjuvant chemoradiation has led to increased survival rates in patients with locally unresectable cancer with otherwise normal hepatic and biliary function and patients with a history of PSC. Patients who have unresectable tumors are usually offered ERCP with stent placement versus percutaneous biliary drainage. This has replaced palliative biliary–enteric anastomosis in most centers. Recent preliminary reports of other palliative treatments (e.g., photodynamic therapy) have been encouraging, but more studies are needed. Chemotherapy and radiation are uniformly ineffective in prolonging survival. Death usually results from recurrent biliary sepsis or liver abscess formation.

KEY POINTS TO REMEMBER

- Of patients with gallstones, 80% remain free of symptoms; therefore, prophylactic surgery is not indicated in asymptomatic cholelithiasis.
- Ultrasonography is the best test for gallstones, with 95% sensitivity and 95% specificity for gallbladder stones. A negative study finding does not rule out common bile duct stones.
- Laparoscopic cholecystectomy is the treatment of choice for biliary pain (commonly referred to as biliary colic) in the presence of gallstones.
- Treatment for acute cholecystitis includes IV antibiotics, bowel rest, and when clinically stable, cholecystectomy or percutaneous cholecystostomy.
- Gallbladder cancer, the most common biliary tract malignancy, usually presents with prolonged abdominal pain, vomiting, and weight loss.
- An ERCP should be performed emergently in all cases of acute cholangitis for biliary decompression.
- Primary sclerosing cholangitis is best diagnosed with direct cholangiography (ERCP or PTC), which demonstrates a "string of beads" appearance. Magnetic resonance cholangiopancreatography is a useful alternative.
- Up to 70% of cases of PSC occur in patients with inflammatory bowel disease (ulcerative colitis much more commonly than Crohn's disease).

REFERENCES AND SUGGESTED READINGS

Bortoff GA, Chen MY, Ott DJ, et al. Gallbladder stones: imaging and intervention. *Radiographics* 2000;20(3):751–766.

Chang KJ. State of the art lecture: endoscopic ultrasound (EUS) and FNA in pancreaticobiliary tumors. *Endoscopy* 2006;38(Suppl 1):S56–S60.

Diehl AK. Epidemiology and natural history of gallstone disease. *Gastroenterol Clin North Am* 1991;20:1–19.

Fogel EL, McHenry L, Sherman S, et al. Therapeutic biliary endoscopy. *Endoscopy* 2005;37(2):139–145.

Freeman ML, Nelson DB, Sherman S. Complications of endoscopic biliary sphincterotomy. *N Engl J Med* 1996;335:909–918.

LaRusso N, Shneider B, Black D, et al. Primary sclerosing cholangitis: Summary of a workshop. *Hepatology* 2006;44(3):746–764.

Holtmeier J, Leuschner U. Medical treatment of primary biliary cirrhosis and primary sclerosing cholangitis. *Digestion* 2001; 64(3):137–150.

Hungness ES, Soper NJ. Management of common bile duct stones. *J Gastrointestinal Surg* 2006;10(4):612–619.

Jones RS. Carcinoma of the gallbladder. *Surg Clin North Am* 1990;70:1419–1428.

Kadakia SC. Biliary tract emergencies: acute cholecystitis, acute cholangitis and acute pancreatitis. *Med Clin North Am* 1993;77:1015–1036.

Kirchmayr W, Muhlmann G, Zitt M, et al. Gallstone ileus: rare and still controversial. *Australian and New Zealand Journal of Surgery* 2005;75(4):234–238.

Lai ECS, Mok FPT, Tan ESY. Endoscopic biliary drainage for severe acute cholangitis. *N Engl J Med* 1992;326:1582–1586.

LaRusso NF, Schneider BL, Black D, et al. Primary sclerosing cholangitis: summary of a workshop. *Hepatology* 2006;44(3):746–764.

Lee YM, Kaplan MM. Primary sclerosing cholangitis. *N Engl J Med* 1995;332:924–937.

Malhi H, Gores GJ. Cholangiocarcinoma: modern advances in understanding a deadly old disease. *J Hepatol* 2006;45(6):856–867. Epub 2006 September 25.

Mela M, Mancuso A, Burroughs AK. Review article: pruritus in cholestatic and other diseases. *Aliment Pharmacol Ther* 2003;17(7):857–870.

Qureshi WA. Approach to the patient who has suspected acute bacterial cholangitis. *Gastroenterol Clin North Am* 2006;35(2):409–423.

Rohatgi A, Singh KK. Mirizzi syndrome: laparoscopic management by sub-total cholecystectomy. *Surg Endosc* 2006;20(9):1477–1481.

Rosen CB, Nagorney DM, Wiesner RH. Cholangiocarcinoma complicating primary sclerosing cholangitis. *Ann Surg* 1991;213:21–25.

Verma D, Kapadia A, Eisen GM, et al. EUS vs. MRCP for detection of choledocholithiasis. *Gastrointest Endosc* 2006;64(2):248–254.

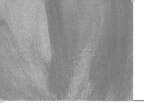

Gastrointestinal Procedures

23

Sanjay Sikka

INTRODUCTION

The ability to perform endoscopic procedures has radically changed the practice of gastroenterology. **Endoscopy** allows for direct visual inspection, tissue sampling, and minimally invasive therapeutic intervention. An endoscopic procedure is worth performing if the benefit for the patient exceeds the risks by a sufficiently wide margin. Preparation for endoscopy involves addressing important issues specific to each patient, such as assessing contraindications and relative contraindications, medication allergies, patient medications, and possible interactions with medicines used for sedation. In addition, the presence of coagulopathy, comorbid factors, and conditions potentially requiring antibiotic prophylaxis must be considered. Furthermore, each patient, or a designated guardian, should understand the benefits and risks associated with the procedure, and informed consent must be obtained before the procedure is initiated. General indications for endoscopic procedures are listed in Table 23-1.

UPPER GASTROINTESTINAL ENDOSCOPY

- Esophagogastroduodenoscopy (EGD) allows high-resolution visual inspection of the upper gastrointestinal (GI) tract from the esophagus to the second portion of the duodenum. At most institutions, examinations are performed using topical anesthetics applied to the oropharynx in combination with intravenous (IV) conscious sedation; deeper, monitored anesthesia can also be used with assistance from an anesthesiologist when conscious sedation fails or is anticipated to fail. EGD can be used for a variety of indications, such as the diagnosis and management of abdominal pain or upper GI bleeding, the screening and diagnosis of esophageal or gastric malignancies, and the palliation of dysphagia resulting from both malignant and benign causes. Various instruments may be passed through the therapeutic channel of the endoscope for use in tissue biopsy, medication delivery, or cauterization for the goal of hemostasis. The only patient preparation required is to avoid oral intake for ≥ 6 hours before the procedure.
- Endoscopy has a small but definite risk of complications, overall estimated to occur in 0.1% having the procedure. Significant bleeding has been reported in 0.025% to 0.15%. Perforation has been reported in 0.02 to 0.2%, and cardiorespiratory complications, mostly attributed to premedication or sedation, can occur in 0.05% to 0.73% of patients. The risk of mortality as a result of upper endoscopy has been estimated to range from 0.005% to 0.04%.

COLONOSCOPY

- Colonoscopy can be used to visually inspect the entire colon as well as the terminal ileum. As with EGD, colonoscopy almost always involves the use of IV conscious

TABLE 23-1	GENERAL INDICATIONS FOR ENDOSCOPIC PROCEDURES

Gastrointestinal endoscopy is generally indicated:

If a change in management is probable based on results of endoscopy

After an empiric trial of therapy for a suspected benign digestive disorder has been unsuccessful

As the initial method of evaluation as an alternative to radiographic studies

When a primary therapeutic procedure is contemplated

Gastrointestinal endoscopy is generally not indicated:

When the results do not contribute to a management choice

For periodic follow-up of healed benign disease unless surveillance of a premalignant condition is warranted

Gastrointestinal endoscopy is generally contraindicated:

When the risks to patient health or life are judged to outweigh the most favorable benefits of the procedure

When adequate patient cooperation or consent cannot be obtained

When a perforated viscus is known or suspected

sedation or monitored anesthesia. Colonoscopy is performed for a variety of indications, including evaluation and treatment of overt lower GI bleeding, evaluation of iron-deficiency anemia, screening for colon cancer, diagnosis and cancer surveillance in inflammatory bowel disease, palliative treatment of stenosing or bleeding neoplasms, and evaluation of clinically significant diarrhea of unexplained origin. Various instruments may be passed through the therapeutic channel of the endoscope for use in tissue biopsy, medication delivery to the colonic mucosa, cauterization or fulguration of tissue, and removal of polyps. Colon preparation is required before the procedure. This usually involves a lavage or purgative method used on the day or evening before the patient's colonoscopy. Acceptable regimens include polyethylene glycol (GoLYTELY or MiraLax) or phospho-soda preparations.

• Colonoscopy also has a small but definite risk of complications, estimated to occur in 0.1% to 1.9% of patients having the procedure. Significant bleeding can be seen in up to 1.9% of patients, and perforation can occur in up to 0.4% of patients. The rate of bleeding complications seen with therapeutic colonoscopy is roughly double that seen with diagnostic colonoscopy. Surgical consultation should be obtained in the event of suspected perforation. Cardiorespiratory complications, which are also a concern, are mostly attributed to the sedation used during the procedure. Mortality has been reported in up to 0.06% of patients.

FLEXIBLE SIGMOIDOSCOPY

Flexible sigmoidoscopy involves a shorter examination compared with colonoscopy and is used to examine the distal colon up to the splenic flexure. This examination is usually performed without sedation, which adds the advantages of decreased cost, fewer complications associated with sedation, and decreased lost work time for the patient. The procedure is more uncomfortable for the patient, however, because no sedation is given. This procedure also eliminates the need for a complete colon preparation. Two enemas given a few hours before the procedure are usually adequate preparation. The risk of perforation during flexible sigmoidoscopy is low (0.01%). Flexible sigmoidoscopy is generally used for evaluation of suspected distal colonic disease when colonoscopy is not indicated, anastomotic recurrence in rectosigmoid carcinoma, and exclusion of infection or immune-mediated processes (e.g., graft-versus-host disease) in certain patient subsets, including those with inflammatory bowel disease or following bone marrow transplantation.

SMALL BOWEL ENTEROSCOPY

- Because standard upper GI endoscopy is limited to the level of the second portion of the duodenum, a special endoscope is needed to examine the upper GI tract beyond the ligament of Treitz. Two types of enteroscopes developed for this purpose are the push enteroscope and the single- or double-balloon enteroscope. Sonde enteroscopy, a procedure involving a long, thin endoscope advanced by small bowel peristalsis, is no longer in use.
- Push enteroscopes are 160 to 240 cm in length and can be used for therapeutic intervention. They allow for controlled insertion and withdrawal. Push enteroscopy is traditionally used after a negative upper endoscopy and colonoscopy. The yield of push enteroscopy in this setting is approximately 60%.
- Balloon enteroscopy utilizes single or double inflatable balloons on the end of the endoscope and an accompanying overtube to grip the intestinal wall and allow deep cannulation of the small bowel. Both transoral and transanal approaches can be used and often the entire length of the small bowel can be examined when both approaches are used in combination. This form of enteroscopy allows biopsy or treatment of lesions noted beyond the reach of push enteroscopes and is replacing intraoperative enteroscopy in some centers.
- Capsule enteroscopy is currently being used in many settings as a means to visualize segments of the bowel previously inaccessible to endoscopy. For this study, the patient swallows a capsule that contains a camera, light source, battery, and radio transmitter. As the capsule traverses the GI tract, it takes pictures and transmits these images to a receiver that the patient wears on the belt. The capsule takes 8 hours of images, usually sufficient time to traverse the ileocecal valve. The images are then loaded onto a computer where they can be viewed in a movie format at up to 25 frames per second. The current indications for capsule endoscopy include evaluation of obscure GI bleeding and persistent occult GI bleeding. The major contraindication is the presence of intestinal strictures which can obstruct passage of the capsule.

ENDOSCOPIC RETROGRADE CHOLANGIOPANCREATOGRAPHY

- Endoscopic retrograde cholangiopancreatography (ERCP) is performed using a specially designed endoscope that involves a side-viewing imaging system. This system allows direct visualization of the major and minor papillae and facilitates insertion of devices into the desired duct.
- An ERCP can be used effectively in detecting and treating choledocholithiasis. Sphincterotomy may be performed at the time of stone removal to reduce the chance of recurrent choledocholithiasis. ERCP may also be used therapeutically to dilate benign and malignant strictures in the biliary tree with or without subsequent stent placement. Brushings for cytology may also be obtained during ERCP to assist in the diagnosis of cholangiocarcinoma and pancreatic neoplasms.

- The ERCP procedure is associated with all the risks of upper endoscopy. Approximately 5% of patients develop postprocedural pancreatitis. The incidence is higher when sphincter of Oddi manometry is performed. This is usually mild and self-limited; however, in a small percentage of cases, this can be life-threatening.

ENDOSCOPIC ULTRASONOGRAPHY

Endoscopic ultrasound (EUS) allows for high-resolution imaging of the luminal GI tract. It uses higher frequencies than transabdominal ultrasound and provides resolution of the GI tract wall into nine distinct layers that correlate closely with histology. This is of great value in the preoperative staging of GI malignancies and the evaluation of intramural and submucosal masses. In addition, diagnostic tissue sampling can be performed under EUS guidance. Specific roles for EUS include the staging of esophageal cancer (including the use of fine-needle aspiration to detect malignant lymphadenopathy), diagnosis of submucosal tumors, staging of pancreatic cancer, detection of small pancreatic and ampullary tumors, and even the staging of certain lung cancers.

LIVER BIOPSY

In some instances, histologic examination of liver tissue is necessary. Common indications for liver biopsy include evaluation of abnormal liver chemistries, assessment of degree of inflammation and fibrosis in chronic liver disease (e.g., hepatitis C), and diagnosis of liver masses. Liver biopsy can be accomplished by several different techniques. Bedside percutaneous liver biopsy is commonly performed by gastroenterologists or hepatologists. The patient is placed supine with the right arm behind the head. With ultrasound guidance or percussion, an appropriate biopsy location is chosen in the right lateral chest wall, usually near the eighth intercostal space. The area is prepared and draped in sterile fashion, and lidocaine is used to infiltrate the skin, subcutaneous fat, intercostal muscles, and liver capsule. A small incision is made, and the liver biopsy needle is advanced to the liver capsule. With the patient held in full expiration, the biopsy needle is advanced into the liver parenchyma, and a core of tissue is obtained. The patient is then observed closely for at least 4 hours for complications. Contraindications to percutaneous liver biopsy include severe coagulopathy, thrombocytopenia, or ascites. If percutaneous liver biopsy cannot be safely performed, or if portal pressure measurements are needed, transjugular liver biopsy under radiologic guidance may be performed. Directed biopsy with ultrasound or computer tomography (CT) guidance may be necessary for sampling of liver masses. Complications of liver biopsy are rare but can be severe. The most common complication is pain at the biopsy site or in the right shoulder. Less common complications are bleeding, pneumothorax, gallbladder perforation, inadvertent kidney biopsy, or death. Most complications are apparent within the first 4 to 6 hours, but they can occur up to 48 hours after biopsy.

CONSCIOUS SEDATION

- Conscious sedation provides adequate analgesia and sedation for most GI procedures while allowing the patient to cooperate with verbal commands. Conscious sedation for endoscopic procedures usually involves a benzodiazepine (i.e., midazolam) and an opiate (i.e., meperidine). Propofol is a short-acting sedative, and its use requires the presence of an anesthesiologist for both the administration of the drug and airway control.
- The American Society of Anesthesiology (ASA) assessment (categories I–V) is useful in evaluating the sedation risk for a patient. ASA category I represents the least risk.

Advanced age, obesity, pregnancy, sleep apnea, a history of substance abuse, or severe cardiac, respiratory, hepatic, renal, or central nervous system (CNS) disease places patients at higher risk for sedation. Patients should be made NPO before their procedure to reduce the risk associated with anesthesia.

• The most common sedation complications include airway obstruction and respiratory depression, oversedation, hypoxia, and hypotension. Patients are monitored during the procedure using continuous pulse oximetry, heart monitoring, and intermittent blood pressure recordings.

ANTIBIOTIC PROPHYLAXIS FOR ENDOCARDITIS

• Bacterial endocarditis is a potentially life-threatening infection. Approximately 4% of patients develop bacteremia associated with endoscopy, but this varies, depending on the specific procedure performed. Prosthetic heart valves, a history of endocarditis, and surgically constructed systemic pulmonary shunts are considered higher-risk cardiac conditions and have traditionally been targeted for antibiotic prophylaxis. Recent guidelines by the American Heart Association, however, no longer recommend antibiotic prophylaxis in conjunction with routine GI procedures. At the time of writing this chapter, The American Society of Gastrointestinal Endoscopy guidelines regarding recommendations for the use of prophylactic antibiotics in endoscopic procedures remain as published in 2003 and are listed in Table 23-2.

TABLE 23-2	AMERICAN SOCIETY OF GASTROINTESTINAL ENDOSCOPY RECOMMENDATIONS FOR ANTIBIOTIC PROPHYLAXIS

Antibiotic recommended:

High-risk procedure (stricture dilation, varix sclerosis, ERCP) in high-risk conditions (prosthetic valve, previous endocarditis, synthetic vascular graft <1 year old, systemic pulmonary shunt, complex cyanotic congenital heart disease)

Acute GI bleeding in the cirrhotic patient

Endoscopic feeding tube placement

ERCP for obstructed bile duct or pancreatic pseudocyst

Antibiotic optional:

Low-risk procedure (colonoscopy, esophagogastroduodenoscopy, varix ligation) in high-risk conditions

High-risk procedure in intermediate-risk conditions (rheumatic disease, mitral valve prolapse with regurgitation, hypertrophic cardiomyopathy, congenital heart disease)

Antibiotic not recommended:

Low-risk procedure in intermediate-risk conditions

Any endoscopic procedure in low-risk cardiac conditions (coronary artery bypass grafting, pacemaker, automatic implantable cardioverter-defibrillator)

Any endoscopic procedure in patients with prosthetic joints

GI, gastrointestinal; ERCP, endoscopic retrograde cholangiopancreatography.

- Antibiotics should be administered 30 to 60 minutes before the procedure but can be efficacious when given as long as 2 hours after the procedure. For upper endoscopy and stricture dilation, give ampicillin 2 g IV 30 minutes before the procedure or amoxicillin 2 g PO 30 to 60 minutes before to the procedure. For all other procedures, give ampicillin 2 g IV. Vancomycin 1 g IV, is substituted for the penicillin-allergic patient. An IV cephalosporin or its equivalent should be administered to patients having percutaneous endoscopic feeding tube placement.

ANTICOAGULATION AND ANTIPLATELET AGENTS

Patients who require chronic anticoagulation or antiplatelet agents pose a challenging problem when a GI procedure is needed. The bleeding risk for GI procedures is increased in the setting of anticoagulation or antiplatelet drugs, especially if polypectomy or biopsy is performed. If possible, warfarin should be discontinued ≥5 days before the procedure, and the international normalized ratio (INR) can optionally be checked on the day of the procedure. The threshold for an acceptable INR is not well established, but most endoscopists prefer the INR to be <1.5. If anticoagulation cannot be stopped for an extended period of time (mechanical valves, atrial fibrillation with known left atrial thrombus), then the patient should be admitted for conversion from warfarin to heparin. Once the INR has decreased to an acceptable level, the procedure can be safely performed by stopping heparin 6 hours before the procedure. The timing for resuming anticoagulation depends largely on what type of procedure is performed. Aspirin and other antiplatelet agents should be discontinued ≥1 week before the procedure. These recommendations are easier to follow for elective procedures. For patients with acute bleeding who require endoscopic therapy, attempts should be made to correct any coagulopathy using a combination of fresh-frozen plasma (FFP), vitamin K, and platelets.

KEY POINTS TO REMEMBER

- An EGD allows visual inspection, sampling, and treatment of lesions in the upper GI tract from the esophagus to the second portion of the duodenum.
- Colonoscopy can be used to inspect and perform interventions in the entire colon and terminal ileum.
- Capsule endoscopy and balloon enteroscopy allow visualization of the entire small intestine.
- An ERCP uses a side-viewing endoscope to examine the major and minor papilla and it facilitates insertion of devices into the biliary or pancreatic ducts.
- Conscious sedation provides adequate analgesia and sedation for most GI procedures.
- Antibiotic prophylaxis is recommended for patients having high-risk procedures with high-risk conditions for bacterial endocarditis. Recent guidelines, however, have called this practice into question.

REFERENCES AND SUGGESTED READINGS

Berner JS, Mauer K, Lewis BS. Push and sonde enteroscopy for the diagnosis of obscure gastrointestinal bleeding. *Am J Gastroenterol* 1994;89:2139–2142.
Carlsson U, Grattidge P. Sedation for upper gastrointestinal endoscopy: a comparative study of propofol and midazolam. *Endoscopy* 1995;3:240–243.

Chong J, Tagle M, Barkin JS, et al. Small bowel push type enteroscopy for patients with occult gastrointestinal bleeding of suspected small bowel pathology. *Am J Gastroenterol* 1994;89:2143–2146.

Froehlich F, Gonvers JJ, Vader JP, et al. Appropriateness of gastrointestinal endoscopy: risk of complications. *Endoscopy* 1999;31(8):684–686.

Groveman HD, Sanowski RA, Klauber MR. Training primary care physicians in flexible sigmoidoscopy—performance evaluation of 12,167 procedures. *West J Med* 1988; 148:221–224.

Kavic S, Basson M, Complications of endoscopy. *Am J Surg* 2001;181:319–332.

Mallery S, Van Dam J. Advances in diagnostic and therapeutic endoscopy. *Med Clin North Am* 2000;84(5):1059–1083.

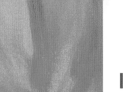

Index

Page numbers followed by *f* refer to figures; page numbers followed by *t* refer to tables.